Palliative Care Nursing

Caring for Suffering Patients

Kathleen Ouimet Perrin, PhD, RN, CCRN
Professor of Nursing
Saint Anselm College
Manchester, New Hampshire

Caryn A. Sheehan, DNP, APRN-BC
Associate Professor of Nursing
Saint Anselm College
Manchester, New Hampshire

Mertie L. Potter, DNP, APRN, PMHCNS-BC
Clinical Professor of Nursing
MGH Institute of Health Professions
Boston, Massachusetts

Mary K. Kazanowski, PhD, APRN-BC, CHPN
Coordinator, VNA Palliative Care
VNA of Manchester and Southern New Hampshire
Manchester, New Hampshire

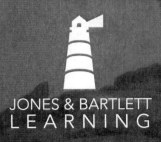

JONES & BARTLETT
LEARNING

World Headquarters
Jones & Bartlett Learning
40 Tall Pine Drive
Sudbury, MA 01776
978-443-5000
info@jblearning.com
www.jblearning.com

Jones & Bartlett Learning books and products are available through most bookstores and online booksellers. To contact Jones & Bartlett Learning directly, call 800-832-0034, fax 978-443-8000, or visit our website, www.jblearning.com.

Substantial discounts on bulk quantities of Jones & Bartlett Learning publications are available to corporations, professional associations, and other qualified organizations. For details and specific discount information, contact the special sales department at Jones & Bartlett Learning via the above contact information or send an email to specialsales@jblearning.com.

Some images in this book feature models. These models do not necessarily endorse, represent, or participate in the activities represented in the images.

The authors, editor, and publisher have made every effort to provide accurate information. However, they are not responsible for errors, omissions, or for any outcomes related to the use of the contents of this book and take no responsibility for the use of the products and procedures described. Treatments and side effects described in this book may not be applicable to all people; likewise, some people may require a dose or experience a side effect that is not described herein. Drugs and medical devices are discussed that may have limited availability controlled by the Food and Drug Administration (FDA) for use only in a research study or clinical trial. Research, clinical practice, and government regulations often change the accepted standard in this field. When consideration is being given to use of any drug in the clinical setting, the health care provider or reader is responsible for determining FDA status of the drug, reading the package insert, and reviewing prescribing information for the most up-to-date recommendations on dose, precautions, and contraindications, and determining the appropriate usage for the product. This is especially important in the case of drugs that are new or seldom used.

Production Credits

Publisher: Kevin Sullivan
Acquisitions Editor: Amy Sibley
Editorial Assistant: Rachel Shuster
Production Manager: Carolyn F. Rogers
Marketing Manager: Meagan Norlund
V.P., Manufacturing and Inventory Control:
 Therese Connell

Composition: Shepherd, Inc.
Cover Design: Kristin E. Parker
Cover Image: © Kurt/Dreamstime.com
Printing and Binding: Edwards Brothers Malloy
Cover Printing: Edwards Brothers Malloy

Library of Congress Cataloging-in-Publication Data
Palliative care nursing : caring for suffering patients / Kathleen Ouimet
Perrin ... [et al.].
 p. ; cm.
Includes bibliographical references and index.
ISBN 978-0-7637-7384-7 (pbk.)
1. Palliative treatment. 2. Nursing. 3. Suffering. I. Perrin, Kathleen
Ouimet.
 [DNLM: 1. Nursing Care—methods. 2. Palliative Care—ethics.
3. Pain—nursing. 4. Terminal Care—methods. WY 152.3]
 RT87.T45P32 2011
 616′.029—dc22
                                  2010037431

6048
Printed in the United States of America
17 16 15 14   10 9 8 7 6 5 4 3

Dedication

We dedicate this book to all of our patients and their families. We have borne witness to their suffering—from psychological distress, from loss and bereavement, from countless and sometimes unfathomable physiological ailments. It is also dedicated to our nurse colleagues and the nursing students who have collaborated with us to provide nursing care. This book originated from our realization that as nurses we are fellow travelers with our patients and their families in their journey through suffering. When we give voice to both their suffering and our own, we can work together to alleviate it.

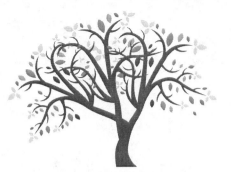

Contents

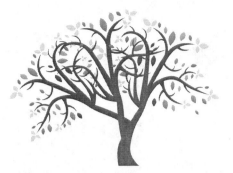

Preface

At some critical juncture in all our professional lives, perhaps while we were students, perhaps as practicing nurses, all of us have realized that our patients are suffering. Sometimes they are suffering from a disease process, sometimes from adverse effects of the treatments we administer, and sometimes from the psychological distress that accompanies a disease.

Jacqueline Merry described how she learned this lesson when as a new nursing student she was assigned to care for a woman who the day before had had bilateral mastectomies. When Jacqui entered the room, the patient was dressed beautifully, knowledgeable about her disease, smiling, and "not in need of a thing." When Jacqui asked her patient how she was coping with her diagnosis of breast cancer and her surgery, the patient responded, "Oh, I'm handling it so well. Everyone keeps telling me that they can't believe how strong I am and how well I am dealing with everything." However, as Jacqui began to assess her patient and prepare her for discharge, a powerful doubt developed: What if the woman she was caring for was presenting a fragile façade covering up being truly terrified? Jacqui was sure there was something that she should be doing and felt she had failed because she could not discover what it was.

As Jacqui wheeled the patient to an elevator and it began to descend to the lobby where the patient's husband was waiting, a great change came over the patient. Her shoulders slouched forward and she cupped her head in her hands. Tears streamed down her cheeks as she wept silently. Jacqui stopped the elevator, put a hand on the patient's shoulder, and just stood there while the patient cried. When she was finished, the patient wiped the tears from her eyes, proudly lifted

Figure F–1

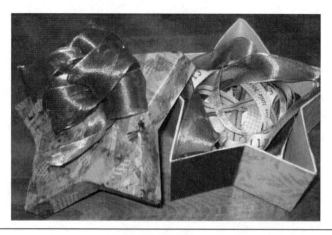

her head, and nodded she was ready. Jacqui opened the elevator doors and wheeled her down the hall to her husband.

After this event, Jacqui wondered what she could have done for her patient? Was having someone "just be there" what the patient needed most? While reflecting on the experience, Jacqui created the box in Figure F–1 to represent this patient. The box is a beautiful star-shaped box with exquisite pink paper and a lovely bow. Yet when you open it, you see ribbons in disarray, each marked with a powerful emotion, in stark contrast to the neat, "perfect" exterior.

Jacqui left the hospital that day fearing that she had failed her patient. How many times have any of us left after a long day wondering what else we might have done if only we had had a chance. In his discussion of nurses and their response to suffering, Jameton (1983) said, "I envision hospitals as places of suffering and I see nurses sweeping it all up. Then I wonder what they do with all that suffering after they have gathered it up." This book is intended to assist nurses to reflect on the suffering, tragedies, and sometimes horror they see in the clinical setting, and to work through some of their own feelings and reactions.

This book was also developed to assist nurses in finding answers to Jacqui's questions. How do we identify a patient who is suffering? How do we assess whether our patient (and/or her family) is coping with the event? How can we identify the sources of our patients' suffering when we believe they are putting up a façade? What can we do to alleviate patient suffering? How can we convey the extent of the suffering to the other members of the healthcare team and advocate excellent palliative care for our patients? This book was developed with the intention of helping nurses improve their ability to recognize the suffering of others and respond to it in such a way as to optimally relieve or alleviate patients' distress.

Reference

Jameton, A. (1983, June). Panel Discussion at the National Endowment for the Humanities Summer Institute in Nursing Ethics, Medford, MA.

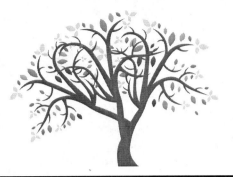

Acknowledgments

We wish to acknowledge our families who have provided us with the love and support that has sustained us throughout our nursing careers, but especially as we worked on this project.

Thank you to my husband, Robin, and my parents, Marie and Charles Ouimet, for challenging me to reach beyond what I thought I could do.

Kathleen Ouimet Perrin

Thank you to all of my family members, who are my greatest inspiration and continued source of love and hope.

Caryn A. Sheehan

Thank you to my husband, Fred, for his continued role modeling of faith, peace, and joy on our journey together, and for his constant encouragement and support of my professional endeavors.

Mertie L. Potter

Thank you to my family, Glenn, Sarah, Olivia, Tim, and my sister Pat and brother Mike, who have provided me so much support in my palliative care work.

Mary K. Kazanowski

We wish to acknowledge our nursing students from whom we have learned so much. We continue to be impressed with their ability to empathize with suffering patients and their families as well as their level of compassion and commitment to alleviate suffering. Specifically, we wish to acknowledge and thank the following former students who allowed their projects and/or papers to be included in this book.

Chapter 1	Sarah Morin	Case study and figure
	Leslie Burnham	Case study
Chapter 2	Erica Lopes	Figure
Chapter 3	Angelina Makarov Skorupski	Poem
Chapter 4	Marysa Morin	Poem
	Kathleen Masterson	Case study
	Meghan Jacques	Case study
Chapter 5	Kristina Michaud	Figure
	Megan McMahon	Case study
Chapter 6	Katie Powers	Case study and figure
Chapter 7	Emily Traicoff	Figure
Chapter 8	Jillian Buratto	Figure
Chapter 9	Kaitlin Farley	Figure
	Shaylin Kirby	Case study
	Erin Latina	Case study and poem
Chapter 10	Madelyn Cantarow	Case study and figure
Chapter 11	Megan McMahon	Figure
Chapter 12	Jessica Cantone	Case study and figure

We also want to acknowledge our colleague Laurie Tyer, who assisted us by writing the exercise for Chapter 5.

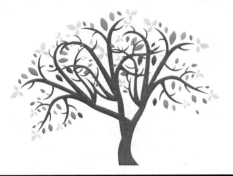

About the Authors

Kathleen Ouimet Perrin, PhD, RN, CCRN, is a professor of nursing at Saint Anselm College, Manchester, New Hampshire, where she teaches courses in critical care nursing, professional nursing, and understanding suffering to baccalaureate nursing students. She received her bachelor's degree from the University of Massachusetts, Amherst; her master's from Boston College; and her doctoral degree from the Union Institute, Cincinnati, Ohio. Her primary areas of interest are critical care nursing, ethical issues, nursing history, and suffering experienced by patients and healthcare providers.

Caryn A. Sheehan, DNP, APRN-BC, is an associate professor of nursing at Saint Anselm College, Manchester, New Hampshire, where she teaches geriatric and medical/surgical nursing to baccalaureate nursing students. She received her bachelor's degree from Saint Anselm College, her master's from Boston College, and her doctoral degree from Case Western Reserve University, Cleveland, Ohio. Her primary areas of publication and interest are men's health, oncology, and chronic pain/quality of life.

Mertie L. Potter, DNP, APRN, PMHCNS-BC, is a clinical professor of nursing at Massachusetts General Hospital Institute of Health Professions in Boston, Massachusetts. She teaches in the direct entry master's program and the accelerated baccalaureate nursing program within the psychiatric-mental health specialty track. Dr. Potter has a consultation/nurse practitioner practice in which she works with nursing staff and sees patients. She received her bachelor's degree from Simmons College, her master's from the University of Michigan, and her doctoral degree from Case Western Reserve University. Her special interest areas are grieving, spirituality, body–mind–spirit health, nursing theory, suffering, medical missions, and team building.

Mary K. Kazanowski, PhD, APRN-BC, CHPN, is a nurse practitioner on the Palliative Care Team at Concord Hospital, Concord, New Hampshire, and Nurse Practitioner, Coordinator of Palliative Care for the Visiting Nurse Association Homecare and Hospice of Manchester & Southern New Hampshire, in Manchester, New Hampshire. She received her bachelor's degree from Saint Anselm College, her master's from Boston University, and her doctoral degree from Boston College. Her special interests are in symptom management and the implementation of palliative and hospice care into the healthcare system.

Chapter Contributors

Maureen M. Gaynor, MSN, APRN, PMHCNS-BC, is a clinical instructor of nursing at Saint Anselm College in Manchester, New Hampshire. She teaches psychiatric-mental health in the baccalaureate nursing program and maintains an independent, private practice. She received her nursing diploma from Pilgrim State Nursing School, her bachelor's degree from the New York Institute of Technology, and her master's from Stony Brook University. Her interests are holistic nursing, depression, and women's issues.

Sylvia M. Durette, MS, PMHCNS-BC, is an instructor of nursing at St. Joseph School of Nursing and a board certified psychiatric clinical nurse specialist. She received her bachelor's degree from Saint Anselm College, her master's degree from Boston University, and a Certificate of Advanced Graduate Study from Northeastern University in psychiatric nursing.

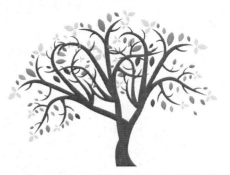

ONE

The Nature of Suffering and Palliative Care

■ Mary K. Kazanowski and Kathleen Ouimet Perrin

Objectives

1. Explore the nature of suffering.
2. Describe various sources of suffering.
3. Recognize the suffering experience as demonstrated by the patient and family.
4. Examine the role of the nurse in assessing for suffering.
5. Identify interventions to prevent and alleviate suffering.
6. Explain the relationship between suffering and palliative care.

Student Project

Figure 1–1 Windspinner

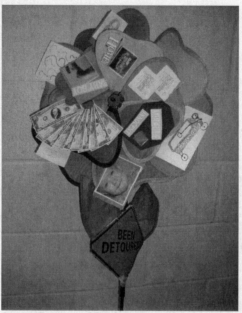

Source: Courtesy of Sarah Morin, student nurse.

Case Study 1–1

Peter was 2 years old and had been a patient on the pediatric unit for most of the summer. He was not a typical patient; the doctors had not been able to make a definitive diagnosis for him. As more and more specialists became involved and more conflicting opinions were given to the family, the family's suffering increased. Although she had three other children at home, Peter's mother was with him almost 24 hours a day. Peter was very irritable, would not eat, and would often just cry.

Peter's mother felt as if their lives were whirling out of control, as depicted in the photo above, the Wind Spinner. She would say that she felt like a bad mother because she could not comfort Peter, manage the care of her other three children, or make sense of the conflicting opinions of the competing physicians. One particular day Peter's mother broke down crying hysterically, and said "I wish he had cancer, so they could just treat it."

Never had I seen a mother suffering so much that she wished her child had cancer.

Source: Courtesy of Sarah Morin, student nurse, 2008.

Questions on the Case Study
1. What behavior is Peter exhibiting that might make you think he is suffering?
2. Likewise, what might make you think his mother is suffering?
3. What do you think about Peter's mother wishing that he had cancer?

Introduction

Definitions provide a basic understanding of the word "suffering" but are limited in their ability to convey the meaning and impact of the suffering experience. The *American Heritage Dictionary* (1992) defines suffering as "the condition of tolerating or enduring evil, injury, pain, or death or the source of pain or distress." Dr. Eric Cassell (1982), in his seminal work on suffering first published in the *New England Journal of Medicine,* described suffering as severe distress associated with events that threaten the intactness of the individual. Cassell described an individual as a complex social and psychologic entity and stressed that "suffering is experienced by persons in their entirety, not merely by their bodies" (p. 639).

Similarly, Wright (2005) defines suffering as physical, emotional, or spiritual anguish, pain, or distress. Experiences that promote suffering include

- serious illness that alters one's life and relationships as one knew them;
- illness that forces exclusion from everyday life;
- the strain of trying to endure;
- longing to love or be loved;
- acute or chronic pain;
- conflict, anguish, or interference with love in relationships.

Wright (2005) further describes suffering as "raw, deep, and personal" (p. 37). Both Cassell and Wright stress suffering as an experience that is unique to an individual, so what constitutes suffering to one person might have a completely different meaning to another.

The Experience of Suffering

Cassell (1991) believes that three kinds of knowledge are needed to understand the impact of suffering on an individual:

- One must understand the "brute facts" of the suffering as experienced by the individual.
- One must have knowledge of the individual's values.
- One must appreciate the aesthetic meaning the individual attaches to the experience.

Thus, to understand the suffering experience, nurses must invite patients to share their experiences of suffering..

Obtaining Private and Personal Information

How does one invite a patient to share personal and private feelings and thoughts, especially about a taboo subject such as suffering? Illness narratives from individuals in their roles as patients or from their families are rich sources of information that can provide insight into the experience. Wright (2007) describes the illness narrative as the story of the experience, the suffering, which includes the effect of suffering on an individual, on her relationships, and on her world. Narratives can be collected formally through the research process or informally, through impromptu or planned conversations. A simple open-ended question, such as "What is causing you to suffer during the course of this illness and your treatment?" can allow patients to begin to describe their experience. Such conversations may occur at the bedside, in the home, or in the hallway of a busy clinic. Providing opportunities for patients to express their illness narratives and listening attentively to these stories is a major nursing responsibility. Sharing in the narrative by attentive listening is also a privilege.

Sources of Suffering

A multitude of sources can lead to a suffering experience. Although it is imperative to remember that the suffering experience is unique to each individual and that a specific source does not lead to suffering in all situations or for every person, knowing the various possible origins can be valuable in recognizing the suffering experience. According to Reed (2003), sources of suffering can be physical, psychological, sociocultural, developmental, or spiritual.

Physical Sources of Suffering

Physical sources are some of the most obvious causes of suffering, with pain being most commonly recognized by healthcare providers as a cause. Ferrell (2008) notes that it is specifically pain without meaning that is associated with suffering. For example, the pain of childbirth is not usually associated with suffering in the same way as the chronic, severe pain of peripheral vascular disease. A study by Lesho and others (2006) showed that healthcare workers across healthcare settings significantly underestimated the extent of suffering their patients experienced from physical, nonpainful symptoms such as nausea, debilitating fatigue, or pronounced dizziness.

Physical sources of suffering may include

- illnesses that cause pain, functional decline, fatigue, dyspnea, nausea, anorexia, and vomiting;
- injuries that cause pain, functional limitations, and fatigue;
- treatments that cause pain and anxiety such as blood draws, dressing changes, suctioning, and insertion of invasive apparatus such as chest tubes, nasogastric tubes, and feeding tubes.

Psychological Sources of Suffering

Cassell (1991) and Ferrell and Coyle (2008) stress that in many instances suffering is associated with either an actual loss or the threat of a loss. Cassell believes that suffering begins not when the loss occurs but when the person becomes aware of the impact of the loss on his future existence. Thus the suffering might begin before the actual loss or a substantial amount of time after the loss has occurred as the reality and future consequences become apparent to the person. The loss may be that of a relationship or a bodily part or function, or it may be the person's realization that his life is nearing its end. Ferrell and Coyle note that the recognition of the loss leaves the person with a "sense of brokenness" (p. 246). Lesho and others (2006) found that just as healthcare providers underestimated the extent of physical, nonpainful conditions as sources of their patients' suffering, they also underestimated loss as a source. In their study, the authors cited examples of patient losses as "not being attractive anymore," "losing my hair and my breast," "not being able to walk," and "not being able to have sex" (p. 776).

Ferrell and Coyle (2008) believe that the sense of loss is usually accompanied by the expression of intense emotions ranging from sadness to anguish or fear and despair. Lesho and others (2006) noted that patients expressed these emotions by statements such as "I'm afraid of what is happening to me" or "I worry I will be a burden on my family" (p.775). However, in several of these areas they found that healthcare providers overestimated the extent of patient suffering. Impaired communication exemplified by the patient's stating "my healthcare provider does not allow time for me—or does not listen to me" was also identified more often as a source of patient suffering by healthcare providers than by patients. These overestimates by healthcare providers could be at least in part because the emotional display and verbal behaviors are more obvious to healthcare providers. Nurses need to be careful to validate with their patients whether the patients are suffering psychologically and assess how much they are suffering. In addition to loss, Flaming (1995) included "being in limbo" as a psychological cause of suffering. In this type of suffering, the future is unknown and the inability to know what is likely to happen can gnaw away at the patient. Being in limbo may be confined to a limited amount of time, such as while a person is waiting for test results, or it may extend over years, as in patients surviving treatment for cancer.

Psychological sources of suffering may also include

- guilt,
- fear,
- anxiety,
- betrayal, and
- erosion of trust.

Sociocultural Sources of Suffering

Ferrell and Coyle (2008) believe that one of the major causes of sociocultural or social suffering is that patients suffering from depression or experiencing the physiological effects of their illness withdraw from their families and social networks. When that occurs, the patient often feels isolated and abandoned. The patient may feel abandoned by family and loved ones, but also by their healthcare providers. The patient's fear of abandonment by a healthcare provider can be triggered by a callous statement such as "There is no more that we can do." There may be no more that can be done to *cure* a patient but there is always some way to *care* for the patient. Communicating a commitment to care can ease a patient's sense of abandonment.

Another sociocultural source of suffering that has an indisputable impact on a large percentage of patients is poverty. Poverty manifests itself in poor health, low educational attainment, neglect, homelessness, violence, and abuse, all of which can lead to suffering. People who are poor and members of minorities have the highest morbidity and mortality rates for most major types of cancer. Williams (2004) examined the ways poverty exacerbated the suffering of young, dying patients. She noted that the dying patients who were in the most distress were those with the most interpersonal difficulties and that patients with lower socio-economic status had more self-reported needs. Patients in her study identified fears of eroding the positive sentiment of others and becoming a nonperson whose life was irrelevant. As their disease progressed, the patients in her study were more likely to withdraw from others by no longer attending family, community, or religious events. She concluded that dying in poverty and experiencing social isolation or even social death contributed to patient suffering.

Harrison and Falco (2005) believe that human suffering is a significant consequence of racial disparity in health care. After reviewing research concerning healthcare delivery to African Americans, they concluded that there was "powerful evidence that even controlling for differences related to access, insurance and socioeconomic status, our healthcare system is deeply racist" (p. 252). The disparities associated with racism provided another obstacle to access to health care and eventually led to some African Americans avoiding receiving necessary care. Harrison and Falco use the term "suffering" to describe the disparities because it puts a "face" on the issue (p. 258). Manifestations of suffering displayed by those African Americans who are receiving inadequate care include mistrust, invisibility, unknowing, and loss of humanity. Harrison and Falco argue that a community health nurse serving as an advocate could reach out to members of minorities, help them access necessary health care, and alleviate some of their suffering.

Sociocultural sources of suffering pertain to relationships that are

- interpersonal,
- family relationships, or
- community relationships.

Developmental Sources of Suffering

Developmental sources of suffering include problems with achievement of central tasks within the various levels of growth. Certain age groups have different risks with regard to suffering, based on their control, independence, and vulnerability. For example, young children are more vulnerable than adolescents.

Flaming (1995) believes that suffering may be incomprehensible to young children because they lack the cognitive ability to understand what is happening to them. Worse, children may believe that the suffering has been inflicted on them as a punishment for misbehavior. They may suffer silently, never telling their parents why they believe they are suffering. Older children may suffer silently, pretending that things are okay in an effort to make a difficult situation more bearable for their parents. As an example of this, the third child in a family of five was born with congenital heart disease. While the baby was hospitalized in a tertiary medical center with the mother staying at her bedside, the two older school-age children were cared for by their grandmother at home. The children were never able to tell their already distraught parents that their grandmother was hearing voices and seeing things. As soon as they returned from school and until their father came home late in the evening, their grandmother locked them in a hallway broom closet, not giving them anything to eat and not allowing them out to use the bathroom.

Older adults are more likely to have multiple sources of suffering than young and middle-aged adults. Many older adults experience chronic pain from physical sources such as arthritis. Yet, studies have indicated that it is existential pain rather than physical pain that is their major source of suffering (Gudmannsdottir & Halldorsdottir, 2009). The existential sources of suffering for older adults may include the loss of their loved ones resulting in a loss of a sense of connectedness as well as the loss of their homes, health, and independence.

Developmental sources of suffering may also include

- education-related pressures such as peer pressure and the pressure to succeed in school,
- changes in physical appearance and body image,
- changes in role with aging, such as retirement or the loss of a job,
- loss of sense of self with the development of Alzheimer's, or
- changes in balance and physical functioning with old age.

Spiritual Sources of Suffering

Spiritual sources of suffering are those that impact whatever or whoever gives meaning or purpose to a person. Religion, which involves affiliation or membership in a particular faith community, may or may not play a role in spirituality, because spirituality is much broader than religion. Examples of spiritual sources of suffering could include a patient's questioning why something is happening to her or wondering what she might have done to deserve such an experience. If the person cannot find an answer that satisfies her, then asking these questions may lead to spiritual distress.

A suffering experience may also be accompanied, rather than caused, by spiritual distress (Ferrell & Coyle, 2008). This may occur for a variety of reasons. The suffering person might fear that the end of her life is approaching and might begin to search for meaning in her life as the end nears. If she is experiencing a sense of hopelessness, the sufferer might call into question what she believed previously about the meaning of life and for better or worse may begin to "re-evaluate her relationship with a higher being" (Ferrell & Coyle, 2008, p. 246).

Flaming (1995) describes three different situations in which patients developed spiritual suffering:

- The patient begins to doubt the validity of his long-held religious beliefs and is no longer comforted by his relationship with his God.
- A patient who has previously not been religious or spiritual begins to explore a faith system wondering if it might make bearing her suffering easier.
- The patient suffers because she believes that she is being punished for lack of faith.

Although these sources of suffering were listed and described separately, suffering seldom affects a patient in only one dimension. Often, multiple sources impact the patient's experience concurrently. Additionally, these sources of suffering can be impacted by gender, culture, limited financial assets, limited knowledge and resources, and the environment, including the culture of health care.

Recognizing Suffering

It is imperative that the nurse be able to identify potential sources of suffering, but merely knowing what can cause suffering does not guarantee that a nurse will recognize patients and families who are suffering. Long ago, Kahn and Steeves

(1986) raised the question, how does a nurse infer suffering? They noted that nurses' inferences of patient suffering were related to the nurse's "own cultural and socioeconomic backgrounds, to patient diagnoses, and to patient ethnicity" (p. 628). However, the nurses' inferences of patient suffering were not related to the nurse's age, educational levels, or years of experience. The authors also noted that nurses' ability to recognize patient suffering might be related to the nurses' beliefs about suffering and suppositions that their patients were suffering.

Silent Sufferers

Recognition of suffering requires an understanding that patients and their families may not choose to communicate their experience to others. For a variety of reasons, many patients and families suffer in silence. Patients may do so because they believe that the topic is not appropriate for polite conversation—even in a conversation with a healthcare professional. Or, they may suffer in silence because they are afraid of how people will respond to them. Silent sufferers may include those with addictions or mental illness who suffer in silence because of embarrassment, or because of fear that others will not understand their plight and/or they will be ostracized. Silent sufferers also include those with illnesses contracted sexually, or by illicit drug use, such as hepatitis B, C, or human immunodeficiency virus (HIV). Individuals who have committed morally reprehensible crimes or made immoral choices such as infidelity often suffer alone. Regardless of the cause, source, and presence or absence of indicators for suffering, it is the role of the nurse to assess for suffering in all patient encounters.

Assessing for Suffering

The perception of suffering held by a healthcare provider to some degree impacts the individuals who depend on the person for care. Depending on the healthcare provider's experience, the word "suffering" can conjure up a host of thoughts, images, and feelings. This perception may enhance quality care and outcomes, but it also may serve as a barrier to accurate assessment of another's experience and to provision of interventions that could impact the suffering experience. For this reason, it is essential that healthcare providers listen for and hear the perspective of suffering held by the patients and/or families whom they are attending. Because nurses spend more time with patients than any other providers, they have the potential to hear, and understand, the many sources of their patients' suffering, the nature of their patients' experiences, and the responses of the patients and families to the suffering experience.

Nurses are taught to assess routinely for signs or symptoms of physical and emotional distress associated with illness and injury. However, a nurse's perception of expected outcomes of disease (e.g., it is supposed to hurt) and a nurse's orientation to treatment (e.g., it is meant to help) will impact her view of a patient's experience. What is essential is that regardless of the nurse's perception of illness or treatment, it is the perception of the patient (or family) that makes the experience what it is. Patient/family experiences are unique, and the presence of suffering is determined by the perception of the patient (or family), not the nurse. It can be difficult for a nurse to assess a patient and family for multiple sources of suffering. When a nurse asks a patient how the patient feels, the patient usually responds by describing his physical condition. Thus, if the nurse wants information about the person's other concerns, the question will need to be phrased somewhat differently. For example, the nurse might ask, "How is this hospitalization going for you and your family?" or "What has been the most difficult thing about this illness for you?" Byock (1997) suggests using the phrase, "How are you feeling within yourself?" since he believes it cuts though the patient's defenses and gets immediately to the heart of the patient's concerns.

Such questions can allow patients to begin to develop their "illness narrative." The illness narrative has been utilized extensively as a qualitative research tool to explore the sources and meaning of suffering to a patient and family. It is important for patients to have an opportunity to develop the narrative since it allows them to take the experience out of a purely medical context and integrate the illness and suffering into their life story.

Tools for quantitative assessment of patient suffering are currently under development by Lesho and others (2006). A variety of other tools that assess concepts related to patient suffering are already available. These include tools such as the Pictorial Representation of Illness and Self-Measure (PRISM), which assesses the burden of suffering because of an illness (Kassardjian, Gardner-Nix, Dupak, Barbati, & Lam-McCullock, 2008). The National Palliative Care Research Center provides links to valid tools for the assessment of pain and symptom management, functional status, psychosocial care, and quality of life. When the nurse assesses the patient for suffering, it is essential that the nurse recall that patients, particularly hospice patients, state that pain and suffering are two different phenomena and that they experience more suffering than pain (Baines & Norlander, 2000). This is important since nurses are more likely to have been educated about pain assessment, utilize a standardized tool to assess pain, and have experience in providing relief of pain. Assessing and alleviating the multiple sources of suffering can be far more complex and difficult.

The Relationship Between Suffering and Palliative Care

A growing body of evidence indicates that there are significant levels of unrelieved suffering for patients within the U.S. healthcare system (Brunnhuber, Nash, Meier, Weissman, & Woodcock, 2008). Some of this suffering is a result of a mismatch between patient needs and the type of care provided within our healthcare system. This is partly because our system is structured to aggressively treat acute illnesses rather than manage the chronic illnesses that many patients suffer with, and eventually die from. Palliative care has evolved in an attempt to better address the needs of individuals with advanced (often chronic) illness. The World Health Organization's definition of palliative care is displayed in Box 1–1.

Palliative care is multidisciplinary care, intended to focus on relief of the patient's symptoms and promotion of the patient's quality of life. In an editorial in the *American Journal of Nursing,* Mason, Coyle, and Ferrell (2004) call for all care to be palliative care, which they define as care that is based on patient need rather than on patient prognosis or diagnosis. This emphasizes the focus of providing care that is individualized for the patient, not the diagnosis. Palliative care is not the "one size fits all care" that is common to each patient with a specific diagnosis in the current healthcare system. In addition, it is also not just for patients with a terminal illness. In fact, the goal of palliative care—relieving suffering and providing the best possible quality of life for patients and their families—is appropriate for all patients and can be provided in conjunction with aggressive or curative care.

How does palliative care work both alone or in conjunction with curative care? Palliative care focuses on the relief of the symptoms and mitigation of the sources of patient suffering. So, rather than focusing on the treatment of heart failure, the palliative care team would help the patient to find relief from the accompanying shortness of breath or extreme fatigue, or help the patient have the strength to carry on with his activities of daily living or cope with his medical

Box 1-1   World Health Organization (WHO) Definition of Palliative Care

WHO defines palliative care as "an approach that improves the quality of life of patients and their families facing the problems associated with life-threatening illness, through the prevention and relief of suffering by means of early identification and impeccable assessment and treatment of pain and other problems, physical, psychosocial and spiritual. Palliative care

- provides relief from pain and other distressing symptoms;
- affirms life and regards dying as a normal process;
- intends neither to hasten nor postpone death;
- integrates the psychological and spiritual aspects of patient care;
- offers a support system to help patients live as actively as possible until death;
- offers a support system to help the family cope during the patient's illness and in their own bereavement.
- uses a team approach to address the needs of patients and their families, including bereavement counseling, if indicated;
- will enhance quality of life, and may also positively influence the course of illness;
- is applicable early in the course of illness, in conjunction with other therapies that are intended to prolong life, and includes those investigations needed to better understand and manage distressing clinical complications" (WHO, 2008).

The WHO definition of palliative care for children states that it "represents a special, albeit closely related field to adult palliative care," with principles related to pediatric chronic disorders. Palliative care for children

- is the active total care of the child's body, mind, and spirit, which also involves giving support to the family;
- begins when illness is diagnosed, and continues regardless of whether a child receives treatment directed at the disease;
- requires a broad multidisciplinary approach that includes the family and makes use of available community resources;
- can be provided in tertiary care facilities, in community health centers, and even in children's homes.

Source: Courtesy of the World Health Organization. *Definition of palliative care for children.* World Health Organization website. http://www.who.int/cancer/palliative/definition/en. Accessed September 16, 2010.

regimen. Additionally, the team would focus on having the patient fully understand his choices for care. In short, symptom management, communication, assistance with goal setting, and clinical decision making while providing support for the patient and the family are the primary goals of palliative care.

To meet their goals, the palliative care team would have to provide these to the patient and family:

- expert management of pain and other symptoms;
- clear communication among patient, family, and team;
- help in navigating the healthcare system;
- detailed practical information and assistance;
- guidance with difficult and complex treatment choices; and
- emotional and spiritual support.

Evidence Base for Palliative Care

Although the experience of suffering is certainly not confined to patients with life-limiting illnesses or even chronic non-life-threatening illnesses, nurses and providers wishing to expand their understanding of the suffering experience and enhance their knowledge of interventions to alleviate suffering would benefit greatly from reviewing the palliative care literature. Because it is a young specialty, there is limited evidence to support all interventions. However, the evidence is building; and many of the interventions that may not be supported by research are supported by respected traditions from the disciplines of psychology, sociology, and theology (Lipman, Jackson, & Tyler, 2009). The principles, philosophy, and practices of palliative care, with its emphasis on interdisciplinary interventions, serve as an excellent model to use in addressing those who are suffering.

Nursing Attributes Needed for Palliative Care

Nurses have traditionally been important members of the palliative care team. They are often among the first healthcare professionals to recognize patient suffering, assess it, and begin to attempt to alleviate it. After recognizing that a patient is suffering, the nurse may begin an assessment by listening to the patient's illness narrative or by doing a more structured appraisal. How the nurse responds to the patient's and family's account of suffering is important as it will allow the nurse to develop an understanding of what they are experiencing, learn about their values and hopes, and understand their goals. As the patient is describing his suffering, the nurse might respond by listening or affirming what is being conveyed. But apathy should never be the response. In fact, an apathetic response by a nurse can increase the burden of patient or family suffering and can be a source of suffering in and of itself. Reich (1989) spoke of the importance of nurses being fully present and listening carefully to patients who are suffering, thus providing them "voice." Ferrell and Coyle (2008), in their article "The Nature of Suffering and the Goals of Nursing," also stated that nurses respond to suffering primarily through their presence.

Pavlish and Ceronsky (2009) surveyed oncology nurses with regard to what they believed were the most important attributes for providing palliative care. They too emphasize the importance of presence and another attribute they call *perceptive attentiveness.* Together these two attributes imply that palliative care nurses should attend to the unique situations and subtle needs of their patients. This means that they need to "tune in" to the patient and see the patient behind the equipment, listening to the needs and concerns of that specific person. When they are with each patient, they should have an aura of peacefulness about them so the patient does not fear that the nurse needs to be running off to attend to something else. As noted earlier, they should be listening attentively to what that patient and family has to say; not thinking where they needed to be next or what they believe should be the patients' greatest concern. Simon, Ramsenthaler, Bausewein, Krischke, and Geiss (2009), in attempting to discover a core attitude for palliative care nurses, identified *authenticity,* which they described as being present, being open, and having unconditional regard for the patient and family. Betty Ferrell (2005) would call this being in relationship with the patient and family and say "that nurses hold an intimate place, perhaps a sacred place, in caring for a patient and family in pain" (p. 86). The nurses in the 2009 study by Simon and others also identified creating a relationship with the patient and family as being at the center of their work.

Another attribute identified by the nurses in Pavlish and Ceronsky's 2009 study was being deliberate, hearing what the patient and family had to say, and considering their options before proceeding. Simon and others (2009) referred to a similar behavior, calling it "creating space." Nurses in their study noted that patients needed the time, knowledge, and space to choose their own way. They believed it was the nurses' responsibility to provide the preconditions.

Palliative care is founded on the principle of a multidisciplinary approach to care of the patient and family—with the patient and family as a single unit of service. Nurses noted that a family orientation and an ability to collaborate were essential attributes for palliative care nurses (Pavlish & Ceronsky, 2009). Nurses need to assist families to develop confidence in their ability to care for patients. More important, they need to work with patients, families, and other healthcare providers so that they understand each other and develop common goals.

Palliative care nurses emphasized the importance of clinical expertise and honesty when speaking with patients (Pavlish & Ceronsky, 2009). Clinical expertise involved being knowledgeable about the disease trajectory, management of illnesses, and alleviation of symptoms, but also knowing the patient. Honesty was seen as the way the nurses were able to convey this information to the patient and family. The palliative care nurses in Pavlish and Ceronsky's study linked honesty to Ferrell's concept of respect, knowing the patient and family, believing that the patient and family were experiencing what they said they were experiencing, and being an advocate for relief or assistance for them (2005). One nurse in Pavlish and Ceronsky's study commented that the most important aspect of palliative care nursing was that "patients want to know they've been heard, that their top priority is being addressed" (p. 406).

The Role of the Nurse in Alleviating Suffering

Researchers (Pavlish & Ceronsky, 2009; Simon et al., 2009) found that nurse attributes such as those described previously are more important than adherence to specific nursing roles when providing palliative care. Nonetheless, there are some roles that nurses providing palliative care are often called to assume, such as the following:

- *Teaching:* preparing patients and their families for decision making as well as for care of the patient—most important, symptom management
- *Caring:* relating to each patient as a unique individual and providing physical, emotional, and spiritual comfort and support
- *Coordinating:* interfacing with the multidisciplinary team, patient, and family to develop shared goals and a cohesive patient-centered treatment plan
- *Advocating:* getting to know the patient and family, learning their needs and quality of life preferences and implementing the treatment plan

- *Mobilizing:* being attentive, assertive, and resourceful when responding to the ever-changing needs of patients and families (Pavlish & Ceronsky, 2009)

The Process of Suffering

Kahn and Steeves believe that "suffering involves the person in a larger process that includes the person's own coping with suffering and the caring of others" (1995, p. 13). They developed a model (see Figure 1–2) with suffering at the apex of a triangle and caring and coping at both bases. Their model emphasized the primacy of the suffering experience to the individual and showed the relationship of suffering with caring and coping. In their model, suffering results in two processes, one that is intrapersonal (coping) and one that is interpersonal (caring). They defined the relationship between suffering and coping as "the process by which the individual who was suffering made meaning of the suffering experience" (1995, p. 23). They defined caregiving as the relationship between caring

Figure 1–2   The Psychosocial Basis of Suffering

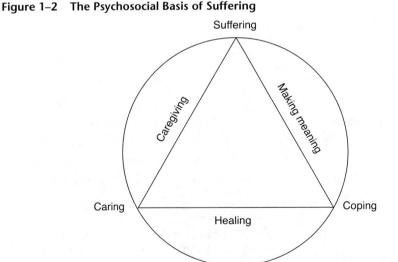

Source: Kahn D. L. and Steeves, R. H. (1996). An understanding of suffering grounded in clinical practice and research (pp. 3–27). In B. R. Ferrell (Ed). *Suffering.* Sudbury, MA: Jones and Bartlett.

and suffering, an "interpersonal process that included efforts made by others to alleviate, ameliorate, or ease the person's suffering" (1996, p. 23).

Kahn and Steeves (1995) believe that nurses are drawn to the suffering person by a caring response. Once in a relationship with a suffering individual, a nurse begins caregiving. Caregiving as provided by nurses includes assessing, goal setting, and planning (with patients) those interventions that are acceptable to them. Nurses would utilize any of the skilled interventions in their repertoire ranging from the use of medications or technologies to the therapeutic use of self. The intervention of facilitating consistent therapeutic communication, from the start of care and throughout, is central to the goal of alleviating suffering. Communication that is therapeutic is based on the underlying principles of respect, genuineness, empathy, and trust (Sheldon, 2009).

While the interpersonal process of caregiving is occurring, the patient would be engaged in the intrapersonal process of making meaning. The base of the triangle in the model describes the dynamic interaction between the individual's ability to cope and the efforts of others to provide care to the individual. When both processes are successful, Kahn and Steeves (1995) believe that the patient's suffering is balanced by healing.

Case Study 1–1   (continued)

The student nurse's response to Peter's mother in the case study at the start of this chapter is an example of how she used her understanding of suffering to identify and implement an intervention that provided some relief: "The only thing that made Peter stop crying was to be pulled around in a red wagon on the unit. His mother would literally pull him around all day, holding the IV pole and wagon in one hand and a book in the other hand. Peter developed a fever one evening. After hours of walking, his mother had finally gotten him to sleep when he needed some IV medication and woke up. Peter started crying, and so did his mother. It was the middle of the night, and neither had slept in days. I took one look at her and said 'I'm going to take Peter in the wagon. You should get some sleep.' I pulled Peter around the unit for 3 hours, while his mother got to sleep."

By recognizing the suffering of the patient and his mother, being aware of the limited number of effective interventions, and embracing the role of alleviating pain for both Peter and his mother, the student nurse facilitated a break their suffering for 3 hours! Nursing interventions to relieve suffering are most often perceived as physical actions such as administering medications, repositioning, massaging, or bathing. But listening, affirming, providing presence, and yes, pulling a wagon should never be underestimated.

Summary

The experience of suffering varies from individual to individual and often involves either the threat of a loss or an actual loss. People usually begin to experience suffering when they realize the impact of the loss on their future existence. Although suffering is often confounded with pain, pain is only one type of physical suffering. Studies indicate that hospice patients say that other sources of suffering are more problematic for them than pain, and that healthcare providers consistently underestimate the suffering associated with symptoms/concerns other than pain.

A variety of tools are available to assess the effects of suffering on a patient's quality of life. Nurses can assess the depth and meaning of suffering for a patient by listening to the patient's illness narrative, a qualitative research technique. Once the sources of suffering and their effect on the patient's life have been identified, nursing care aimed at alleviating the suffering may be instituted. Palliative care is multidisciplinary care of suffering patients and their families with the goal of alleviating patients' suffering and improving their quality of life.

Key Points

1. Suffering often involves a loss or the threat of a loss.
2. Suffering can involve physical, emotional, developmental, or spiritual anguish, pain, or distress.
3. The experience of suffering is unique to each person; therefore, suffering cannot be presumed to be present or absent in any specific situation. The person must be asked what he or she is experiencing.

4. Listening to a patient's illness narrative can help the nurse to understand the source and extent of a patient's suffering.
5. Palliative care is multidisciplinary care, intended to focus on relief of the patient's symptoms and promotion of the patient's quality of life.
6. Nurses have important roles in the alleviation of suffering and the provision of palliative care.

Exercise

Recall a past experience either in your professional life or in your personal life when an individual was suffering.

1. Identify barriers that interfered with your ability to confidently respond to the person's suffering.
2. Given your current understanding of suffering, how would you respond differently now?
3. Based on Kahn and Steeves's model of suffering, draw a diagram depicting the suffering, coping, caring, and ideal healing aspects of this experience.

Questions for Reflection and Journaling

What do you think of when you hear the word suffering?

1. Do you think of an incurable illness, which is accompanied by pain?
2. Do you think of death, and the sorrow of those left behind?
3. Do you think of your own suffering, or the suffering of others?
4. Is suffering physical and constant, or emotional and intermittent?
5. Does it linger and haunt you, or does it resolve itself, and let you move on?

Case Study 1–2: "Dylan"

As we entered the elementary school that day, the staff alerted the school nurse that "Dylan" had abdominal tenderness and a high fever, and he had vomited the day before. Dylan was wearing the same clothes as the day that he had vomited; they had a nauseating odor. He had not bathed, as evidenced by the emesis present in his long hair. Upon examination, Dylan still had a slight fever and complained that he had not eaten since the previous day. Because the school mandates that students remain at home for 24 hours after vomiting or high fever, the nurse tried to call home several times to alert Dylan's mother, but received no response. Since there were no emergency contacts for Dylan or his 5-year-old sister, the nurse and I drove him home.

Upon arriving, Dylan called out for his mother to answer the door. Although a television could be heard inside no one responded to the calls or our knocking on the door. After several minutes, Dylan remembered that he had a key in his backpack and began to unlock the door, whereupon his mother hastily opened the door, almost knocking her child over. The house was filled with grocery store plastic bags filled with clothing and toys. The television still blared in the background. When the nurse calmly explained to Dylan's mother why he could not be in school, she glared at him and said, "He did what?" She refused financial assistance from the nurse for cab fare to take Dylan to a clinic saying, "I don't want it, I'm not taking it. When I was sick with an ear infection, I walked to the clinic. I did it and he can do it." When the nurse continued to suggest he needed medical care, Dylan's mother responded, "Well, I'll just keep him out of school for the rest of the week, I don't need you." Then she slammed the door, keeping Dylan inside.

When Dylan returned to school several days later, he had a bruise on his face, which he told the teachers was from "walking into a wall." The school photographed his face and reported the entire incident to the authorities. However, they determined that there was inconclusive evidence of abuse and Dylan's situation continued.

When I returned from clinical, I spent the day crying. I was upset at the thought that because I had helped bring Dylan home, perhaps I was part of the catalyst that caused his mother to escalate her abuse. I cried because I felt overcome with guilt at being unable to rescue this child and his sister who desperately needed a good, safe, clean home. Later, I comforted myself by realizing that although Dylan might not be able to escape from his mother, he could seek refuge in the school setting.

Source: Courtesy of Leslie Burnham, student nurse, 2006.

Questions on the Case Study

1. What are the physical, psychological, sociological, developmental, and spiritual sources of suffering in this case study?
2. What other factors could be involved that would impact this child's suffering?
3. How else might the nurse have tried to assess the suffering present in the situation?
4. Were the nurse and student able to validate any of the sources of suffering—why or why not?
5. Do you believe there are situations when a nurse might unintentionally make a patient's suffering worse?
6. Do you believe there are situations when there is very little that the nurse can do to alleviate the patient's suffering?
7. What other interventions might the nurse and student have considered?

References

Baines, B., & Norlander, L. (2000). The relationship of pain and suffering in a hospice population. *American Journal of Hospice and Palliative Care, 17*(5), 319–326.

Brunnhuber, K., Nash, S., Meier, D. E., Weissman, D. E., & Woodcock, J. (2008). *Putting evidence into practice: Palliative care.* London: BMJ Publishing Group.

Byock, I. (1997). *Dying well: Peace and possibilities at the end of life.* New York: Riverhead Books.

Cassell, E. (1982). The nature of suffering and the goals of medicine. *New England Journal of Medicine, 306*(11), 639–645.

Cassell, E. (1991, May–June). Recognizing suffering. *Hastings Center Report,* 24–31.

Ferrell, B. (2005). Ethical perspectives on pain and suffering. *Pain Management Nursing, 6*(3), 83–90.

Ferrell, B. R., & Coyle, N. (2008). The nature of suffering and the goals of nursing. *Oncology Nursing Forum, 35*(2), 241–247.

Flaming, D. (1995). Patient suffering: Taxonomy from the nurse's perspective. *Journal of Advanced Nursing, 25,* 1120–1127.

Gudmannsdottir, G. D., & Halldorsdottir, S. (2009). Primacy of existential pain and suffering in residents in chronic pain in nursing homes: A phenomenological study. *Scandinavian Journal of Caring Sciences, 23*(2), 317–327.

Harrison, E., & Falco, S. (2005). Health disparity and the nurse advocate: Reaching out to alleviate suffering. *Advances in Nursing Science, 28*(3), 252–264.

Kahn, D. L., & Steeves, R. H. (1986). The experience of suffering: Conceptual clarification and theoretical definition. *Journal of Advanced Nursing, 11,* 623–631.

Kahn, D. L., & Steeves, R. H. (1995). The significance of suffering in cancer care. *Seminars in Oncology Nursing, 11*(1), 9–16.

Kahn, D. L., & Steeves, R. H. (1996). An understanding of suffering grounded in clinical practice and research. In B. R. Ferrell (Ed.), *Suffering* (pp. 3–27). Sudbury, MA: Jones and Bartlett.

Kassardjian, C., Gardner-Nix, J., Dupak, K., Barbati, J., & Lam-McCullock, J. (2008). Validating PRISM (Pictorial Representation of Illness and Self-Measure) as a measure of suffering in chronic non-cancer pain patients. *Journal of Pain, 9*(12), 1135–1143.

Lesho, E., Udvari-Nagy, S., Laszlo, R., Saullo, L., & Rink, T. (2006). How accurate are health care workers' perceptions of patient suffering: A pilot study. *Military Medicine, 171*(8), 774–778.

Lipman, A. G., Jackson, K. C., & Tyler, L. S. (Eds.). (2009). *Evidence based symptom control in palliative care.* New York: Haworth Press

Mason, D., Coyle, N., & Ferrell, B. (2004). Why isn't all care palliative care? *American Journal of Nursing, 104*(11), 11.

National Consensus Project Task Force. (2009). *Clinical practice guidelines for quality palliative care* (2nd ed.). Philadelphia: National Consensus Project for Quality Palliative Care.

Pavlish, C. & Ceronsky, L. (2009). Oncology nurses' perceptions of nursing roles and professional attributes in palliative care. *Clinical Journal of Oncology Nursing, 13*(4), 404–412.

Reed, F. C. (2003). *Suffering and illness: Insights for caregivers.* Philadelphia: F. A. Davis.

Reich, W. (1989). Speaking of suffering: A moral account of compassion. *Soundings, 72*(1), 83–108.

Sheldon, L. K. (2009). *Communication for nurses: Talking with patients* (2nd ed). Sudbury, MA: Jones and Bartlett.

Simon, S., Ramsenthaler, C., Bausewein, C., Krischke, N., & Geiss, G. (2009). Core attitudes of professionals in palliative care: A qualitative study. *International Journal of Palliative Care, 15*(8), 405–411.

Williams, B. (2004). Dying young, dying poor: A sociological examination of existential suffering among low-socioeconomic status patients. *Journal of Palliative Medicine, 7*(1), 27–37.

World Health Organization. *Definition of palliative care.* Retrieved from World Health Organization website: http://www.who.int/cancer/palliative/definition/en.

World Health Organization. *Definition of palliative care for children.* Retrieved from World Health Organization website: http://www.who.int/cancer/palliative/definition/en.

Wright, L. (2005). *Spirituality, suffering, and illness: Ideas for healing.* Philadelphia: F. A. Davis.

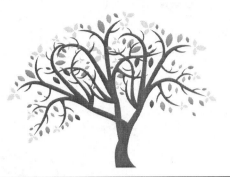

TWO

Suffering in Special Populations

■ Mertie L. Potter

Objectives

1. Compare and contrast suffering in different cultures.
2. Describe suffering in relation to a child's developmental needs.
3. Distinguish sources of suffering for the patient with mental illness and his or her family/significant others.
4. Examine sources of suffering more common late in life with individuals who have experienced cognitive deficits or impairments.
5. Clarify sources of suffering for student nurses and nurses.

Student Project

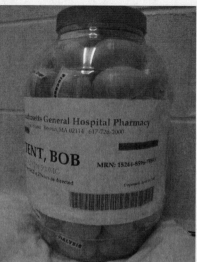

The student described the suffering she witnessed while turning an 84-year-old gentleman in the Intensive Care Unit and looking into his eyes. His eyes conveyed a deep level of suffering that the student had not previously considered when performing other "routine" tasks. It occurred to her that this task was not "routine" to this older patient. In fact, it was yet one more reminder of the suffering, pain, and loss of health and independence that patients have to endure. She used the analogy of a pill bottle to demonstrate how nurses often consider many of their interventions to be therapeutic, while patients may perceive them as a source of suffering.

She labeled "pills" to indicate the suffering she observed in this patient. Some were labeled anasarca (generalized edema), psychosis, pain, amputation, acute respiratory distress syndrome, chest tubes, intra-aortic balloon pump, precautions, postoperative medications, multisystem organ failure, dialysis, psychosis, central line, chest tube, cardio-pulmonary resuscitation (CPR), adult respiratory distress syndrome (ARDS), pneumonia, lack of sleep, and sepsis.

Source: Courtesy of Erica Lopes, student nurse.

Case Study 2–1: Loss of Pet "Rainbow"

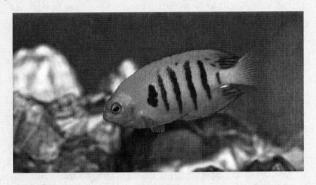

David received Rainbow on his sixth birthday. It was his very first pet, and he was determined to take good care of him. David still was adjusting to the loss of his mother's presence due to divorce. David took great pride in watching over his newfound friend. Rainbow only lived 2 weeks. David was devastated when Rainbow died. David's little body convulsed as he sobbed for about 20 minutes. His father was surprised at his son's strong reaction to this loss.

David asked if he could use his grandmother's Mary Engelbreit garden marker as a gravestone for Rainbow. David and his grandfather buried Rainbow ceremoniously in semifrozen, snow-covered ground near the back steps of their house. The colorful "HOME SWEET HOME" garden marker signifies where Rainbow is buried. On the back of the "gravestone" in black magic marker Rainbow's death is memorialized with these words:

Rainbow

February 11, 2008

Questions on the Case Study

1. What differences/similarities do you think may exist among a 3-year-old diagnosed with a terminal illness, an 8-year-old who lost his first pet, a 20-year-old diagnosed with a chronic mental illness, and an 85-year-old diagnosed with dementia?

2. Which individual would be most difficult for you to care for and why?

Introduction

Suffering is a theme contemplated in various arenas, including health care, politics, law, philosophy, and religion. In spite of great strides made to relieve it, much suffering continues, and in some cases it is seemingly "more outrageous, unjust, and unbearable than ever before" (Gonzalbo, 2006, p. ix). Why is that? Is it because our world seems smaller, more accessible, and more connected, making us more aware of suffering on a worldwide scale—and does this broaden and deepen our awareness and concern? Are we on "suffering overload," because we are confronted daily with humanity's suffering through many forms of media? Is it because we as nurses see new technology and treatments that allow us to alleviate some forms of suffering but perhaps may generate others?

Gonzalbo (2006) asserts that each culture must decide how it will deal with the concept of suffering in its many different forms as well as determine what meaning to give to the suffering. Furthermore, Gonzalbo suggests that meaning attribution strongly correlates with feelings and causes one to decide if suffering "is related to the will of the gods or fate" or is "a form of punishment or a means of purification" (2006, p. 2).

Questions for Journaling
1. Why do you think suffering exists?
2. Does mankind have any control over suffering?

Each individual's suffering is unique and special to that individual, and in most cases, it is interpreted through the individual's cultural perspective, both past and present. Most groups of individuals who experience a common type of suffering or experience the same difficulty together might consider that their group is "special." Any individual or population can be considered "special" in relation to suffering. The purpose of this chapter is not to detract from the significance of suffering experienced by any individual or group. It is hoped this chapter will help the reader learn how to identify and understand the suffering of an individual or group and learn ways to alleviate it or provide comfort in relation to the suffering—both that witnessed by the nurse and that experienced by the nurse.

Children, those diagnosed with mental illness, and older adults diagnosed with cognitive deficits are selected as special populations for a number of reasons. First, it can be challenging to obtain evidence-based data from all three of these populations. Children may or may not be able to express their suffering verbally and/or clearly. Likewise, someone diagnosed with a severe mental illness may face similar difficulties in terms of self-expression of suffering and willingness to share. Additionally, older adults who have cognitive deficits or impairments may face comparable struggles. All three groups may face similar challenges in expression of their suffering and in obtaining comfort in relation to their suffering. Although the three groups may have some likenesses, they will be explored separately because of their unique considerations. Factors related to each of these groups can be applied to other individuals or groups experiencing suffering.

Suffering is defined as "the condition of one who suffers: the bearing of pain or distress" (*American Heritage Dictionary*, 2006, p. 1730). Gonzalbo relates suffering to "pain, sickness, separation, abandonment, death." Suffering often impacts an individual physically, emotionally, spiritually, culturally, and psychologically (2006, p. 2). Ferrell and Coyle (2008, p. 243) depict suffering as having three core dimensions: (1) subjection to violence, (2) sensation of being deprived or overwhelmed, and (3) living in apprehension.

Råholm points out that the words "patient" and "suffering" come from similar Latin roots, as both mean "to bear"; furthermore, to be a patient means "to suffer" (2008, p. 64). Suffering not only involves bearing some level of distress and pain but also may be worsened through alienation and loneliness. Therefore, the need is paramount for the nurse to connect with patients, as well as bear with them through their suffering. Part of this bearing may involve the nurse's presence and willingness to listen to patients' stories in order to give meaning to their experience of suffering and to assist them through the ordeal (Råholm, 2008).

Sources of Suffering: Cultural Considerations

Culture

Suffering occurs within the context of an individual's historical, cultural, sociopolitical, religious/spiritual, and economic perspectives (Barton-Burke, Barreto, & Archibald, 2008). Within those perspectives, individuals will have their own unique experiences that define the suffering experience for them. Each individual suffers differently and uniquely. How people journey through suffering arises from a blend of their traditions and styles (Gonzalbo, 2006, p. 16).

Kirmayer (2001, p. 22) asserts that culture is not merely a trait displayed by patients but rather a transient and transforming concept involving interrelationships that take place between individuals, communities, and larger philosophies and organizational practices. Part of the grieving process or journey for an individual involves redefining and reintegrating the self into life (Shapiro, 2008, p. 41). An individual's cultural background and present cultural environment and experience can impact that redefinition and reintegration greatly.

Another important factor related to culture that will influence an individual along the journey is resilience. Resilience is the ability to bounce back and persevere through challenging times (Engel, 2007). When individuals are suffering or experiencing adversity, concentrating upon their strengths may foster resilience. Resilience involves facing stress and dealing with it in a manner that enhances confidence and social competence (Rutter, 1985).

Likewise, hardiness is a trait that can help sustain individuals through suffering. Hardiness is considered to have three main components: (1) commitment (meaning and purpose), (2) control (sense of autonomy over one's life), and (3) challenge (zest for life that perceives change as an exciting opportunity for growth) (Ablett & Jones, 2007, p. 737). Thus, the characteristic of commitment aids individuals in their journey through suffering by affirming meaning and purpose to what they are experiencing. Although individuals who are suffering may not feel in control of the actual circumstances, they can have a sense of control in how they respond to the suffering. Finally, for hardy individuals, change is embraced as a normal attribute of life that presents opportunities rather than problems.

Although certain experiences may be universal, expression of such experiences can vary greatly. Furthermore, care providers and clients often have very different backgrounds and experiences that impact their perspectives on culture (Kirmayer, 2001). In addition, care providers' ethnocultural background, professional education, and work environment will affect how they view clients and culture. Tension exists between what is universal and what is unique. Each patient a nurse encounters is unique; individuality must be acknowledged. At the same time, the nurse must look for aspects common to others' suffering to assist the patient in realizing the universality of suffering.

One's culture provides examples and cues related to resilience or lack thereof. For example, studies with African Americans have indicated that during stressful periods, African American families often have a strong social network to draw upon, tend not to seek help of professionals, and are more likely than other cultural groups to offer and receive intergenerational help (Laurie & Neimeyer, 2008). Some additional factors to note about African Americans are that they (1) live on average 6 years fewer than Caucasian males and females, (2) often have lost a loved one prematurely and possibly due to homicide, and (3) frequently have endured racism, poverty, and oppression (Laurie & Neimeyer, 2008). Having understanding and empathy for a patient whose background may encompass any of the aforementioned is crucial if the nurse is to foster an effective relationship that builds trust and helps the patient with suffering.

Another example of cultural diversity nurses may encounter is the way Chinese immigrants face end-of-life issues. Lin (2008) explored how United States (U.S.)-resident Chinese immigrants seek meaning when diagnosed with metastatic cancer. Cancer is one of the leading health issues for U.S.-resident Chinese immigrants. It is commonly considered bad luck in Chinese culture to discuss dying and death. Lin found that the 12 participants in this qualitative study felt meaning in their lives helped them journey through their suffering. The specific areas in which nurses can support meaning to life include helping patients who are suffering sense love and compassion, joy and value, hope and faith, readjustment and transcendence, and empowerment and peaceful dying (Lin, 2008, p. 256). Nurses can support these areas by listening to patients' life stories, promoting support and caring from families and religious practices, and ensuring good symptom control (Lin, 2008, pp. 256–257).

People in Western culture tend to avoid suffering and find little value in it. In a grounded theory study by Sacks and Nelson (2007), 18 chronically ill patients participated. The study explored nonphysical suffering and what might be helpful in dealing with it. Although each individual's suffering was different, trust was a common theme and pivotal to the suffering experience. The study supported the importance of nurturing trust in the nurse-patient relationship, especially during a time of vulnerability for the patient. Patients valued talking with nurses about their suffering to get perspective on the suffering situation, provide meaning within the context of the suffering, and reframe the suffering experience. Patients also increased their trust and appreciation for nurses who demonstrated competence in clinical skills, knowledge and trustworthiness, comfort care, and understanding of how a symptom affected the patient (Sacks & Nelson, 2007, p. 688).

Shapiro (2008) contends that families play an important role in helping individuals regain a degree of normalcy and routine when overwhelming circumstances arise. This process is (1) multifaceted, (2) takes place on many levels and dimensions, and (3) involves individual, relational, and cultural expectations. She further asserts that individual as well as family strengths can be stimulated by nursing interventions that support grief and growth (Shapiro, 2008).

Healthcare Disparities

Conditions, such as being diagnosed with cancer, can be an "equalizer"—that is, cancer affects people of all ages, races, genders, and economic states. It also results in a multicultural experience (Barton-Burke *et al.*, 2008, p. 235). In regard to treatment of cancer, however, it becomes evident that there is an unbalanced aspect in relation to culture. Those who have language barriers or are without sufficient economic resources carry a heavier burden of suffering. Therefore, the equalizing effect of a diagnosis such as cancer is negated by disparities related to treatment among those with language or monetary difficulties.

Given the increasing diversity of culture within the United States, nurses are challenged to provide culturally sensitive care to clients as well as information and education that are readily understandable. Nursing education programs and healthcare facilities vary greatly in how they provide information to assist nursing students and nurses to become familiar with different cultural groups for whom they provide care. Adequate resources must be provided to increase nursing skills and confidence in working with culturally diverse populations (McHenry, 2007).

Sources of Suffering for Children

Concerns

What makes the suffering of children unique? Children are considered a vulnerable population based upon their developmental level, immature coping resources, and subjection to adult authority. Being a vulnerable population puts children at risk for suffering. Young children often have not had many life experiences or developed cognitive systems with which to process and handle suffering. They have not lived long enough to "bank" coping experiences that would allow them to respond with maturity and seasoning. Children (infants will be included here as

Case Study 2–2: Cross Culture

The short-term medical mission team from the United States to Guinea has been working since 7:30 A.M. Overloaded minibuses, trucks, and cars have driven long distances from very remote villages and arrived at the mission compound with many individuals expecting to receive free dental, eyeglass, and medical care. It is 5 P.M. Many are walking up to team members and pointing out what is hurting them or what they need or would like done for them. Some want cosmetic repairs on their teeth rather than health-promoting and life-saving extractions or fillings.

Communication outside the clinic is mostly nonverbal, as most of the mission team members do not speak the native languages. There are people from four different language groups who arrived for treatment. Coordination is done by the full-time missionaries who live in the area and can speak one or more of the languages represented. The medical team pressures the team leader to keep the clinics open one extra hour to try to accommodate more people. The team leader is not in agreement with the team but decides to go with their request. The clinics stay open the extra hour. One hour later, many still go unseen, are turned away, and return to their villages without treatment. Team members are saddened and overwhelmed, but agree that they are too tired to suggest any further extension today.

At the daily debriefing, expression of feelings is encouraged. The team leader then makes a strong recommendation: all clinics should open and close as previously scheduled for the remainder of the team's time there.

Questions on the Case Study

1. What difference does it make and to whom how long the clinics are kept open?
2. What factors would impact your decision in such a situation to keep the clinics on schedule or extend the hours?

children) most likely will experience some form of suffering for the first time while still young. Numerous factors impact how children will face suffering:

- genetics,
- birth order,
- gender,
- environment,
- support systems,
- family mobility,
- individual health,
- family health, and
- experience with loss.

Although sometimes considered and treated as "mini-adults," children are not small grownups but are impacted on many of the same planes as adults—physical, emotional, sociocultural, spiritual, and/or psychological—in relation to suffering. A person's genetic makeup helps determine what internal resources that individual may have to deal with suffering experiences. A child may have a strong physical, psychological, and emotional disposition inclined toward resilience and hardiness, or be more fragile and susceptible to stressors. Children most frequently learn and reflect the values and spiritual belief systems of their primary caregivers. The social and cultural behaviors of children, whether positive or negative, are greatly influenced by their peers.

Placement within the family, also referred to as birth order or ordinal position, determines in many ways how a child will be treated by others within and outside the family. Older children often are expected to be courageous and protect younger siblings whereas younger children may be treated as needing more care and protection. Similarly, gender may affect the way boys suffer, given that some boys, because of the physiological differences from girls, are raised to stifle emotions as a sign of being strong and coping with suffering. This is particularly true of more traditional cultures (Dunlap, 2004).

Environmental influences include local environmental health concerns related to water, air, and sanitation. Social, economic, and cultural environmental factors have implications for how a child may respond to suffering. In addition, regional and global environmental issues may impact a child's personal environment.

Family mobility and stability shape children's views of their environment. Some children face multiple moves while in their family of origin. Level of

Table 2–1   Potential Problems for Children Who Have Been Abused

Academic difficulties	Lying
Aggressive behavior	Malnutrition
Alcohol and/or other drug abuse	Oppositional behavior
Anxiety	Panic attacks
Attention problems	Physical symptoms such as headaches
Bad dreams	and stomachaches
Bed wetting	Repeated self-injury
Behavior problems	Risky sexual behaviors
Chronic pain	Running away
Compulsive sexual behaviors	Self-neglect
Concentration problems	Separation anxiety
Dangerous behavior such as speeding	Sexual dysfunction
Dehydration	Sleep disorders
Depression	Social withdrawal
Dissociative states	Stealing
Eating disorders	Stuttering
Failure to thrive	Substance abuse
Fear or shyness	Suicide attempts
Fear of certain adults or places	Thumb-sucking or any age-
Frequent injuries	inappropriate behavior
Insomnia	Truancy
Learning problems	

Source: Adapted from Newton, 2001.

involvement of extended family or friends for support may be affected by family mobility and stability also. Such support may be increased or decreased depending upon family circumstances. Children who have caregiver relationships with high levels of responsiveness, warmth, and consistency in discipline may have an enhanced ability to handle uncontrollable and controllable life stressors (Wolchik, Ma, Tein, Sandler, & Ayers, 2008).

Some children will face acute and/or chronic illnesses. Some acute conditions are more prevalent in children—for example, pediculosis (headlice), varicella (chickenpox), otitis media (middle ear infection), impetigo (skin infection), and Henoch-Scholein Purpura (auto-immune illness). Likewise, some chronic illnesses may occur initially in childhood. Some examples of these conditions are epilepsy, sickle cell disease, asthma, rheumatic heart disease, cystic fibrosis, and autism. Such illnesses, whether acute or chronic, place a strain on the individual and the individual's family system because of the unpredictability of the illness and the seriousness and/or length of time the family system must cope with the child's illness.

In addition, one or more members in a child's family may experience health challenges, such as conditions that are hereditary or conditions involving substance abuse or dependency. The latter may not only involve interfacing with medical systems but also may involve interactions with legal systems.

Children can suffer many types of losses, including

- pet(s),
- safety and trust,
- familiar environment,
- parents(s),
- sibling(s) or extended family member(s)/significant other(s), and
- health.

For many, especially children, pets are a member of the family. Loss of a pet from natural causes, accident, or euthanasia can result in feelings of tremendous loss, guilt, negativity, withdrawal, anger, depression, and illness. The loss of a pet may be the first loss a child experiences. If pain and/or death of the pet were witnessed or compounded by previous suffering, it can be particularly trying for the child (see Case Study 2–1).

Safety and trust are foundational hierarchical needs in Maslow's theory (Maslow, 1943). Abuse and violence are not unique to children. However, children are particularly defenseless because of inequities between perpetrator and victim related to size, age, and often dominance in relationship. Children who experience abuse, either physical or sexual, may acquire various maladaptive, antisocial, and self-destructive behaviors and thoughts while struggling with abuse and trying to grasp why it is occurring (see Table 2–1). Children may be threatened and told to keep the abuse a "secret." Carrying "the secret" can be additionally overwhelming, cause further stress, and impede the child from being able to develop trusting relationships. Multiple exposure to abuse raises a child's risk for experiencing autonomic and endocrine hyperarousal and numerous conditions (see Case Study 2–3) (Newton, 2001).

Children can experience suffering from causes unrelated to illness. Bullying and school violence are traumatic for children. Teasing that is constant, hurtful,

Case Study 2–3: Loss of Health in Child, "Cassandra and Her Mother"

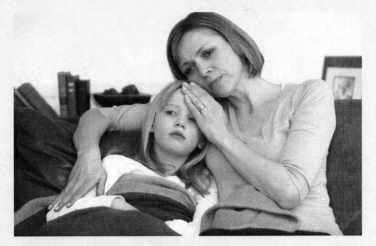

Cassandra was diagnosed with an unusual form of the auto-immune disease Henoch-Schonlein Purpura (HSP) at age 7. Most children who are diagnosed with HSP have a resolution of symptoms within about 4 weeks.

She had classic purpura, joint pains, and arthritis, as well as severe abdominal pain and mild kidney involvement. There was no cure—only symptom management. Included in Cassandra's history was a 3-month period of physical abuse by a childcare worker when Cassandra was a toddler. Her family had a strong faith but wondered why a young child had to endure so much pain and why God allowed Cassandra (and them) to suffer so. Cassandra was the youngest of three children. Her siblings responded differently to Cassandra's illness; one cared for her in tangible ways; the other often withdrew or was angry that medical care was not delivered sooner.

With the condition of HSP, Cassandra and her family experienced aspects related to both acute and chronic illness. Cassandra had had 17 hospitalizations. The family developed some "fire drill routines" when Cassandra's HSP pain symptoms returned and exacerbated. For over 2.5 years between purpura outbreaks and worsening episodes, the family held a guarded hope that Cassandra would be healed—and then one day, she was.

> ### Questions on the Case Study
> 1. Compare 2–3 differences and similarities that occur in acute and chronic illnesses.
> 2. Discuss the different aspects of suffering experienced by Cassandra, her mother, and her siblings.
> 3. How might faith help or hinder a family such as Cassandra's? Support your answer with evidence based data.

and unkind constitutes bullying. Children can feel helpless, unprotected, and alone if they experience either bullying or school violence. Bullying is on a continuum of various forms (see Table 2–2; *Helping Kids Deal with Bullies*, 2009).

School violence, although less frequent than bullying, has major implications for children who witness or are subjected to it. Children who are victims of bullying are at greater risk for involvement in greater and extenuated violence (Dunlap, 2004).

Moving, for whatever reason, may be distressing for a child. Leaving the familiar, even if the previous environment was unpleasant or disruptive, represents change and loss of the known. Leaving a familiar environment may occur rapidly, for example, because of disaster or some other event. Children often perceive a

Table 2–2   Forms of Bullying

Hitting
Shoving
Name-calling
Threats and mocking
Extorting money and treasured
   possessions
Shunning
Spreading rumor
Using e-mail, chat rooms,
   instant messages, social
   networking websites, and
   text messages to taunt or
   hurt feelings

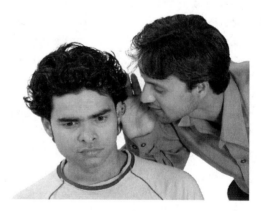

Source: Adapted from *Helping kids deal with bullies*, 2009.

change in routine as loss, as routine provides a level of comfort, regardless of the circumstances (Dunlap, 2004).

Loss of siblings, parents, and extended family/significant others may occur because of moving; divorce; military service; missionary service; business responsibilities; incarceration; and suicide, homicide, accidents, or other causes of death. Children can begin experiencing separation anxiety any time from age 6 months to 8 months (Durso, 2001). By 2 years of age, or the end of the sensorimotor stage in Piaget's theory, a child generally has developed object permanence and realizes and expects that the caregiving figure will return (Piaget, 1932).

Younger siblings in a family in which a child has died may experience more difficulty in coping than older siblings. Older siblings often have more life circumstances, developmental maturity, and additional support systems through relationships, such as marriage (Dyregrov & Dyregrov, 2005). Death of a sibling can result in survivor guilt, with remaining siblings wondering why they were spared or if they could have prevented the loss of their sibling.

In 2007 (Melhem, Moritz, Walker, Shear, & Brent, 2007), a sample of 129 children and adolescents who were 7 to 18 years of age and had experienced the loss of a parent by suicide, accident, or sudden natural death were assessed for complicated grief. Complicated grief was found to be a significant syndrome even after the researchers controlled for current depression, anxiety, and posttraumatic stress disorder. This sample also demonstrated significant functional impairment and correlation with suicidal ideation.

Circumstances that result in separation from a caregiver for an extended period can result in a sense of grave loss for children. Examples of such situations are boarding school for the child; business responsibilities; military commitment of one or more parents; missionary or other service-related responsibilities; parental relocation or prolonged travel due to employment; accidents; marital separation or divorce; or loss of parent(s) to death or other circumstances, such as incarceration. These circumstances also may result in the loss of care by and contact with extended family members/significant others. In the case of divorce, children by and large have to deal with the loss repeatedly. Losing parents because of incarceration or suicide carries additional burdens of stigma and negative legacy for a child.

Children whose parents are incarcerated, on death row, or have been executed carry a unique burden (Beck & Jones, 2007). These children face stigma; an impeded, if not terminated, parental relationship; and in some cases, the anticipation of a gruesome death for their parent. Similarities of imprisonment of a parent to the divorce of one's parents *may* include these:

- no resolution or ending;
- presence of distorted grief reaction;
- intense emotions and higher rates of depression;
- high levels of distress, disorganization, and prolonged grieving;
- nonfinite loss and disenfranchised grief;
- desire to have the absent parent in some form;
- limitations of the parent–child relationship and visits (due to barriers of either institutional glass or distance);
- experience of social isolation;
- boundaries of the relationship dictated by a legal system;
- loss of childhood;
- increased role of caretakers in a child's life.

Children may be impacted with acute and/or chronic health issues. Impaired health may lead to disability and/or long absences from family or school. Health issues have a bearing upon a child's physical, emotional, sociocultural, spiritual, and psychological health.

Nursing Interventions

Recognizing a child's developmental level is critical when assessing needs, concerns, and requests; children cannot be treated as "little adults." Children are known for resilience—the ability to rise above or bounce back from aversive events and maintain relative equilibrium in functioning amid the events (Bonanno, 2004; Engel, 2007). Capitalizing upon this resilience is helpful when formulating nursing interventions. Following are possible interventions for children dealing with suffering:

- Remembering positive and good characteristics about the lost figure or situation; focusing upon positive rather than negative is helpful.
- Providing ceremony to help deal with loss.
- Supporting an individual's faith and culture to enhance healing.
- Recommending bibliotherapy, that is, helping select books that might relate to the individual's suffering circumstances.

- Using creative therapies (art, music, play therapy, etc.) according to the child's abilities and desires to help express and process feelings.
- Considering individual and group interventions at school where children spend a good deal of their time and can share with their peers.
- Exploring benefits of summer camps that might assist the child in dealing with suffering.

Fortunately, research bears out the finding that children, as well as adults, generally follow a pattern of resilience without professional intervention when grieving; only a small percentage of children experience lasting complications from grief (Currier, Holland, & Neimeyer, 2007). Interventions can help ease children's suffering when done in a time-sensitive manner and with specific intervention criteria. Complicated grief in children and how best to intervene still needs to be explored (Currier et al., 2007).

Sources of Suffering for Individuals Diagnosed with Mental Illness

Case Study 2–4: Suffering from Mental Illness, "Mariah"

Mariah Porter is a 20-year-old sophomore student attending a large urban university in the northeast. Her college is about 400 miles from home. She recently had a psychotic episode and was admitted to a private psychiatric facility near her parents' home in a small suburban town. She has two older brothers and one younger sister. Growing up, Mariah was known for her intelligence and having her "head in a book." She never had many friends and tended to spend time with her siblings rather than others. She was considered "shy" and "reserved."

Her parents regret that they did not take Mariah for counseling at the school's urging when she was a senior in high school. During the spring of her senior year, Mariah exhibited bizarre behaviors and was convinced that other students were against her. Her primary care provider recommended a psychiatric evaluation. Her parents did not want Mariah "labeled" as mentally ill so did not take her for an evaluation. They struggled with Mariah's strange behaviors for about 1 month and helped her keep up with schoolwork by hiring a tutor. Mariah had been admitted early to college because of her high test scores and consistently high grades throughout school. This "episode" resolved somewhat, and she was able to graduate. However, she never quite fit back in with her peers after being tutored at home.

Adjusting to city life was very difficult for Mariah. Two of her three roommates were from foreign countries and spoke to one another in their native tongue whenever they were in the college dorm suite. Her third roommate was away from the dorm often with her boyfriend and succeeded in college despite not studying much. Although studying had come easily to Mariah in high school, now she was struggling to maintain her grades and scholarship and lost much sleep trying to do so. She felt isolated and wondered if "others" were trying to make her fail by placing her with these three roommates.

Mariah's parents feel they have "failed" her. They are unsure what the future will hold for Mariah and if she will be able to make it on her own. Mariah has made comments to her parents, such as "You'd be better off if I were dead." She used to be meticulous about her appearance but since her psychotic episode has not paid attention to her hygiene and appearance. The hospital is planning to discharge Mariah within a few weeks. Mariah does not want to go back to college, and her parents do not know how she is going to function anywhere independently.

Questions on the Case Study
1. What kind of "suffering" do you think Mariah may be experiencing?
2. What suffering might her parents be encountering?
3. Are any of them "screaming in pain"?
4. How does Mariah's "suffering" make you feel?

Concerns

An individual diagnosed with mental illness faces suffering in many forms. Probably one of the most painful aspects involves stigma. Stigma for the individual diagnosed with mental illness involves "a collection of negative attitudes and beliefs that lead people to fear, reject, avoid, and discriminate against people with mental illness" (Fontaine, 2009, p. 43). At the end of the continuum on stigma is ostracism, a point at which the individual is totally rejected. Additionally, individuals suffering from mental illness may perpetuate stigma by internalizing negative stereotypes and becoming immobilized to the point of rejecting help being offered to them (Fontaine, 2009).

Economics impacts treatment options for those diagnosed with mental illness. In many parts of the United States there is a shortage of healthcare providers and healthcare options to treat mental illness. Many people diagnosed with mental illness are uninsured.

Having a family member diagnosed with mental illness may affect the other family members, resulting in lost dreams, relationships, income, and social status as well as other important aspects of family life. Mental illness often involves cycles of acute and chronic episodes. Such cycling can be very disruptive for both the individual, the family, and/or significant others. Battles may ensue over treatment and possible hospitalizations. Involvement with the legal system may result if the individual knowingly or unknowingly breaks laws. Sometimes, those diagnosed with severe mental illness no longer have families who feel able or willing to support them after becoming worn out or angry with dysfunctional behaviors.

Interestingly, 40 to 50% of Americans diagnosed with mental illness return to their families after discharge from acute care (Fontaine, 2009). This places a tremendous caregiving burden on the family.

Nursing Interventions

There is no current cure for mental illness. The best treatment option is management of symptoms through medication and various therapies. Many with mental illness can lead productive stabilized lives.

Maximizing support systems for both the individual and the family will be important. Sharing resources that are a fit for the individual and family is most helpful. Assisting individuals to function at their highest level possible is an optimal goal. Enlisting the individual's partnership on this journey is crucial to its success. Demonstrating genuine care and compassion for the patient's suffering with a mental illness will enhance the likelihood of initiating a partnership on this challenging journey.

Sources of Suffering More Common Late in Life

Case Study 2–5: Suffering in the Older Adult, "Mary Salerno"

Mary Salerno, an 88-year-old widow and mother of four adult children, was diagnosed with late onset Alzheimer's disease at 80 years of age. She has lived with her 60-year-old daughter Janine for the last 5 years.

Janine and her husband have become increasingly concerned about Mary. In the past 10 months, Mary wandered from the house on five occasions. All five times, neighbors called to tell Janine that they saw her mother walking down the road. On two of these occasions, the temperature outside was below freezing and Mary was not properly dressed for the weather. Janine has begun to keep the doors locked so that her mother will not wander away.

On the sixth occasion, Mary climbed out of a window onto the porch, went to a neighbor's home, told the neighbor Janine was abusing her, and said she no longer wanted to live with Janine because she is being held as a prisoner. Mary stuck out her arm and said, "See these bruises? That woman is abusing me." The neighbor could not see any marks on Mary's arm and called Janine.

Janine came to the neighbor's house and was devastated when her mother started saying, "I'm not going with her. She abuses me. I have bruises all over my body." The neighbor took Janine aside and told Janine that she did not believe she had done anything to Mary. The neighbor suggested they call the police to get some assistance. A police car with two young police officers arrived at the neighbor's house. Mary would not answer their questions and sat rigidly on the neighbor's lawn chair with her arms folded over her chest.

After numerous attempts to talk with Mary, the police officers called for Sergeant Smith, an older officer who frequently handled domestic issues. Mary seemed to like Sergeant Smith and after some time agreed to get into his police car. When they arrived at Janine's home, Mary said she was not getting out of the police car because she only felt safe if Sergeant Smith were there. Sergeant Smith told Mary he would come back tomorrow to make sure everything was okay if she would go into the house with him now. Mary reluctantly agreed.

Sergeant Smith escorted Mary to Janine's house. He quietly told Janine he would not be back tomorrow but wanted to make sure he could get Mary into the house. He listened to Mary's description of the past few months. He gave Janine names and numbers of potential caregiving facilities. Janine made it clear to him she had no intention of placing her mother in any facility.

Questions on the Case Study
1. What types of suffering are depicted in this case study and who is experiencing it?
2. What do you think about Sergeant Smith's telling Mary he would return the next day when he had no intention of returning?
3. Given that Janine is committed to keeping her mother in her home, what type of interventions might be helpful for this family?

Concerns

Older adults often experience multiple losses. These losses increase in impact and number as one grows older (Lewis & Trzinski, 2006). Some examples include

- spouses/significant others;
- friends;
- roles;
- economic status;
- health;
- home;
- familiar places.

In the case study about Mary Salerno, she had lost someone or something from each of the areas listed above. Her biggest challenge of late and that of her family had been dealing with her Alzheimer's disease.

Alzheimer's disease is the most common of the dementia disorders. There is a 25% occurrence rate in females age 90 years and 21% in males; at age 95 years, it increases to 41% for females and to 36% for males age (American Psychiatric Association [APA], 2000, p. 156). Dementia may be "static, progressive, or remitting" (APA, 2000, p. 152). In Mary's case, it was progressive.

Deficits that occur with dementia include

- memory;
- language function;
- motor abilities;
- executive function.

The areas in which Mary was most affected were her memory and executive function. She enjoyed excellent physical health and had no impairment in her language function or motor abilities. About a year ago, her oldest adult son died. She had difficulty realizing he was gone. Recently, she had become more agitated and depressed, exhibiting behavioral problems such as wandering.

Janine, on the other hand, was physically exhausted keeping up with her mother and was grieving the loss of the close relationship she had once shared with her. She had little time to spend alone with her husband. Janine actually was depressed and experiencing anticipatory grieving regarding further "loss" of her mother.

Nursing Interventions

In spite of difficulty expressing grief, older adults with cognitive impairment appear to undergo similar types of grieving as those who are cognitively intact although loss for them may result in more complicated grief processes. Depending upon level of impairment and stage of dementia, individuals respond differently (Lewis & Trzinski, 2006). Those who are in the early stages of dementia with short-term memory loss and cognitive issues may have more anxiety if each time they hear about a loved one's death is the "first time" for them. Those in advanced stages of dementia may have difficulty grasping the permanence of death and be missing support and understanding from a caregiver who may have died (Lewis & Trzinski, 2006).

Support and understanding are key factors in helping those with cognitive impairment. However, two innovative approaches—spaced retrieval and group buddies—help individuals with dementia deal with death and are specifically targeted to assist individuals with dementia who are grieving (see Box 2–1 and Box 2–2).

Student Nurses/Nurses and Suffering: Evidence-Based Practice Examples

For students, experience with helping patients who are suffering often is limited. Furthermore, they may have had personal suffering experiences they have not

Box 2–1   Helping Individuals with Dementia Deal with Death: Spaced Retrieval

Spaced Retrieval

- Used with individuals having mild to moderate dementia.
- Involves implicit learning—motor learning and repetition priming—retained longer in individuals with dementia—presented in everyday social context.
- Given information targeted for recall.
- Asked about information.
- Given positive reinforcement for correct answer.
- Allowed an interval of time.
- Re-tested.

Source: Lewis & Trzinski, 2006, pp. 779–780.

Box 2–2   Group Buddies

- Taking spaced retrieval to another level—therapeutic play activity.
- Implemented by Trzinski and Higgins (2001) in pilot study with older adults having varied cognitive levels of functioning.
- Manipulate play by use of stuffed animals, that is, "group buddies."
- Viewed by group members as confidants, supports, memory tools, and sources of comfort (Higgins & Trzinski, 2001).
- Increases socialization, fosters creativity, and enhances discussion and exploration of feelings.

Source: Adapted from Lewis & Trzinski, 2006, p. 783.

processed. A phenomenological study done with 11 Taiwanese nursing students explored their reactions and responses to the death of peers (Jiang, Chou, & Tsai, 2006). Themes that emerged from this study indicated that these 11 nursing students experienced

- morbid anxiety;
- helplessness after death;
- fear of disappearance after death;
- thinking of one's own future.

Table 2–3   The Experience of Hospice Nurses Working in Palliative Care

1. An active choice to work in palliative care
2. Past personal experience influences caregiving
3. Personal attitudes to caregiving
4. Personal attitudes toward life (and death)
5. Awareness of own spirituality
6. Personal attitudes toward work
7. Aspects of job satisfaction
8. Aspects of job stress
9. Ways of coping
10. Personal/professional issues and boundaries

Source: Adapted from Ablett & Jones, 2007, p. 735.

To help patients grieve, student nurses who may not have had much experience with grieving could benefit from support. They also need support to increase their ability to handle the death of patients.

Nurses meet patients at points of vulnerability. Nurses must confront the many different faces of suffering in patients: physical, emotional, psychological, spiritual, cultural, social, economic, and others. They have the distinct privilege of being positioned to help patients do the "the work of suffering," namely, move through pain to healing (Råholm, 2008, p. 64).

The words "patient" and "suffer" have the same Latin roots meaning "to bear" (Råholm, 2008, p. 64). Helping patients find a voice in their suffering, even if they cannot speak, is important. Amidst silent suffering, the presence of an attentive nurse may provide the patient a voice, lighten the patient's burden, and begin to bind up the patient's wound (Råholm, 2008).

Interestingly, those working in palliative care with cancer patients do not show higher levels of psychological distress and additionally, demonstrate lower levels of burnout than staff working in other areas of care (see Table 2–3; Ablett & Jones, 2007). With that in mind, it is helpful to try to determine what factors and processes assist nurses in promoting resilience and sustaining a sense of well-being. Ablett and Jones (2007, p. 235) conducted interviews with 10 palliative care nurses and determined that the "job-person fit" was critical, as was the nurses' sense that they

- had chosen to work in this specialty area;
- could make a difference in their patients' lives;
- were aware of their own mortality and spirituality.

Self-transcending Through Suffering

Self-transcendence, or the sense of going beyond and outside of one's self, can come about through suffering; an individual can be "opened, deepened, and spiritually changed" during a suffering experience (Wayman & Gaydos, 2005, p. 264). In a study by Wayman and Gaydos (2005, pp. 265–269), these themes of self-transcendence through suffering emerged:

- turning point;
- pause;
- confrontation;
- surrender;
- extraordinary experiences;
- touchstones;
- change;
- valuing life;
- unfolding wholeness;
- meaningful work;
- gratitude;
- humility;
- an elemental experience—use of metaphors.

When nurses explore self-transcendence with patients who are suffering, they can enhance healing when a cure is not possible.

Summary

Each individual's suffering is unique. This chapter examined suffering within a number of special populations, such as the impact of different cultural considerations; different types of suffering experienced by children; unique features related to those diagnosed with mental illness; challenges presented to older adults impaired cognitively; and the importance of student nurses and nurses getting support with their own personal suffering.

Key Points

1. The potential for "suffering overload" exists today as we become more aware than ever before of suffering on a worldwide scale.
2. Children are not "mini-adults" but are impacted in many of the same areas as adults in relation to suffering: physical, emotional, sociocultural, spiritual, and/or psychological.
3. Those diagnosed with mental illness may face unique areas of suffering, such as stigma, financial strain, restricted healthcare access, lack of support systems, and legal concerns.
4. Older adults with cognitive deficits or impairments often face compromised memory, language function, motor abilities, and executive function.
5. It is beneficial if student nurses and nurses can process their own suffering to help themselves and patients journey through a patient's suffering.

Exercise

Answer the following questions.

1. Think about someone you have observed who handled suffering differently from the way you do. What was different? Were there any ways in which the individual demonstrated values and expressions of suffering similar to yours?
2. How would you feel if you were caring for a patient who was screaming in pain? What would you say to the person or do for the person?

References

Ablett, J. R., & Jones, R. S. P. (2007). Resilience and well-being in palliative care staff: A qualitative study of hospice nurses' experience of work. *Psycho-Oncology, 16*, 733–740.

American Heritage Dictionary of the English Language (4th ed., new updated edition). (2006). Boston, MA: Houghton Mifflin.

American Psychiatric Association. (2000). *Diagnostic and statistical manual of mental disorders* (4th ed., text rev.). Arlington, VA: Author.

Barton-Burke, M., Barreto, R. C., & Archibald, L. I. S. (2008). Suffering as a multicultural cancer experience. *Seminars in Oncology, 24*(4), 229–236.

Beck, E., & Jones, S. J. (2007). Children of the condemned: Grieving the loss of a father to death row. *Omega, 56*(2), 191–215.

Bonanno, G. A. (2004). Loss, trauma, and human resilience: Have we underestimated the human capacity to thrive after extremely aversive events? *American Psychologist, 59*, 20–28.

Currier, J., Holland, J., & Neimeyer, R. (2007). The effectiveness of bereavement interventions with children: A meta-analytic review of controlled outcome research. *Journal of Clinical Child and Adolescent Psychology, 36*(2), 253–259.

Dunlap, L. (2004). *What all children need.* Lanham, MD: University Press of America.

Durso, B. (2001). *Separation anxiety. Your child's development.* Retrieved from http://www.keepkidshealthy.com/development/separation_anxiety.html

Dyregrov, K., & Dyregrov, A. (2005). Siblings after suicide: "The forgotten bereaved." *Suicide and Life-Threatening Behavior, 35*(6), 714–724.

Engel, B. (2007). Eagle soaring: The power of the resilient self. *Journal of Psychosocial Nursing, 45*(2), 44–49.

Ferrell, B. R., & Coyle, N. (2008) The nature of suffering and the goals of nursing. *Oncology Nursing Forum, 35*(2), 241–247.

Fontaine, K. L. (2009). *Mental health nursing* (6th ed.). Upper Saddle River, NJ: Pearson Education.

Gonzalbo, F. E. (2006). *In the eyes of God: A study on the culture of suffering.* Austin: University of Texas Press.

Helping kids deal with bullies. Retrieved from http://kidshealth.org/parent/emotions/behavior/bullies.html.

Jiang, R-S., Chou, C-C., & Tsai, P-L. (2006). The grief reactions of nursing students related to the sudden death of a classmate. *Journal of Nursing Research, 14*(4), 279–284.

Kirmayer, L. J. (2001). Cultural variations in the clinical presentation of depression and anxiety: Implications for diagnosis and treatment. *Journal of Clinical Psychiatry, 62* (supplement 13), 22–30.

Laurie, A., & Neimeyer, R. (2008). African Americans in bereavement: Grief as a function of ethnicity. *Omega, 57*(2), 173–193.

Lewis, M., & Trzinski, A. (2006). Counseling older adults with dementia who are dealing with death: Innovative interventions for practitioners. *Death Studies, 30*, 777–787.

Lin, H. (2008). Searching for meaning: Narratives and analysis of US-resident Chinese immigrants with metastatic cancer. *Cancer Nursing, 31*(30), 250–258.

Maslow, A. H. (1943). A theory of human motivation. *Psychological Review*, *50,* 370–396.

McHenry, D. M. (2007). A growing challenge: Patient education in a diverse America. *Journal for Nurses in Staff Development, 23*(2), 83–88.

Melhem, N. M., Moritz, G., Walker, M., Shear, M. K., & Brent, D. (2007). Phenomenology and correlates of complicated grief in children and adolescents. *Journal of the American Academy of Child and Adolescent Psychiatry*, *46*(4), 493–499.

Newton, C. J. (2001). Effects of child abuse on children: General abuse. Retrieved from http://www.findcounseling.com/journal/child-abuse/child-abuse-effects.html

Piaget, J. (1932). *The moral judgment of the child.* London, UK: Routledge and Kegan Paul.

Pilkington, F. B. (2006). Developing nursing knowledge on grieving: A human becoming perspective. *Nursing Science Quarterly, 19*, 299–303.

Råholm, M-B. (2008). Uncovering the ethics of suffering using a narrative approach. *Nursing Ethics, 15*(1), 62–72.

Rutter, M. (1985). Resilience in the face of adversity: Protective factors and resistance to psychiatric disorder. *British Journal of Psychiatry, 147*, 598–611.

Sacks, J., & Nelson, J. (2007). A theory of nonphysical suffering and trust in hospice patients. *Qualitative Health Research, 17*(5), 675–689.

Shapiro, E. (2008). Whose recovery, of what? Relationships and environments promoting grief and growth. *Death Studies, 32*, 40–58.

Wayman, L. M., & Gaydos, H. L. (2005). Self-transcending through suffering. *Journal of Hospice and Palliative Nursing, 7*(5), 263–270.

Wolchik, S. A., Ma, Y., Tein, J-Y, Sandler, I. N., & Ayers, T. S. (2008). Parentally bereaved children's grief: Self-system beliefs as mediators of the relations between grief and stressors and caregiver-child relationship quality. *Death Studies, 32*(7), 597–620.

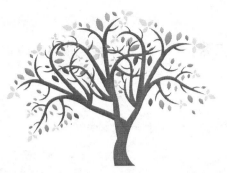

THREE

Grieving and Suffering

■ Mertie L. Potter

Objectives

1. Compare and contrast traditional and contemporary grief models.
2. Utilize one of the grief models when completing the exercise, "Reflecting upon Personal Loss."
3. Articulate different needs of individuals experiencing loss and grief at various developmental stages related to different losses.
4. Differentiate between feminine grieving and masculine grieving.
5. Explain complicated bereavement.
6. Incorporate professional communication skills in a simulated grief scenario, address ethical and moral values involved, state professional skills needed, and demonstrate critical thinking when completing the exercise, "Bearing the Grief of Others."

Student Project

The following poem was put to music and translated from Russian to English by student nurse Angelina Makarov Skorupski.

Where the Road of Life Ends

Verse 1
I see lights from a palace where the Father resides,
Where the end of life's road is.
All wounds will be healed, there we'll find peace,
Where the end of life's road is.

Chorus
After the end of a long day's battle, I'll finally be home
Where my loving Saviour will greet me
Where the end of life's road is.

Verse 2
I'll look back and smile at all my suffering,
Where the end of life's road is.
I'll forget my enemies forever
Where the end of life's road is.

Verse 3
I'll enter with my friends, into my promised home,
Where the end of life's road is.
All that I've longed for, with faith I've only dreamed of—
Where the end of life's road is.

The final definitive version of this poem has been published in the *Journal of Holistic Nursing, 25*(3). Sage Publications Ltd./Sage Publications, Inc. All rights reserved.

Source: Courtesy of Angelina Makarov Skorupski, student nurse, 2005.

Case Study 3–1

Thirty-five-year-old Dan is a devoted father of three children and esteemed nurse anesthetist. Dan has a 7-year-old son, a 5-year-old daughter, and a 3-year-old son. His wife died in an airplane crash 1.5 years ago. Dan has struggled to keep things going on the home front while maintaining his busy and demanding work schedule. His family and friends keep trying to introduce him to female friends they think would be good for him and good for his children. Dan insists he is not ready to date and does not know if he ever will be. Dan is the older of two siblings. His 33-year-old sister who is an attorney is single and lives about 10 hours away. Dan lost his mother 2 years ago to cancer. His father lives nearby, is retired, and tries to help Dan as much as he can.

Recently, Dan's 3-year-old son was diagnosed with Wilms' tumor, a cancer of the kidney. His son is scheduled for surgery in 1 week. Dan's family, friends, and co-workers are very supportive. However, Dan is exhausted and not sure how he is going to sustain the pace he has been keeping. The youngest son does not remember his mother.

Dan's oldest son complains that his friends' mothers go on school outings with his class. He does not want to talk about his own mother.

Dan's daughter still asks, "When is Mommy coming back?" She talks of her mother often, looks at her picture, and occasionally has episodes of enuresis.

He recently went to a grief support group at the suggestion of his co-workers and sister. His co-workers told Dan they felt he was not himself at work because he seemed on edge and irritable. His sister noted that Dan was taking his frustration out on his oldest son. However, with the additional stress of his youngest son's condition, Dan does not know how he will be able to keep up with all the necessary medical appointments. His children's pediatrician recently suggested family counseling.

Questions on the Case Study

1. How does Dan's story make you feel?
2. Although it would be important to get Dan's input, how would you prioritize Dan's greatest needs?
3. In what ways do you think Dan may be experiencing suffering?

Introduction

Cassell's (1982) work defined suffering as both an individual's experience of a particular circumstance and the meaning the individual assigns to the experience. Cassell (1991) asserted that it is important to treat human suffering as well as physical injury and disease. The body of this work is intended to help nurses address human suffering—their own and that of their patients. Much of the suffering experienced by nurses and by the patients for whom nurses care relates to loss and grieving, because loss and grieving are closely intertwined with suffering.

Suffering engulfs one's body, mind, and spirit. Allmani (2007) contends that suffering is "the simultaneous experience of bodily and mental pain" and the feeling of being "a distance from the spiritual dimension" (p. 240.) Suffering is tied to the essence of being human (Lin, 2008). Suffering is all-encompassing and, as described by one study participant, "is like being hit by an earthquake; always have tremors, wondering what the next tremors are going be like because you know it can come back" (Sacks & Nelson, 2007, p. 680).

Interweaving of Suffering and Grieving

Loss is "the condition of being deprived or bereaved of something or someone" (*American Heritage Dictionary*, 2006, p. 1034). Actual, potential, physical, emotional, social, spiritual, or symbolic losses may occur. Loss may arise from a number of specific areas, such as health, relationships with significant others, safety, freedom, independence, finances, home, beliefs and values, sense of control, body image, objects, pets, roles, identity, control, and hope. With suffering defined as "the bearing of pain or distress" (*American Heritage Dictionary*, 2006, p. 1730), the previously mentioned losses logically may frequently include bearing of pain or distress.

Grief is "deep mental anguish, as that arising from bereavement" (*American Heritage Dictionary*, 2006, p. 772). Cowles and Rodgers (1991) reviewed nursing and medical literature related to grief; they conceptualized grief to be "a dynamic, pervasive, highly individualized process with a strong normative component" (p. 121). An individual's grief is unique.

Although each person goes through grief in his or her own way, a number of factors affect how an individual experiences grief (Table 3–1) Examining these factors with those journeying through grief can help elucidate to some degree what

Table 3–1   Factors Impacting an Individual's Grief

1. Circumstances of the death
2. Relationship to deceased
3. Characteristics of bereaved
4. Interpersonal support

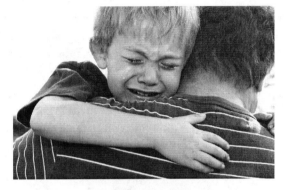

5. Sociocultural factors
6. Professional roles
7. Attitudes toward death and dying
8. Demoralized or disenfranchised losses

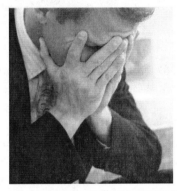

Adapted from Breen & O'Connor, 2007, p. 200.

they are experiencing and how they can best be helped. Some of these factors are listed here (Breen & O'Connor, 2007, p. 200):

- Circumstances of the significant other's death—Was the death anticipated, was it the result of violence, did it occur after a lengthy illness, or was it preventable?
- Relationship to the deceased—How close was the bereaved to the deceased?
- Qualities of the bereaved—What are the bereaved's age, gender, coping style, cognitive strategies, spirituality/religiosity, earlier life history, and possible concurrent crises?

- Support—Does the bereaved have interpersonal support available? What type of support is it, and what is the extent of the support?
- Sociocultural factors—Does the bereaved practice any rituals, customs, or traditions and do they have relevance for the bereaved?
- Professional roles—What is the impact of professionals, such as morticians and counselors, in relation to the bereaved's experience of death and grief?
- Attitudes—What are the bereaved's attitudes toward death and dying?
- Demoralized or disenfranchised losses—Has the death experienced been treated as though it were an immoral or unapproved of loss?

In addition, there are a number of assumptions within traditional grief theories. These assumptions assert that grief

- follows a distinct pattern;
- is short term and finite;
- runs its course through specific stages/phases/processes involving shock, yearning, and recovery;
- needs to be worked through;
- involves an anticipatory aspect when terminal illness occurs;
- must involve finding meaning and/or positives gained from the death;
- results in detachment from the deceased loved one;
- is abnormal if continued (Breen & O'Connor, 2007, pp. 199–200).

Traditional and Contemporary Models of Loss and Grieving

A number of models have been developed in an attempt to explain loss and grieving. Traditional models present grieving as having specific stages that an individual may progress through, either directly or with vacillating movements, from stage to stage. Breen and O'Connor identified characteristics of traditional models (2007, pp. 200–201):

- Grief follows a distinctive prototype.
- Grief is time-limited and runs a relatively short course.
- The journey of grief is a somewhat linear process of various stages, phases, tasks, or processes involving shock, yearning, and recovery.
- "Working through" grief to resolution is necessary.

- Anticipatory grief begins prior to death if the significant other has a terminal illness.
- Death must involve meaning and/or positive outcomes.
- Resolution occurs when the bereaved lets go of or releases the deceased.
- Continuation of grief is not considered abnormal and unhealthy.

Contemporary models contrast in a number of ways to traditional models. Contemporary models portray grief as an ongoing process that never ends but continues to evolve. Bereaved individuals sustain a relationship with the deceased in some manner. Major traditional and contemporary models are discussed next.

Traditional Models

As stated, traditional models incorporate staging. Individuals are thought to process loss by journeying through distinct stages, resolving the loss experienced, and releasing the lost loved object or person.

Lindemann (1944) studied survivors and grieving family members of the Boston Cocoanut Grove Club Fire in 1942. His work provided the foundation for grief research. He described the grieving experienced by family members and survivors, focusing on acute and traumatic loss. Lindemann described symptoms and emotional responses as occurring in typical sequences. He also was the first to suggest the concept of anticipatory grief in relation to women expecting to lose male family members in World War II.

Kübler-Ross (1969) studied persons diagnosed with terminal illness and their emotional responses. She developed a five-stage grief model:

- DENIAL—"No, not me!" During this stage, individuals are in shock or feel numb, resist accepting the loss, and remain in denial.
- ANGER—"Why me?" Individuals begin to realize and understand the loss is real, feel angry that it has happened to them, and question *why* this loss *has* happened to them.
- BARGAINING—"Yes, me, but . . ." Individuals struggle with and question how they might have prevented the loss and attempt to bargain with God or themselves for recovery. Guilt is a common feeling during this stage.
- DEPRESSION—"Yes, me . . ." Reality sets in, individuals become extremely sad about the loss, and may experience physical changes.

- ACCEPTANCE—"Letting go and saying good-bye." Individuals adjust to the loss, release the lost object (e.g., health, loved one, or object), and incorporate the terminal condition into their lives.

Bowlby developed an attachment theory based on observations of infants and children separated from their parents. Along with a colleague, he delineated four phases of grief during adult life (Bowlby & Parkes, 1970). They defined them as

- numbing—shock and disbelief related to the loss;
- yearning and protest—preoccupation with the deceased and an attempt to regain the lost object;
- disorganization and despair—giving up the search for the lost object;
- reorganization—completion of mourning, cessation of searching for the lost, and formation of new relationships.

Pattison (1977) was the first to explore the period of time occurring between living and death, referred to as the living-dying interval. This time period is the interval between knowing death is approaching and the definite time of death. Pattison describes three phases:

- acute crisis phase
- chronic living-dying phase
- terminal phase

What is unique about this concept is that individuals who know they have a terminal illness or know they are going to die because of some other condition almost are "caught" in time. Namely, they have a different perspective on life, as they often become more focused on the specific time period they have left to live rather than on an open-ended "lifetime" ahead of them. The living-dying interval also can be a time of great uncertainty.

Worden (1991) depicted four tasks of mourning to assist individuals in counseling and therapy.

- Accept the reality of the loss—overcoming denial that the lost object will come back
- Experience the pain of grief—giving oneself permission to feel the pain at all levels, including physical and emotional
- Adjust to an environment in which deceased is missing—restructuring one's life and determining new life skills and roles

■ Withdraw emotional energy and reinvest it in another relationship— experience release from or release the lost object so that energy can be invested and relocated in something or someone else

Rando (1984) described grief work and mourning as encompassing six processes. Rando also asserted that grieving might become complicated if one of the six processes of "Rs" became compromised, distorted, or failed. These six processes are

■ recognizing the loss;
■ reacting to the separation;
■ recollecting and re-experiencing the deceased and the relationship in a realistic way;
■ relinquishing old attachments;
■ readjusting to move adaptively in a new world while not forgetting the old; and
■ reinvesting.

The Universal Model is an adaptation of many of the traditional grieving models. It depicts the stages as follows (McCall, 2004, p. 307):

■ attachment—close connectedness to people who are important in one's life;
■ shock—physiological response (eyes open wider, jaw drops slightly);
■ denial—protective response that modulates feelings/thoughts that come later;
■ feelings—sadness, fear, anger, regret, and many more;
■ depression—a comprehensive sorting process that normally culminates with a sense of a need to "go on";
■ reorganization—the learning or skill phase of recovery that focuses on changes in one's life as a result of the loss;
■ recovery—making new attachments and investing more energy in ongoing relationships.

Most of the early Western grief and loss models were based primarily on studies done with Caucasians and especially with Caucasian women who lost spouses through divorce or death or lost a child (Laurie & Neimeyer, 2008). Studies have focused on the populations of those who experienced (1) divorce, (2) loss of child, or (3) loss of spouse.

Contemporary Models

Contemporary models present a different view of grieving. These models challenge traditional models in several ways including (Breen & O'Connor, 2007)

- lack of transferability to other populations;
- paradox of an individual's grief being unique rather than on a timeline (or staged);
- question of complicated grief versus normal grief.

There are key differences between traditional and contemporary models:

- Traditional: expectation of resolving and forgetting the loss after going through distinct stages of grieving
- Contemporary: expectation of movement and healing related to the loss while continuing on a journey of grieving (Råholm, 2008)

Complicated Grief

If uniqueness of grieving is accepted, the question arises, "Is there a difference between 'normal' and 'complicated' grief?" Namely, if an individual grieves at his or her own pace and in his or her own way, what would constitute labeling an individual's grief as complicated? Should complicated grief be classified as a mental disorder in the fifth edition of the *Diagnostic and Statistical Manual of Mental Disorders (DSM)* (American Psychiatric Association, 2000; Breen & O'Connor, 2007)?

General consensus has been reached around the different characteristics of complicated grief. Complicated grief can be prolonged, delayed, or exaggerated. Rein (2006) describes grief as often occurring in "waves" (p. 242). If an individual is unable to recover from one wave to the next, and if the intensity of the symptoms do not resolve, the individual's grief may become prolonged and complicated. For those denying the reality of a loss, avoiding the pain, being unable to adapt to life without the lost loved one or object, and being unable to have other loving relationships, grief may be delayed and become complicated. Delaying grief can be more strenuous than the actual grief work. For the individual who already has ongoing challenges and stresses, grief may become exaggerated and complicated (Rein, 2006).

Florczak (2008) suggests, "Grieving the loss is always there, never gone and the meaning everchanging" (p. 7); also, grieving the loss is "persistent sorrow arising with weaving familiar-unfamiliar patterns anew" (p. 8). Contemporary models assert that grieving is not a stage or premorbid condition to be reached but a journey of moving, healing, and remembering (Råholm, 2008). The work of suffering is part of this movement through pain that needs to occur. Resolution and forgetting are not part of this journey for an individual, but enduring, struggling, and becoming are (Råholm, 2008).

Chronic Sorrow

Chronic sorrow describes normal responses to various losses related to chronic illness. Chronic sorrow consists of grief that has a cyclical and recurring nature and varies in intensity at different times. The term was first coined by Olshansky (1962) as an emotional response observed in parents having children diagnosed with learning difficulties. Burke et al. (1992) later recognized the same phenomenon in individuals with chronic illness. Eakes, Burke, and Hainsworth (1998) later developed a middle-range theoretical model of chronic sorrow. Later studies have demonstrated the presence of chronic sorrow in individuals diagnosed with multiple sclerosis (Isaksson, Gunnarsson, & Ahlstrom, 2007; Isaksson & Ahlstrom, 2008), individuals testing positive for human immunodeficiency virus (HIV) (Lichtenstein, Laska, & Clair, 2002), individuals diagnosed with diabetes (Hayes, 2001), and spouses of those diagnosed with Alzheimer's disease (Mayer, 2001).

Questions for Reflection
1. What feelings are evoked within you when you hear the word "grieving?"
2. Do you think individuals go through "stages" of grieving? Why? Why not?
3. Do you think any differences exist between men and women when they grieve?

Developmental Needs

Normal growth and development necessitate movement of an individual from dependency to interdependency and, hopefully, to independency. Some individuals may return to dependency or interdependency prior to death. Life involves change, and that change often involves loss and suffering. Type of loss and the developmental stage impacts how an individual will respond to loss and grieving.

Table 3–2   Developmental Views of Death

Age	Stage of Development	Task/Area of Resolution
Birth–2 years	Infancy	Sense of separation; no concept of death
2–5 years	Early childhood	Death is transient, not permanent state
6–10 years	Late childhood	Beginning awareness of the reality of death
13–25 years	Adolescence–young adulthood	Similar to adult view—realization of mortality and eventual death; death anxiety more evident; death perceived as a future event
26–65 years	Middle-aged and older adults	More aware and accepting of death

Source: Adapted from McIntier, 1995, and Rando, 1984.

Used with permission. Reprinted from Potter, M. L. (2010). Loss, suffering, grief, and bereavement. In M. Matzo & D. Sherman (Eds.). *Palliative care nursing: Quality care to the end of life* (3rd ed., pp. 199–226). New York: Springer.

Infancy and Toddlers

Birth is a traumatic event for a newborn. Transitioning from dependency and nurture inside the womb to dependency and nurture outside the womb brings many challenges for the infant. Protection, sustenance, rest, warmth, and survival are no longer a given. Granted, some infants are challenged in utero if the mother's health is compromised in any number of possible ways. However, suffering and loss have potential to become part of the infant's new environment once "thrust out" or "removed" from the womb. The infant is helpless and defenseless at this point of life and totally dependent upon others for survival. For example, some infants may develop a condition known as failure to thrive in which the infant does not advance as expected due to various organic or nonorganic causes: physical, psychological, social, or economic. Thus, the infant may have to deal with suffering and loss in different contexts.

Infants usually develop an acute awareness of separation from their mother or mother-figure around the sixth month. This state is called separation anxiety. It has been suggested that this keen awareness of loss may indicate a beginning awareness of death (Backer, Hannon, & Gregg, 1994). Bowlby's (1980) model of attachment between mother and infant and the infant's experience of separation from the mother provides a basis for this hypothesis. As development continues, additional suffering and loss occur (see Table 3–2).

Early Childhood

Children under the age of 2 usually sense separation but do not have a full understanding of the concept of death. Children between 2 and 5 years of age view death as a transient state but not a permanent event. Between the ages of 6 months and 1 year, individuals begin to have a sense of object constancy, that is, they sustain the memory of their adult caregiver; they can internalize a representation of their adult caregiver (Geis, Whittlesey, McDonald, Smith, & Pfefferbaum, 1998).

Research has indicated that children as young as 4 years of age may express grief although not always in ways similar to adult expressions of grief (International Work Group on Death, Dying, and Bereavement, 1999). Grief may be exhibited in children as

- regression;
- exaggerated fears;
- guilt;
- ambivalence;
- denial;
- fear for own well-being;
- increased vulnerability;
- temper tantrums;
- difficulty concentrating;
- physical symptoms;
- clinging;
- whining;
- bedwetting;
- expectation that deceased will return; and
- mood swings (Kirwin & Hamrin, 2005; Potter, 2006).

Late Childhood

Around age 5, a child begins to be able to differentiate between temporary separation and permanent loss (Black, 1998). Between 5 and 11 years of age, children recognize the reality of death and that the body goes through changes with death (Kirwin & Hamrin, 2005). During this age period, children may

- give death a personality, such as the "boogie man";
- show no emotion, slight emotion, or great emotion; or
- feel responsible for an individual's death (Roper, 2006).

Adolescence to Young Adulthood

The conceptualization of death by adolescents is similar to that experienced by adults. An increasing awareness of one's own mortality arises as adolescents move toward their individuality and independence. The main difference between adolescents and more mature adults is that adolescents view death as future-oriented, namely, they will not experience death until well in the future.

According to Piaget (1972), young adolescents begin to display formal logical thought processes that enable them to reflect upon their own deaths. Unlike younger children, adolescents may experience death anxiety, namely, negative stress, in relation to thoughts about death. Ens and Bond (2007) found that grief resulting from bereavement was a significant predictor of death anxiety in their study with 226 adolescent participants. Their findings suggest that an adolescent's strength of relationship with the deceased is an important factor that impacts an adolescent's bereavement (Ens & Bond, 2007).

Middle-aged and Older Adults

Middle-aged adults and older adults are more aware and accepting of death. They usually have had more experience with loss and grieving than youth and young adults. Adults generally are better able to see loss and grieving as a part of the flow and rhythm of life. Older adults often have to contend with grief overload as they may be experiencing numerous losses all at once.

Cultural Considerations Related to Loss and Grieving

Culture refers to "the customary beliefs, social forms, and material traits of a racial, religious, or social group" (*Merriam Webster Online Dictionary*, 2009). The importance of culture in relation to health is demonstrated in Canadian research that took place with five ethnolinguistic groups (Simich, Maiter, Moorlag, &

Ochocka, 2009). The ethnocultural communities were Latin American, Mandarin-speaking Chinese, Polish, Punjabi Sikh, and Somali. Several themes arose from this research (Simich et al., 2009, p. 210):

- functioning within various social settings;
- making decisions;
- coping with stress;
- maintaining financial stability;
- addressing family and work responsibilities.

Shapiro (2008) recommends considering both cultural context and developmental level of an individual or family when assisting them in bereavement. This process involves valuing self-determination that is appropriate for the bereaved's age. Shapiro advocates shifting the focus of bereavement intervention from decreasing distress in individuals and families to promoting positive coping and resilience within individuals and families. Grieving often is intergenerational, and there are strengths that the different generations can draw from one another. For example, young grievers may receive benefits from older grievers who have developed some resilience and protective factors from other grieving experiences. Those who are older may redirect the focus of their grief to providing care for those who are younger and grieving. Relationships and environments promoting grief and growth are powerful and can be positive resources when used to assist those who are bereaved.

Extraordinary Losses

Extraordinary losses are just as described, namely, extra ordinary or beyond that expected under usual or ordinary life circumstances. These types of losses do not happen to every individual in a lifetime. They are not common developmental or situational experiences. Extraordinary losses usually are extremely difficult and/or traumatic to experience, process, share, and express. Categories and examples of extraordinary losses include

- sudden traumatic loss through suicide, homicide, accident, heart attack, or stroke;
- anticipatory grieving due to loss of health, prolonged grief, or chronic illness, such as schizophrenia and diabetes;

- disenfranchised loss when being the lover of a married individual, a partner within a gay couple, an individual diagnosed with AIDS, or a survivor of a suicide (either the actual survivor or the significant others related to the survivor);
- public tragedy after a plane crash, flood, hurricane, volcano, tsunami, tornado, act of terrorism; or
- unexpected loss resulting from the death of child, an accident, or a divorce.

Shunning, shaming, stigmatizing, or social rejection may occur in cases of chronic illness and disenfranchised losses.

Feminine and Masculine Grieving

Initially, the belief was that men and women grieve differently. Doka and Davidson (1998, p. 140) examined masculine grievers and found the following characteristics among them:

- shelving of thoughts and feelings to meet obligations and then dealing with the thoughts and feelings at a more appropriate time;
- expressing grief through activities;
- using humor to manage anger and aggression;
- seeking companionship rather than support;
- using solitude to reflect and adapt; and
- reading and maintaining a journal.

Dyregrov and Dyregrov (2004) studied Norwegian men and women to explore differences in grieving. They found that grief literature was dominated by an exploration of spousal grief and that the majority of those previously studied were widowed American women.

Thomas (2004, pp. 259, 264) wanted to validate men's grief and found that there was a masculine way of expressing emotions during grief. Thomas determined that masculine grieving involved a pattern in which individuals

- moderated their feelings;
- focused on thinking;
- immersed themselves in activity; and
- desired solitude.

Thomas (2004, pp. 259, 264) also found that males tended to have

- poorer health;
- a higher risk of mortality than females;
- a link between emotion and disease that demonstrated health-damaging emotional states and behaviors (such as suppressing emotions) connected to gender role socialization rather than sex differentiation; and
- alcohol use as the drug of choice with a tendency to abuse alcohol five times higher than that of females.

Baum (2003) found several other differences between males and females:

- Timing of mourning occurs earlier in females than in males.
- Who and what they mourn is different since males mourn children, home, family life, and routine, and females mourn more loss of the marital relationship.
- How they mourn is dissimilar, because males tend to act out grief with increased activity, somatization, and/or self-medicating with alcohol and/or other drugs; females verbalize their grief through depression, other emotional and verbal expression, and/or help-seeking.

Evidence-Based Practice

Recent research findings have stressed the need to broaden the participant base of grief studies, examine bereavement interventions, and share information, with these recommendations:

- Explore grief education.
- Examine grief in historical, social, cultural, spiritual, and political contexts.
- Perform more qualitative studies—exchange of ideas among researchers, clinicians, and bereaved.
- Examine current interventions.
- Disseminate findings more effectively (Breen & O'Connor, 2007, pp. 207–212).
- Examine bereavement therapy (Leighton, 2008).

Communication and the Role of Nursing

Råholm (2008) advocates the use of a narrative approach when responding to patients in their suffering. Encouraging patients to share their stories about suffering provides meaning to the experiences, is freeing, helps transform the suffering, and helps the individual find a way out of the suffering.

Educators need to provide an environment in which student nurses take time to listen to their patients' stories, have time to reflect upon the suffering they witness, and recognize the vulnerability nurses may experience when providing presence for another who is suffering. According to Råholm, presence may occur in silence, always occurs at the invitation of the patient, and is a privilege for the nurse (2008, pp. 66–67).

It is important to help individuals maintain a capacity to love, sustain hope in the presence of loss and dying, draw upon intergenerational supports, and nurture meaningful relationships (Shapiro, 2008). Providing compassion and promoting companionship also is important (Potter, 2006).

Case Study 3–1   (continued)

Dan's sister took a family leave of absence to help Dan through his 3-year-old son's surgery. Dan was greatly relieved to have his sister come and help. The children love their aunt and have always looked forward to her visits. Dan has agreed to allow his deceased wife's family, consisting of her parents and two sisters, to come and help also. They had done so initially, but Dan had wanted to show them he could handle everything on his own.

Dan's father has been having the two older children over to his house twice a week to give Dan time to attend appointments with his youngest son. Dan's neighbors and parish have set up a list of volunteers to make meals for Dan's family during the next month.

Family counseling became a priority for Dan, and he decided to step out of his bereavement support group while in therapy with the family. Dan's levels of anxiety, guilt, and depression have lessened; he is more hopeful. The two older children seem to be functioning better, have been asking Dan questions about their mother, and seeking Dan out more for hugs. The youngest son came through his surgery well, has been declared "cured," and is glad to be home again.

Dan's sister is with Dan and the children for 1 more month. His mother-in-law and two sister-in-laws will be taking turns after that to come and assist Dan and the children. The household seems to be in more of a "flow," and each person is journeying and being affirmed in his or her own unique journey through the loss of their beloved family member.

Summary

Suffering most often involves loss and grieving of someone or something. Traditional models of grieving have been utilized the longest, are based upon research done with specific groups, and remain widely used today. Contemporary models differ from traditional models in suggesting that resolution and forgetting the loss do not occur and that grieving is an ongoing journey. How one experiences loss and grieving varies across the life span and is dependent upon developmental stages and life circumstances. Depending upon the type of loss, especially if the loss were considered disenfranchised or involving chronic illness, the grieving individual may experience painful responses related to stigma. Concern may arise if an individual's grief becomes complicated through prolongation, exaggeration, or delay of grieving.

Individuals experience grief uniquely. The manner in which an individual grieves relates to circumstances, relationships, characteristics of the bereaved, support, sociocultural factors, professional contacts, attitudes, and the type of loss (Breen & O'Connor, 2007, p. 200). Differences between masculine and feminine ways of grieving have been demonstrated. Masculine grieving involves more introspection and independent working through grief. Feminine grieving involves more sharing and connecting in working through grief.

Nurses can be helpful to individuals who are grieving by validating the individuals' experiences and assisting them in telling their stories to help provide meaning to suffering. Instilling hope and encouraging connections that promote connectedness are key interventions also.

Key Points

1. Traditional grieving models contend that resolution and forgetting the loss should occur and that an end point results after the person has gone through distinct stages of grieving.

2. Contemporary models assert that movement and healing are the important factors in grieving and that grieving is a continual journey.

3. Grieving is experienced differently across the life span and is unique to each individual.

4. Complicated grieving involves delay, exaggeration, or prolongation.

5. Chronic illness and disenfranchised losses may involve associated "shunning," "shaming," "stigmatizing," or "social unacceptability."

6. Research has demonstrated differences in masculine and feminine patterns of grieving.

7. Encouraging patients to tell their stories may help transform their suffering and provide meaning to their experiences.

Exercises

Reflecting upon Personal Loss

1. Describe the following:
   a. Your first recalled loss, including your age, your loss, and your reaction.
   b. Your most difficult loss, including your age at the time of your loss, your loss, and what at the time you perceived you needed to help you cope with this loss.
   c. In what way(s) you feel your "suffering" was or was not understood by others during either of the two events you just described in "a" or "b."
2. Illustrate the following:
   a. Describe how your experience depicted in "a" or "b" above relates to one of the grief models discussed in this chapter.
   b. Cite reference(s) from which you obtained the information.

Bearing the Grief of Others

Part I

Write out (approximately one page) how you as a nurse would relate to the client in one of the "Loss Situations" listed in Part II of this exercise. Write out what you would say to the person for whom you were providing nursing care. Identify communication skills you need to employ, address ethical and moral values involved for you in the situation, state professional skills you think are required to provide nursing interventions to the survivor if needed, and reference the resource(s) you used to assist you in your decision making about this situation.

Part II: Group project
    a. Discuss with a work group the conclusions you reached while considering how you would provide care to the person in your assigned loss situation in Part I.
    b. Pool the strengths of all group members' thoughts from a discussion of their written assignment.
    c. Select the best communication example from each group member related to how each would approach the individual in his or her scenario.
    d. Share it with the class and note the contribution from each group member.

Loss Situations

    a. Sudden traumatic loss through suicide, homicide, accident, heart attack, or stroke
    b. Anticipatory grieving due to loss of health, prolonged grief, or chronic illness, such as schizophrenia and diabetes
    c. Disenfranchised loss when being the lover of a married individual, partner within a gay couple, an individual diagnosed with AIDS, or survivor of a suicide (either the actual survivor or the significant others related to the survivor)
    d. Public tragedy after a plane crash, flood, hurricane, volcano, tsunami, tornado, act of terrorism
    e. Unexpected loss resulting from the death of child, an accident, or a divorce

References

Allmani, A. (2007). Suffering, choice, and freedom. *Substance Use and Misuse, 42*, 225–241.

American Heritage Dictionary of the English Language (4th ed., new updated edition). (2006). Boston, MA: Houghton Mifflin.

American Psychiatric Association. (2000). *Diagnostic and statistical manual of mental disorders* (4th ed., text rev.). Arlington, VA: Author.

Backer, B. A., Hannon, N. R., & Gregg, J. Y. (1994). *To listen, to comfort, to care: Reflections on death and dying.* Albany, NY: Delmar.

Baum, N. (2003). The male way of mourning divorce: When, what, and how. *Clinical Social Work Journal, 31*(1), 37–67.

Black, D. (1998). Coping with loss: Bereavement in childhood. *British Medical Journal, 316*(7135), 913–933.

Bowlby, J. (1980). Attachment and loss: Volume III: Loss, sadness and depression. London, UK: The Hogarth Press and the Institute.

Bowlby, J., & Parkes, C. M. (1970). Separation and loss within the family. In E. J. Anthony & C. Koupernick (Eds.), *The child in his family: International yearbook of child psychiatry and allied professions* (pp. 197–216). New York, NY: Wiley.

Breen, L. J., & O'Connor, M. (2007). The fundamental paradox in the grief literature: A critical reflection. *OMEGA, 55*(3), 199–218.

Burke, M. L., Hainsworth, M. A., Eakes, G., & Lindgren, C. L. (1992). Chronic sorrow: An examination of nursing roles. In S. G. Funk (Ed.), *Key aspects of caring for the chronically ill* (pp. 231–236). New York, NY: Springer.

Cassell, E. J. (1982). The nature of suffering and the goals of medicine. *New England Journal of Medicine, 306*(11), 639–645.

Cassell, E. J. (1991). *The nature of suffering and the goals of medicine.* Oxford, UK: Oxford University Press.

Cowles, K. V., & Rodgers, B. L. (1991). The concept of grief: A foundation for nursing research and practice. *Research in Nursing and Health, 14*(2), 119–127.

Doka, K. J., & Davidson, J. D. (1998). *Living with grief.* New York: Routledge Taylor & Francis Group.

Dyregrove A., & Dyregrove, K. (2004). *Living with loss over time—Bottle it up or talk it through?* Plenary session conducted at Sudden Infant Death Syndrome International Conference held at Edmonton, Canada.

Eakes, G. G., Burke, M. L., & Hainsworth, M. A. (1998). Middle-range theory of chronic sorrow. *Image: Journal of Nursing Scholarship, 30,* 179–184.

Ens, C., & Bond, J. (2007). Death anxiety in adolescents: The contributions of bereavement and religiosity. *Omega, 55*(3), 169–184.

Florczak, K. L. (2008). The persistent yet everchanging nature of grieving a loss. *Nursing Science Quarterly, 21*(1), 7–11.

Geiss, H., Whittlesey, S., McDonald, N., Smith, K., & Pfefferbaum, B. (1998). Bereavement and loss in childhood. *Child and Adolescent Psychiatric Clinics of North America, 7*(1), 73–78.

Hayes, M. (2001). A phenomenological study of chronic sorrow in people with type 1 diabetes. *Practical Diabetes, 18*(2), 65–69.

International Work Group on Death, Dying, and Bereavement. (1999). Children, adolescents, and death: Myths, realities, and challenges. *Death Studies, 23,* 443–463.

Isaksson, A., & Ahlstrom, G. (2008). Managing chronic sorrow: Experiences of patients with multiple sclerosis. *Journal of Neuroscience Nursing, 40*(3), 180–191.

Isaksson, A. K., Gunnarsson, L. G., & Ahlstrom, G. (2007). The presence and meaning of chronic sorrow in patients with multiple sclerosis. *Journal of Clinical Nursing, 16*(11c), 315–324.

Kirwin, K. M., & Hamrin, V. (2005). Decreasing the risk of complicated bereavement and future psychiatric disorders in children. *Journal of Child and Adolescent Psychiatric Nursing, 18*(2), 62–78.

Kübler-Ross, E. (1969). *On death and dying.* New York, NY: Macmillan.

Laurie, A., & Neimeyer, R. A. (2008). African Americans in bereavement: Grief as a function of ethnicity. *Omega, 57*(2), 173–193.

Leighton, S. 2008. Bereavement therapy with adolescents: Facilitating a process of spiritual growth. *Journal of Child and Adolescent Psychiatric Nursing, 21*(1), 24–34.

Lichenstein, B., Laska, M., & Clair, J. (2002). Chronic sorrow in the HIV-positive patient: Issues of race, gender, and social support. *AIDS Patient Care and STDS, 16*(1), 27–38.

Lin, H. (2008). Searching for meaning: Narratives and analysis of US-resident Chinese immigrants with metastatic cancer. *Cancer Nursing, 31*(3), 250–258.

Lindemann, E. (1944). Symptomatology and management of acute grief. *American Journal of Psychiatry, 101*, 141–148.

Mayer, M. (2001). Chronic sorrow in caregiving spouses of patients with Alzheimer's disease. *Journal of Aging and Identity, 6*(1), 49–60.

McCall, J. B. (2004). *Bereavement counseling.* New York, NY: Haworth Pastoral Press.

Merriam-Webster Online Dictionary. (2009). Culture. Retrieved from http://www.merriam-webster.com/dictionary/culture

Olshansky, S. (1962). Chronic sorrow: A response to a mentally defective child. *Social Casework, 43*, 190–193.

Pattison, E. M. (1977). *The experience of dying.* New York, NY: Simon and Schuster.

Piaget, J. (1972). *The psychology of the child.* New York, NY: Basic Books.

Potter, M. L. (2006). Loss, suffering, bereavement, and grief. In M. L. Matzo & D. W. Sherman (Eds.), *Palliative care nursing* (2nd ed., pp. 273–318). New York, NY: Springer.

Råholm, M-B (2008). Uncovering the ethics of suffering using a narrative approach. *Nursing Ethics, 15*(1), 62–72.

Rando, T. A. (1984). *Grief, dying, and death.* Champaign, IL: Research Press.

Rein, M. (2006). It's the journey, not the destination—Grief and its complications. *Association of Women's Health and Neonatal Nurses, 10*(3), 241–243.

Roper, J. (2006). Understanding sudden loss and traumatic grief at school. *School Nurse News, 23*(1), 36–40.

Sacks, J., & Nelson, J. (2007). A theory of nonphysical suffering and trust in hospice patients. *Qualitative Health Research, 17*(5), 675–689.

Shapiro, E. (2008). Whose recovery, of what? Relationships and environments promoting grief and growth. *Death Studies, 32*, 40–58.

Simich, L., Maiter, S., Moorlag, E., & Ochocka, J. (2009). Taking culture seriously: Ethnolinguistic community perspectives on mental health. *Psychiatric Rehabilitation Journal, 32*(3), 208–214.

Thomas, S. P. (2004). Men's health and psychosocial issues affecting men. *Nursing Clinics of North America, 39*(2), 259–270

Worden, J. W. (1991). *Grief counseling and grief therapy: Handbook for the mental health practitioner.* New York, NY: Springer.

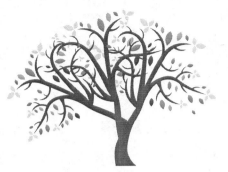

FOUR

Ethical Responsibilities and Issues in Palliative Care

■ Kathleen Ouimet Perrin

Objectives

1. Discuss why it is important that palliative care providers exhibit the virtues/values of respect for human dignity, veracity, nonmaleficence, and fidelity.
2. Compare and contrast ethical dilemmas with tragic circumstances and moral distress.
3. Explore ways to resolve ethical dilemmas.
4. Analyze how the three most common ethical dilemmas identified by nurses, truth telling, right to choose or decline treatment, and prolongation of life relate to palliative care.

Student Project: The Winding Road

Navigating this life really isn't about speed or skill.
Sometimes it's up and then downhill.
There are plenty of speed bumps and potholes along the way
That test you and obstruct your path.
Set your cruise control, stay under the radar.
Head toward the sunset wherever you are.
Keep your fuel tank full and you will go far.
Keep your eyes on the road; keep your lights on
'til you find your destination.
Whether you travel fast or slow
Keep steady on that winding road.

Source: Courtesy of Marysa Morin, student nurse, 2010.

Case Study 4–1

Late one evening, an African American male in his forties arrived in the Emergency Department of a community hospital in respiratory distress related to chronic pulmonary hypertension. Immediately after arrival, he stated that under no circumstances did he want to be intubated. He had been on a ventilator before and was not willing to go through it again. Arterial Blood Gasses were drawn that revealed serious hypercapnea and he was put on BiPap. However, his carbon dioxide levels continued to rise and the physician persuaded him to be intubated despite his previously stated wishes. When I met him in the ICU, he had already been there for several days on a ventilator. He was receiving high doses of sedation but still awoke to verbal and physical stimuli. During report, the nurse informed me that he had had one instance of serious desaturation during the night but had been relatively stable since so the plan was to try to start weaning him during the shift. He was on contact precautions for Hepatitis C and had recently been tested for human immunodeficiency virus (HIV). He was in soft restraints to prevent him from pulling out his endotracheal tube, which he had repeatedly been trying to do.

When I first entered the room, the patient was asleep but awoke when I started to talking to him while doing my assessment. When he opened his eyes for the first time while I was introducing myself to him, I could see the suffering in them. It was undeniable. Within his eyes, I saw such exhaustion and hopelessness; they told me that he would have rather died there in the ED than go through the afflicting process of intubation again. I can't remember who suctioned him first, but I remember standing there while it was happening, holding my patient's hand while he cried. Watching anyone cry is hard for me, but watching a 250 pound black man cry as he tugged at his restraints and coughed as the tube passed down into his lungs was excruciating. I watched as he struggled to defend himself from the invasiveness of the treatment until he finally gave up and just lay there helplessly, his cheeks stained by tears.

Questions on the Case Study
1. What ethical concerns can you identify in this case study?
2. Does the student recognize any ethical issues? What are they?
3. How does she describe the way the decision to intubate the patient was made?
4. What, if any, ethical responsibilities do the healthcare providers have in this situation?

Source: Courtesy of Kathleen Masterson, student nurse, 2009.

Introduction

As the poem and project suggest, making appropriate and wise decisions for very ill patients is not easy and does not always proceed in the way the patient, family, and healthcare providers intend. Decision making in palliative care is like a winding road. It calls for all those involved to pay attention to what is happening to the patient and family and to respond to the patient's most pressing needs while keeping in mind that the goal for this patient will most likely not be a cure for the disease but maintenance of comfort and function for as long as reasonable followed by a peaceful death.

Virtues of Palliative Care Nurses

Cody (2007) believes that bearing witness to a patient's suffering is a moral act because while bearing witness, the nurse is enacting specific virtues. He suggests that when a nurse chooses to bear witness to a person's suffering, the nurse is committing to the values of respect for human dignity (also known as respect for persons), veracity, nonmaleficence, and fidelity. Armstrong (2006) notes that vulnerable patients recognize high-quality nursing care by the virtues the nurses display. These virtues are character traits such as honesty, beneficence, and fidelity that are internal to the nurses' identity and help them to act, think, and feel in morally excellent ways. He argues that to exhibit a virtue, the nurse must learn to "hit the mean," that is, to strike a balance between the excessive and deficient extremes of the character trait. Palliative care nurses consistently say they are required to very carefully balance virtues such as truthfulness and find a way to "hit the mean."

Respect for Persons

Respect for persons implies that each individual matters and should be provided compassionate care. Further, it means that each individual should receive full consideration of her concerns and be autonomous when healthcare decisions are made. Cody (2007) writes specifically about the commitment to respect suffering patients when he says "The commitment to bear witness affirms the dignity and worth of those cared for . . . prompts the nurse to attend closely to the other's reality and to refuse to forget, and inspires the nurse to choose to be faithful to the person unconditionally in upholding the person's truth as the basis for care" (p. 19). His statement emphasizes how essential it is that the suffering patient's needs and concerns should be the most important factors when decisions are made about her health care. In words often used by ethicists, if the patient is to be autonomous, she should be able to express her needs and be the primary decision maker about her care.

Mahon and Sorrell (2008) caution that even when the person is damaged, we should consider what remains. Even when there are limitations from a chronic disease such as Alzheimer's, we should look for what the person has the capacity to do. Patients who are not fully competent may still have the capacity to understand some issues and make authentic decisions in these areas. The healthcare providers in the previous case study should have attempted to understand the concerns of their patient in the ED before persuading him to accept intubation and ventilation again.

Over the past 30 years, encouraging people to make their own healthcare decisions has become a cornerstone of medical ethics in the United States. This is based on the assumption that people who are autonomous and take responsibility for their lives and actions on a daily basis should not become subservient only because they are ill. Benjamin and Curtis (1992) in a classic nursing discussion of autonomy stated that there are both technical and conscience elements of any medical decision. An example of a technical element of a medical decision would be what specific antibiotics are likely to cure a particular infection. For this technical element of the decision, the healthcare provider would most likely be the expert (Benjamin & Curtis). However, it is the patient who must live with the effects of the treatment. Perhaps one of the antibiotics is too costly for the patient to afford, whereas another causes the patient severe diarrhea. Thus, the decision of whether it is possible to live with the effects and side effects of the treatment is a decision that should be made by the person most affected, the patient. According to this principle, it is the patient who should decide what action is most likely to offer her the most benefit and to choose not to accept treatments that do not appear to be in her best interests.

In the United States, a competent adult has the legal right to decline treatments, even those treatments that are deemed to be medically necessary, unless the refusal to accept treatment affects the health and welfare of others. So the patient in the first case study would have had the right to decline intubation and ventilation if he had persisted in refusing them. But how is a nurse to know if the decision is more than a statement made in a frightened moment? The palliative care nurse, who is respecting a patient's autonomy or, as Cody says, "upholding the person's truth as the basis for care" (2001, p. 19) should consider the following questions when caring for the patient:

- Does the person have the capacity to make a decision about health care at this time?
- Has the person stated a preference for the management of her care either in the past (advance directive) or currently?

- To whom or how was the preference stated?
- What is the person's expressed preference?

Veracity

Veracity may be defined as adherence to the truth, truthfulness, or honesty. In their study of honesty in palliative care nursing, Erichsen, Danielsson, and Friedrichsen (2010) differentiate between honesty and truthfulness. They believe that truthfulness and truth telling are the essence of an open and trusting relationship while honesty refers to facts, metaphors, ethics, and communication.

The nurses in Erichsen's study defined honesty as a way of behaving and emphasized that it was essential to be truthful with patients. These nurses believed that it was necessary to be truthful in part because dishonesty would be exposed in the end. But, more important, the nurses believed that honesty was essential for trust to develop and the optimum nurse/patient relationship to ensue. Even though the nurses stated that it was indispensable to a caring relationship for the patient and family to believe that they could ask the nurse any question and receive an honest answer, many of the nurses maintained that they could still be honest by expressing "half of the truth, not telling the patients and/or their family members exactly everything" (Erichsen et al., p. 43). The tension for these nurses was how to be honest in the face of a grim prognosis and still maintain the patient's and family's hope. Hodkinson (2008) reflects a similar concern noting that there may be danger in making truth telling a moral absolute in all cases because there are times when telling the truth might do more harm than good. A nurse who was trying to decide how truthful to be with a patient or family might consider the following questions that Jameton (1984) raised:

- Is the staff (family) successfully hiding things?
- Is the information really harmful?
- Does the harm of disclosure outweigh the good?
- For whom is this bad news?

Because determining how truthful to be with a suffering patient is one of the major ethical dilemmas for all providers of palliative care, it will be discussed in more detail later in the chapter.

Beneficence

Bergdahl, Wikstrom, and Andershed (2007) found that the "will to do good," also known as beneficence, was identified as an essential ability by all participants in their study of abilities of expert palliative care nurses. In fact, the focus of the nurses in the study on doing good permeated all of the interviews, accounting for 59% of the meaning units identified in nurses' interviews. Although this finding is stated slightly differently from Cody's statement that bearing witness ensures a commitment to nonmaleficence, it is really quite similar as many ethicists consider nonmaleficence to be the first and most essential component of beneficence.

Nonmaleficence, the principle of avoiding or preventing harm, is thought to take precedence over the principle of beneficence, attempting to do good for others. Ethicists argue that it is more important to avoid doing harm to patients than it is to attempt to benefit them. Stated another way, most ethicists argue that there is a stronger moral duty to remove or prevent harm than to do good. Examining the case study at the beginning of the chapter provides an example. The physician undoubtedly believed that he was "doing good" by intubating the patient and placing him on a ventilator. In doing so, the physician limited the patient's suffering from respiratory distress and obviously prevented him from dying at that time. Yet, when the student cared for the patient in the ICU several days later, he was suffering both physically and emotionally. Additionally, although the patient had not died in the ED, nothing had been done or could be done to correct his underlying pulmonary hypertension, so his current treatment was only prolonging his suffering and his inevitable demise.

This situation highlights another concern about the principle of beneficence. Who should decide what is in a patient's best interests? If the answer is the patient, then we should be respecting the patient's wishes and autonomy. Therefore, the principle of beneficence may be most appropriate when dealing with vulnerable people who do not have the capacity to make reasoned decisions for themselves. This group of people might include young children, unconscious individuals, some mentally ill people, and others temporarily without the capacity to make a rational, reflective decision for themselves. A person with a healthcare proxy or durable power of attorney for a patient might act out of the principle of beneficence.

A nurse who was espousing the virtue of beneficence or utilizing the principle of nonmaleficence might consider the following questions when caring for a patient:

- Would the proposed action or actions result in physical, emotional, or moral harm to the patient?
- What action would result in the least harm to the patient?
- If none of the actions were likely to result in foreseeable harm, what action would offer this patient the most benefit or would be in this patient's best interests?

Deciding what would benefit another person or be in that person's best interests can be very difficult. Healthcare providers and family members may hold different conceptions of what would benefit the patient most or what moral values are most important. For example, there may be a disagreement about whether a longer, perhaps more painful life, or a shorter, perhaps higher quality of life, would be the greater good.

Fidelity

Cody (2007) states that the nurse should be unconditionally faithful in upholding a suffering patient's truth as the basis for care. Some would describe this as upholding the virtue of fidelity by being faithful to what the patient desires even when there is disagreement. Others would call this the virtue of courage. Arman (2007) says that palliative care nurses need to know their patients and have the courage to act with fidelity to carry out what their patients desire. She notes that courage is required for the nurse to enter into a deep, existential caring encounter with a patient, to learn who the patient really is, to face the abyss of the patient's suffering and not to run away. Courage is also required to be faithful to the patient and convey to the healthcare team the patient's desires even if the family or other healthcare providers do not agree. Another way to explain this virtue might be to say that palliative care nurses need to assume the role of patient advocate.

A nurse considering being an advocate for a patient might consider the following questions:

- Have I formed a deep connection with this patient?
- Do I know what this experience means to him?

■ Do I know what the patient really wants to be done?

■ Do I have the courage to act in the way I believe is necessary?

Ethical Dilemmas

It can be exceedingly difficult for a nurse to "hit the mean" and strike the balance between virtues as described by Armstrong (2006). When a nurse encounters a situation when he cannot determine what he ought to do, he should wonder, "Is this an ethical dilemma?" Ethical dilemmas may exist when there is a conflict between the rights or values/virtues of the people involved in the situation. They may occur when those involved believe that different principles ought to motivate their behavior or when they believe that considerations of the consequences of their actions should drive their decision making. An ethical dilemma might be defined as a situation that gives rise to conflicting moral claims, resulting in disagreements about choices for action. A cue that a nurse is dealing with an ethical dilemma is the language used to describe the situation. Ethical dilemmas are usually described in terms of right or wrong, duty or obligation, rights or responsibilities, and good or bad. They are commonly identified by the question, "What should be done?"

Being able to identify and focus on the moral issues in a situation has been called moral sensitivity. A nurse who is morally sensitive would identify the moral elements in a difficult situation and realize he had a role in the outcome. Some authors equate moral sensitivity with the development of conscience. Others believe that the development of moral sensitivity is the first step in ethical decision making.

Nurses often have difficulty focusing on moral issues and identifying ethical dilemmas. They may fail to note the ethical elements of a situation and proceed according to their usual pattern of behavior. Or, they may misinterpret the problem as a communication, legal, or institutional one and never recognize the ethical component. In the past it was common for nurses and other healthcare providers to define only major life-threatening events, such as euthanasia, as ethical while not recognizing the ethical elements of some of their everyday challenges (Varcoe et al., 2004). With the realization that failure to identify and respond to the ethical elements of any situation may be associated with an increase in a nurse's frustration and burnout, attention is being focused on these everyday events.

Tragic Circumstances

At other times, nurses confound ethical dilemmas with tragic circumstances. A tragic circumstance is one when nothing can be done to alleviate the situation. In such a case, a good choice or solution may be lacking. The sadness of the situation may make the nurse wish that there was something that could be done, but there are often no further options for treatment. An example is the case study described at the beginning of Chapter 8. An 8-year-old boy with leukemia was being considered for a bone marrow transplant. Just as a donor was found, he developed an infection that would not respond to the most potent antibiotics, and donation was no longer a possibility. He died within a few days. The sadness inherent in a tragic circumstance may cause the nurse to experience emotional turmoil and wish there was some way she or he could intervene to improve the situation, but it does not create an ethical dilemma.

Moral Distress

In 1984, Jameton was the first to describe a circumstance that he called "moral distress." In this situation, the nurse may believe she knows the right thing to do. Unfortunately, institutional constraints such as lack of resources or authority prevent her from doing it. Moral distress has been associated with burnout in nursing. Weissman (2009) suggests that moral distress is common in palliative care when providers in the care team fail to communicate with one another. One member or group in the care team might still be pursuing the goal of prolonging a patient's life while other providers might believe that discontinuation of some life-prolonging modalities and an emphasis on comfort care of life would best support the patient's autonomy, dignity, and quality of life. These concerns will be discussed further later in the chapter.

Approaches to Decision Making in Ethical Dilemmas

Once it seems apparent that an ethical dilemma exists, the first essential step is the identification of significant information. Consider the patient in the case study at the beginning of the chapter. The healthcare team will need to take into account the severity and potential for treatment of his pulmonary hypertension, his current and previously expressed wishes, and his current level of suffering. Without a clear understanding of the particulars of the situation, the nurse and the healthcare team will not be able to fully understand the dilemma or choose an action wisely.

What Information Should Be Considered When Making a Decision?

It is important that the nurse understand the person's medical condition. In order to limit potential confusion, it is helpful if the person, family, and all healthcare providers share an understanding of both the person's disease state and the goals for his treatment. Disagreement about a person's prognosis, disease progression, and likely outcome is frequently the reason healthcare providers, the patient, and family members are unable to agree on a treatment plan. As will be discussed later in the chapter, this is especially a problem when a patient's remaining length of life is unclear or when a healthcare team member, a family member, or the patient does not want to acknowledge that the patient's life may be reaching its end.

The nurse should gather data from a wide variety of sources and perspectives, not just medical information. The more accurate and complete the picture, the more clearly the dilemma can be described and appropriate decisions can be reached. Although information about a patient's medical status is essential, the nurse should gather information about the patient's psychological and interpersonal resources as well as his sociocultural background, values, and religion. The nurse would also want to discover if there were any laws or policies that governed her action in the situation.

It is also important that the nurse consider the time frame for making a decision. Many situations allow time for adequate reflection and consideration, but other decisions, like the decision to intubate the patient in the case study, must be made immediately and irrevocably. The amount of information it is possible to gather may be dependent on the immediacy of the decision.

Who Should Be Involved in Making the Decision?

Next, the nurse might consider who should be involved in making the decision. Does the patient have a voice? In the case study, should the patient's previous expressions speak for him? Should the family or primary healthcare provider be involved? Are there any reasons that an administrator or lawyer might be needed? The nurse should determine her role in the decision-making process.

Nurses may be represented in the decision-making process in several ways. First, they may represent their ethical perspective on the situation, carefully explaining their rationale. More commonly, nurses serve as the intermediary between patients, families, and healthcare providers, helping each group to understand the concerns of the others. Nurses often translate the ethical perspectives of their patients for other healthcare providers and clarify what the providers are saying to patients and families. Less frequently, nurses may act independently on their own moral decisions.

How Should One Make a Decision and Choose a Course of Action?

Most people will state that making any decision should involve clear thinking and consideration of the implications of each of the alternatives. Kuhse (1997) writes that making an ethical decision is at least reflective, a social activity, a matter of sound reasoning, impartial, and universal. Moreover, according to Kuhse, making such a decision should not be a matter of religion, a matter of obedience to authority, what comes naturally, social practice, or just a matter of feelings.

Unfortunately, many people view resolving a dilemma as choosing between two options. Consider how the phrase "on the horns of a dilemma" captures the feeling of being caught between two impossible choices. An alternative would be to view moral decision making as exploring a maze or traveling on a winding road. Both experiences involve considering many possibilities, trying a variety of pathways, being open to various possibilities, and remaining flexible. In a maze or on a winding road, as in healthcare decision making, the consequences of each choice are not always readily apparent, and there are usually at least several alternatives and often a series of decisions to be made. Using these analogies reminds people that the choice of a direction (or an ethical viewpoint) is only the beginning of the process. The progression through the maze or along the road will necessitate action (actual movement) and possible future decisions, especially if the consequences are different from those envisioned.

In the winding road poem and in finding a way out of the maze, there is a defined goal. Sometimes healthcare decision making focuses on choosing a particular action and neglects deciding on a goal. Identifying both the goal of health care and proposed actions to meet that goal helps to clarify the decision making. In palliative care, the primary goal is most likely apparent: What can the healthcare team do that is acceptable to all those involved to alleviate the patients' suffering? However, as Gillick (2005) notes, patients will likely want to balance this primary goal with optimization of the length of their lives and their level of function.

When involved in ethical decision making, the nurse might ask herself the following questions:

- What ethically justified goals can be identified?
- What are the ethically justified alternatives for action?
- Are there practical constraints to following any of them?
- What arguments can be constructed in favor of these alternatives (this includes considering the probable consequences)?
- How can these arguments be evaluated?
- What ought to be done?
- Is this decision reflective of sound thinking, or is it based on pressures from society, authority, religion, or purely on emotions and feelings?

What Follow-up Is Necessary After a Decision Is Made?

Most philosophers and ethicists assume that once the decision has been made, the process is complete. However, that is rarely the case for nurses involved in ethical decision making. When questioned about what it is to be ethical, nurses clearly indicate that "one has to follow through in action" (Varcoe et al., 2004, p. 320). In addition, nurses rarely act alone, so making a personal decision may be only a preparatory step for the nurse before convincing others of the soundness of the choice. Also, it is usually the nurse, patient, and family who must implement and live, or die, with the decision. As Jameton (1984) says, this phase is often full of surprises. Or to return to the analogy of the maze, the pathway does not always lead in the direction that was envisioned, and the decision may have to be reconsidered. Monteverde (2009) describes these unforeseen turns in the maze as critical junctures. He believes that each time one is encountered the team should reconsider where it is going and how it plans to get there. He suggests nurses ask at each juncture:

- Have we set the right priorities?
- Are they of the same importance to the patient?
- If not, what consensus can we reach?
- How can we plan for future critical junctures?

Finally, the nurse should evaluate what she learned from the situation. By systematically evaluating all phases of the decision-making process, future decision making might be less complicated. The nurse should consider the following:

- Did an ethical dilemma really exist, or had the nurse been caught up in a difficult or tragic circumstance?
- Was the nurse able to obtain necessary information in a timely fashion?
- If additional information would have been useful, how could the nurse obtain that information for future decisions?
- Were the appropriate people involved in the decision making? Were there others who should have been consulted?
- Was the nurse able to use ethical theories to develop alternatives for action and explain the rationale for her or his chosen intervention? Was this helpful?
- Would the nurse advocate the same action again in a similar situation, or were there unforeseen issues that would cause the nurse to recommend another course of action in similar cases in the future?

Ethical Dilemmas Frequently Encountered by Nurses

Although the order and specific phrasing of the dilemmas have varied from study to study over the past 30 years, three themes have been identified as the most common sources of ethical dilemmas for nurses. These common sources of ethical dilemmas for nurses include truth telling, the right to choose/decline treatments, and the prolongation of life.

Hermsen and Have (2001) analyzed the scholarly palliative care literature to identify the moral issues discussed by the palliative community. They concluded that the proportion of articles related to ethical issues had been increasing steadily over the past 25 years. The most common moral issues in palliative care journals were

- prolongation of life (euthanasia/assisted suicide, nontreatment decisions, and medical futility combined) accounting for 25% of the articles;
- the right to choose/decline treatments (quality and quantity of care/life, terminal sedation, force-feeding/tube feeding, use of morphine and principle of double effect), accounting for 24% of the articles;
- truth telling (communication, autonomy/informed consent, and truth telling disclosure), accounting for 10% of the articles;

- pastoral care/spirituality/meaning, accounting for 13% of the articles; and
- the concept of palliative care, accounting for 8% of the articles.

Spirituality is discussed in Chapter 7 and issues related to palliative care are discussed in Chapters 1 and 5 of this book.

Truth Telling

Ethical decision making often focuses on a dramatic moment or event, such as whether the patient in the case study at the beginning of the chapter should be taken off the ventilator. But the undramatic issues and moments are often pivotal in patients' and families' understanding of the illness, prognosis, or treatment. Owing to the nurse's proximity to the patient and attention to details, it is often the nurse who is present when a question or concern about treatment arises. Monteverde (2009) notes that it is in these undramatic moments when questions about treatment goals and priorities arise that truthfulness becomes important and occasionally is a dilemma for the nurse.

Truth Telling as the Standard of Care

Most ethicists and healthcare providers will argue that the covenant of trust between provider and patient is central to the practice of medicine and "the candid disclosure of information fosters and helps to maintain that trust" (Hebert, Hoffmaster, Glass, & Singer, 1997, pp. 225–228). As noted previously, palliative care nurses are emphatic that honesty is essential for the development of their nurse/patient relationship. Yet, telling the truth, especially when it means providing bad news to a patient, has only become the professional standard within the past 30 years. In a study conducted in 1961, 90% of American physicians would not disclose a diagnosis of cancer to their adult patients (Oken, 1961). When a similar study was conducted in 1979, a complete reversal had occurred and 97% of American physicians stated that they would inform their patients of their disease (Hebert et al., 1997). During that time period, ethicists began to emphasize the importance of truth telling and full disclosure so that patients could make autonomous decisions about their care.

Cultural Bias of Truth Telling

The reliance on truth telling and full disclosure appears to have a cultural bias. American physicians are somewhat more likely than European physicians to say they will reveal the entire truth. Patients from some cultural backgrounds have indicated preferences not to be fully informed. Studies indicate Hispanic women and Korean families are less likely to want to know the full truth. "Second order autonomy" is what ethicists call a rational decision by a patient not to receive full disclosure about his or her medical condition and to abdicate decisions to another person (usually a family member). Because the patient is making the decision not to be involved in her care, the patient is believed to be exercising a form of autonomy. Under such circumstances, truth telling may not be necessary and may even not be appropriate.

However, the cultural norms favoring nondisclosure are changing. In Japan, where physicians traditionally withheld bad news, physicians are now calling for full disclosure, and 97% of patients ask to be given complete and truthful information about their condition (Seo et al., 2000). For these reasons, nurses may feel uncertain about how to deal honestly with patients from different cultures (Erichsen et al., 2010). One way for the nurse to determine how much information the patient wishes to receive is to ask. The nurse might inquire:

- "How much do you want to know about your condition?" or
- "Who do you want to know what is happening to you and to make decisions about your care?"

Avoidance of Truth Telling

Some families may explicitly tell nurses not to inform dying patients how serious their illnesses are (Erichsen et al., 2010). The families may dread how the patient will respond to the grim news or may wish to protect the patient from pain. This places the nurse in a dilemma when she is asked to choose between acting honestly and respecting the request of the family. There are, however, several reasons in favor of telling the truth:

- Concealing painful truths is not usually beneficial to the patient. If the patient does not know her prognosis, she may fail to continue appropriate treatment or may make life choices that she would not have made if she had been fully informed (Gillick, 2009).
- Most adult patients insist that they, not their family members, should receive the bad news and that they should be able to determine who else is told.
- Adult patients have a clear legal right to full information about their diagnosis and prognosis.

■ It is usually not possible to keep the patient from suspecting the bad news, so nurses find themselves utilizing half truths while not actually lying to their patients (Tuckett, 2004).

Another reason that truth telling represents a dilemma for palliative care nurses is that it is usually the physician's responsibility to initially outline the diagnosis, treatment, and prognosis to the patient and family (Erichsen et al., 2010). This can result in problems for a nurse when the nurse knows the patient's prognosis but does not know how much the patient has been told by the physician. This is a major problem if the physician deliberatively withholds diagnostic or prognostic information from the patient. To some degree the nurse is obligated to follow the plan of care as ordered by a patient's physician. Nurses feel dishonest when patients ask them direct questions and they are unable to provide honest, complete answers, especially when they are unsure of what the physician is willing or able to explain.

Sustaining Hope While Still Telling the Truth

When families ask healthcare providers not to tell a patient the truth about an illness, they are identifying something that concerns healthcare providers deeply: how to convey the truth of a grim prognosis to a patient while sustaining hope (Daugherty, 2004). Clayton and others (2008) confirm that the majority of terminally ill patients want their healthcare providers to be honest when discussing prognosis and end of life care. They found that patients desired information that was accurate without being blunt, honest yet not too hard and factual or detailed. Clayton found the use of a communication style that was honest but sensitive fostered realistic hope in the patient and family. On the other hand, patients found it confusing and developed unrealistic expectations when a healthcare provider said something like "there's always hope" because the phrase could be interpreted as hope for survival, a miracle, or a cure. When the patient and family are confused about the prognosis for the patient's illness, it becomes almost impossible for them to rationally consider treatment options.

Right to Choose or Decline Treatment at End of Life

Georges and Grypdonck (2002) identified inappropriateness of medical treatment as an important source of "moral difficulty for nurses" caring for terminally ill patients (p. 163). Nurses' problems arose primarily from three different sources:

disagreement with decisions about end-of-life care, the continued use of advanced technologies when patients were dying, and the lack of consideration of patient dignity at end of life. Rees, King, and Schmitz (2009) noted that families of older adults often caused ethical conflict for nurses because the families could not support the patient's right to refuse treatment. Families might seek extreme forms of treatment despite the older adults' suffering and clearly stated wishes, or they might insist on force-feeding when the older adult was no longer willing or able to eat. Nurses' distress was compounded by "physicians over- and under treatment of patients, focusing on cure and being unable to attend to patients' wider needs" (Rees et al., 2009, p. 443).

When Is a Patient Dying?

It can be difficult to determine when a person is dying. Chronic illnesses such as multiple strokes, degenerative neurologic conditions, cancer, coronary artery disease, heart failure, or chronic lung disease can result in slow deterioration of health over a long period of time. Thus, many people die following long-term dwindling of function, needing years of personal care from a physiological challenge that may have just been an annoyance earlier in life. These patients develop acute illnesses, such as pneumonia, which worsen their underlying heart failure or pulmonary disease. Some patients recover from the acute illness with minimal medical interventions, such as antibiotics; some recover following aggressive treatment, such as ventilators, and some patients die with or without medical intervention. A patient with multiple chronic illnesses may have several episodes of acute illness during the long period of slow deterioration of health that precedes eventual death.

Thus, the miracles of modern medicine have made it difficult to identify and determine when a person is actually dying. In fact, there is evidence that until patients are within about 48 hours of death, physicians are relativity inaccurate at predicting time of death. Additionally, many oncologists tend to overestimate the length of probable patient survival and that is believed to contribute to continued aggressive care and late referral of a patient for palliative or hospice care (Daugherty, 2004).

Jakobsson and others (2006) studied 229 patients in an attempt to identify indicators of a turning point, the time when care was no longer directed toward cure and had been redirected at the relief of suffering. Indicators of a turning point in this study were

- sporadic confinement to bed,
- pain,
- fatigue,
- deterioration in condition,
- breathlessness,
- urinary incontinence, and
- eating disturbances.

In the majority of patients (63%), this turning point was not identified until the last week of life. If the time period was extended to the last month of life, then a turning point was identified for 82% of patients. Clearly, waiting until the last month, or in most circumstances, the last week or days of life to switch from aggressive care to providing comfort to a dying person is waiting too long.

When patients are deteriorating and may be dying, whether in long-term care, home care, hospice, or hospital settings, it is important to identify the goal of care and determine what interventions are appropriate to meet that goal. Perhaps, it is time for us to recognize that there should not be a turning point when the care swiftly shifts from a focus on cure to a focus on palliation. Rather, care should be like a seesaw, at the extremes the care may be focused primarily on curing or on palliation but most of the time the care delivered to patients needs to be a balance between the two.

Gillick (2005) agrees, stating that it is a false dichotomy to say that treatment needs to be directed only toward a goal of cure or one of comfort. She argues that palliative care should be adjunctive therapy that complements the active treatment of the underlying, progressive disease. For example, a patient with severe cardiovascular disease and angina that limited his function could have cardiac stents placed to enhance his functional ability, yet he could also receive assistance in managing his dyspnea and fatigue. Gillick believes that most patients approaching the end of their lives are trying to optimize their function, comfort, and length of life. She believes that by providing interventions simultaneously that might be labeled curative and "carative," we are most likely to help the patient balance these three goals at the end of life. As the illness progresses, the balance will likely shift. At first, the patient may be willing to give up some length of life to maintain function. However, as death approaches, the patient may be willing give up both some function and some length of life to attain comfort. How to balance these three goals ought to be the patient's choice, and the balance the patient chooses should guide the choice of curative/carative therapy whenever possible.

Dilemmas in Pain and Symptom Management

Pain is a common symptom at the end of life, and its management may create mis-understandings and confusion for patients, families, and healthcare providers. Emanuel (1998) estimated that with aggressive use of pain medications, 95% of patients should be pain-free during their dying process. However, many patients, healthcare providers, and family members are ignorant of essential information about how to provide adequate pain relief. Patients may be concerned that they will be less responsive if they take adequate pain medication. This may be par-tially counteracted by central nervous stimulants such as methylphenidate. Other patients and healthcare providers are concerned that the patient will become addicted to the narcotic used to relieve pain. This is not a realistic concern because research has demonstrated that the threat of addiction from commonly prescribed opiates is very small in the patient experiencing pain. Health professionals have expressed fear of prosecution if they prescribe the amounts of narcotics occasion-ally required for pain relief in dying patients. However, prosecution of physicians prescribing pain relief for dying patients is very rare. Finally, caregivers may fail to realize the importance of maintaining a baseline level of pain medication and pain relief. When a patient or caregiver waits to administer pain medication until pain is intense, there is little possibility of adequate and consistent pain relief.

Perhaps one of the most significant fears of caregivers is that by administering an adequate amount of pain medication, they might be morally accountable for the patient's death. Caregivers fear that the pain medications may depress the patient's respiration and hasten her or his death. Actually, adequate pain medication and relief of pain may slightly prolong a dying patient's life. However, caregivers, whether nurses or family members, need to realize that administering medication within the patient's dose range (which may be above the normal dose range for the medication) with the intent of relieving pain is morally acceptable even if it does hasten the patient's death.

A traditional ethical principle, double effect, is invoked in this instance. When an action has two effects, one good (relieving pain) and one bad (hastening death), it has been considered morally permissible to take the action if certain conditions, listed here, are met:

- The act itself (giving pain medication to relieve pain) is either good or morally neutral.
- Only the good effect (pain relief) is intended.

- The good effect is not achieved through the bad effect (the patient's pain is not relieved because the patient dies).
- There is no other means of attaining the good effect (other alternatives for pain relief are not possible or are ineffective).
- There is a good reason for assuming the risk of the bad effect (relief of severe pain).

Dilemmas Surrounding Intractable Pain and Palliative Sedation

For a small percentage of imminently dying patients, it is not possible to alleviate the physical pain and suffering. When their suffering becomes intolerable and refractory, the National Hospice and Palliative Care Organization (NHPCO) supports making the option of palliative sedation available (Kirk & Mahon, 2010). Palliative sedation is the purposeful rendering of the dying patient unconscious so that the person no longer suffers. The goal is symptom relief and not unconsciousness necessarily, so sedation is titrated to reduce consciousness to the minimum level necessary to render symptoms tolerable. For most patients this will mean they are resting quietly and comfortably and can be aroused with verbal stimuli or touch. For a few, deep sedation may be necessary and the patient may be unconscious.

Initiating palliative sedation requires prior consent of the patient and a multidisciplinary team that is skilled in providing standard palliative care. It is only when the normal modalities to relieve pain and physical suffering have been exhausted that NHPCO recommends convening a multidisciplinary team conference specifically about the use of sedation. In all cases, care must be patient and family centered. If the needs of the patient and family differ, the primary focus should be the needs of the patient. Patients may experience existential suffering as well as physical suffering at the end of life, and most patients seem to experience a balance of both. Pure existential suffering is possible but unlikely. At this time NHPCO does not have a position on the use of palliative sedation for pure existential suffering. Instead, NHPCO strongly urges providers to carefully consider the issue and supports further ethical discussion.

Whatever the situation, the initiation of palliative sedation should not be undertaken lightly. Magnusson (2006) categorizes it as a "devil's choice, a choice coerced by circumstances beyond one's control and made all the more terrible by the conviction that tragedy will follow, whichever option is taken" (p. 559). NHPCO states that it is appropriate only for patients who are terminally ill, who are actively dying, and whose death is expected imminently (within 2 weeks).

Since these patients have been receiving palliative care and their symptoms have not responded to appropriate therapy, Carr and Mohr (2008) believe that it is the end point of justifiable palliative care. Supporters of palliative sedation note that when properly administered, palliative sedation is not the proximate cause of a patient's death, nor is death a means of achieving symptom relief. Therefore, the principle of double effect would make it allowable and palliative sedation is distinct from euthanasia and assisted suicide. Magnusson states that it is clear when the intention of the provider is to help the patient without causing death because the

- sedatives and analgesics chosen have established therapeutic properties, and
- dosage of the medications administered are proportional to the suffering the patient is enduring.

In 2003, the Hospice and Palliative Care Nurses Association stated: "The ethical justification for palliative sedation is based on precepts of dignity, autonomy, beneficence, nonmaleficence, and the rule of double effect. These principles endorse the right of the individual to make healthcare decisions based on personal values and quality of life considerations and the responsibility of clinicians to provide humane and compassionate care that is consistent with professional and societal norms" (p. 1).

Nurses are intimately involved in the provision of palliative sedation. They administer and monitor the medications, assess the effectiveness of the treatments, and provide support and comfort for the patient and family. When Gran and Miller (2008) examined nurses' views on whether palliative sedation posed an ethical dilemma, they identified the following concerns:

- Although most of the time, patients and their families both decided that the patients' suffering was intolerable and requested sedation, there were some circumstances when the patient did not/could not participate in the decision. Nurses found that ethically difficult.
- More than 60% of the nurses said that deep palliative sedation was more ethically challenging for them than light sedation.
- Almost half of the nurses said palliative sedation was ethically challenging because it is always serious to interfere with patients' responsiveness and ability to communicate with their families.

■ Slightly more than 10% of nurses believed it complicated caring for the patient since patients had no way of conveying their needs.

Dilemmas Surrounding Nutrition and Hydration at the End of Life

As the end of life approaches, many patients reduce their oral intake. This is caused by a variety of factors such as anorexia/cachexia syndrome, generalized weakness, nausea, bowel obstruction, and decreased level of consciousness (Brunnhuber, Nash, Meier, Weissman, & Woodcock, 2008). When van der Riet, Good, Higgins, and Sneesby (2008) reviewed a series of studies on hydration at the end of life, they found that providing additional hydration had mixed results at best. Although some patients experienced improved sedation when they were hydrated, many experienced discomfort from fluid retention manifested as edema, ascites, incontinence, urinary retention, pleural effusion, or pulmonary secretions. Many palliative care nurses believe that the natural process of the patient not wanting to eat or drink at the end of life is helpful in relieving or preventing this constellation of symptoms. There is also evidence that dehydration, which may occur at end of life, does not cause suffering, provided that good oral hygiene is maintained (van der Riet et al., 2008). A Cochrane review conducted in 2008 by Good and others could not find sufficient evidence to make any recommendation concerning the use of artificial hydration in adult palliative care patients.

Most dying patients do not suddenly stop taking food and fluid but rather decrease their intake slowly over time, experiencing neither hunger nor thirst (van der Riet et al., 2006). Thus, van der Riet recommends that when a dying patient becomes uninterested in food or has difficulty swallowing that food and fluid should be offered but not forced. The patient should be encouraged to consume as little or as much food and fluid as he desires, which often means the person consumes very little.

However, as Gillick (2009) notes, there is such a widespread association between nourishment and nurturing that many families cannot be persuaded that they are not abandoning their family member when they do not force-feed them or provide them with artificial forms of nourishment. Families often feel that they should strongly encourage their loved ones to eat because food and fluids are normal components of care. Families may also believe that their loved ones should be provided with artificial forms of nourishment through tube feedings or total parenteral nutrition. When a person is approaching death, most ethicists and religious leaders agree that force-feeding and artificial nutrition are not appropriate, especially if they are increasing the patient's discomfort or the patient finds them burdensome.

Palliative care specialists stress that it is more important to manage symptoms such as thirst and hunger of the patient than to adhere to any general formula. Byock (1997) includes in his promises to dying patients, "We will always offer you food and water." This accentuates the importance of offering oral feedings but permits the patient to determine whether he can tolerate them. When the patient is unable to swallow or does not desire food and fluids but is complaining of thirst or a dry mouth, the nurse may teach caregivers to moisten the mouth and lips or provide ice chips.

Since the goal of palliative care is the best quality of life for the patient near death, the healthcare team should reevaluate a situation in which the patient seems to be experiencing distress from lack of food or fluids. In the rare circumstance when a patient is suffering from dehydration-induced delirium, artificial hydration might be considered. Palliative care nurses are often required to assist patients and their families in determining whether they should attempt artificial hydration or whether dehydration and natural progression of the process is more appropriate.

Prolongation of Life

Weissman (2009) states that the most common cause of moral distress in palliative care practitioners is conflict with other healthcare providers about the discontinuation of potentially life prolonging treatments. Conflict may result when the palliative care team's underlying goal of alleviating discomfort and providing care is in opposition to a referring physician's perceived professional duty to preserve life. The conflict can be worsened by the emotional impact some healthcare providers experience when withholding or withdrawing care and the unrealistic fear of malpractice.

Cardiopulmonary Resuscitation (CPR) and Do Not Resuscitate (DNR) Orders

Do not resuscitate orders warrant special discussion because CPR, unlike other medical interventions, is required for all patients who die in a hospital unless there is a physician's order stating that the patient is not to be resuscitated. Despite the fact that it is required for all patients, CPR is usually unsuccessful, with only 13% to 18% of patients surviving to hospital discharge, many with neurological impairments. Additionally, resuscitation is most likely a painful or at least an uncomfortable process. The patient's ribs may be broken, endotracheal intubation is performed, and electric shocks may be delivered. Finally, as the 1995 SUPPORT study discovered, nearly half of the patients who wanted CPR to be withheld did not have a DNR order written during their hospitalization. Nearly one third of those patients died before discharge and likely had CPR performed.

Therefore, if a patient is in the hospital, either the patient or the patient's surrogate ought to be asked if CPR should be performed or withheld if the patient experiences cardiac or respiratory arrest. Since CPR has a small chance of being successful, it is not clearly futile. Thus, the decision about resuscitation is value-laden, not purely medically determined, and one in which patients and families should participate. Resuscitation is clearly an intrusive, expensive, and possibly painful medical intervention. Given this information, patients and families may decline CPR if they believe it will offer only minimal benefits or be too burdensome.

Unfortunately, many physicians are uncomfortable and unwilling to initiate discussions about forgoing treatment, for example discussing DNR orders (Smith & O'Neill, 2008). Often, it is the nurses who have been listening to the patients' and families' concerns about prognoses and treatment choices, who alert the physicians to the patients' and families' willingness to discuss resuscitation. Nurses may need to spend a significant amount of time explaining the concept of DNR in understandable terms to patients and families so that they can give informed consent.

How the patient and family are approached also has an impact on their decision. If they are asked, "Do you want everything done?" They will almost always say yes. Saying they do not want everything done for a dying family member makes people feel as if they are abandoning the person (Gillick, 2009). However, the response to the following question may be very different. "Unless there is an order saying not to attempt it, when a patient's heart stops, we must try to restart it again. I don't believe we could successfully restart your (family member's) heart and since trying to do that can be painful, I would prefer not to try. Do you agree?"

Nurses should emphasize to patients and families that consent to a DNR order does not imply consent to withdraw other medical interventions or a decision to switch to a goal of comfort rather than cure (Smith & O'Neill, 2008). These are separate issues that may be discussed simultaneously or at a later time. Consenting to a DNR does not imply that the patient will receive less care. Studies indicate that patients with DNR orders in ICUs usually receive more nursing time and nursing care than those ICU patients who do not have DNR orders.

Withholding and Withdrawal of Life-Sustaining Technologies

Most medical ethicists, physicians, and nurses consider both the withholding and the withdrawal of burdensome or extraordinary interventions to be ethically justifiable. When a patient is deteriorating and dying from the disease process and the proposed medical interventions are unlikely to prevent the patient's inevitable death but could prolong suffering and the dying process, the interventions offer minimal benefit and may be withheld or withdrawn. Thus, aggressive medical interventions such as CPR, mechanical ventilation, chemotherapy, or hemodialysis may be justly withheld or discontinued in the dying patient. Additionally, if an intervention is too burdensome (painful, costly, or having excessively unpleasant side effects) for a patient to tolerate, the patient may choose to decline or discontinue the procedure. Forgoing, withdrawing, or withholding medical treatment, which offers minimal benefit or is excessively burdensome, is classified as passive euthanasia.

To understand why such a position is ethically justifiable, one must acknowledge that modern medicine is not capable of curing all conditions and that it can impose inordinate suffering on patients in attempts to prolong their lives. The principle of autonomy might be invoked to justify the patient's being able to determine when the benefits of a slightly longer life are outweighed by the burdens of physical and emotional suffering. Since the treatment is not capable of curing the patient, it is not the withdrawal of the intervention that directly causes the patient's death but the relentless progress of the patient's disease. That is why withdrawal and withholding are classified as passive euthanasia.

When a patient is deteriorating and possibly dying, many patients and families prefer a trial of aggressive medical management. Withholding or withdrawing medical interventions may be discussed before medical therapy is initiated, after a predetermined trial of aggressive therapy, or any time medical interventions do not appear to be benefiting the patient. Listed here is a sequence that might be followed for withholding or withdrawing medical interventions:

- Initiation of a do not resuscitate order
- No further additional aggressive or heroic treatment such as intubation or ventilation to be provided
- No further curative treatment to be provided
- Withdrawal of probably discomfort-producing technology
- Provision of comfort measures, without invasive procedures such as blood draws

Patients and their families need to be reassured that the patient will still be cared for when aggressive medical interventions are stopped. The designation of comfort measures, like the institution of palliative care, should be a cue that aggressive nursing care is required to maintain patient comfort and control patient symptoms. Nursing and pharmacological interventions to manage the symptoms people experience at the end of life are described in more detail in Chapter 5. Nurses should reassure patients and families by both their words and their actions that they will continue to provide quality nursing care after life-sustaining interventions are withdrawn. In an effort to promote rest, peace, and privacy, nurses may forgo routinely checking vital signs. However, they need to continue certain assessments (e.g., respiratory, gastrointestinal, and genitourinary) so as to identify and treat symptoms of distress.

Active Assistance with Dying

Some terminally ill patients request healthcare providers to hasten their deaths. Because either the patient or provider is taking an action that has the direct effect of shortening the patient's life, this process is known as active euthanasia. Active euthanasia is legal in only a few places, yet patients around the world request healthcare providers assist them in dying. When Mak and Elwyn (2005) investigated the reasons that patients already receiving hospice care would consider assisted death, they uncovered the following reasons. The patients were

- aware that their disease was progressing, death was inevitable, and their situation was hopeless;
- experiencing multidimensional suffering and knew that their significant others were suffering as well;
- anticipating a future that was worse than death with continuing suffering and poor communication from their healthcare providers;

■ hoping for good quality end-of-life care and an escape from their present suffering.

Hurst and Mauron (2006) argue that the values of palliative care and active euthanasia are similar, in that they both reduce physical and emotional suffering. Yet they differ in the amount of control the patient has over the timing of the end of life. A majority of providers believe that choosing death should not be in human hands, whereas those advocating active euthanasia say that a good death should be at the time of the patient's choosing. There are three forms of active euthanasia: assisted suicide, voluntary active euthanasia, and involuntary active euthanasia. In the first two, the person has requested a hastened death. In the third, someone else has chosen that the person should die.

Assisted Suicide

When an individual knowingly provides the means for a patient to commit suicide but the patient completes the act, it is termed assisted suicide. Assisted suicide is legal in the states of Oregon and Washington in certain situations, and in the Netherlands. Advocates of assisted suicide state that suicide allows terminally ill patients to control the time and situation of death. Supporters of assisted suicide declare that just as a medical intervention that has become too burdensome may be withdrawn, so may a life that has become too burdensome be ended. They maintain that if patients are able to control the time of their death, they may complete all necessary business, and death will be both timely and peaceful.

Supporters of assisted suicide also argue that dying by medication overdose is a far more humane method of death then dying naturally. They believe that by committing suicide, the dying patient does not experience any discomfort at the end and is not forced to endure a protracted, painful dying experience. Supporters of assisted suicide may declare, "We treat our dogs and cats more humanely at the end of life than our relatives." Some physicians will agree and argue that assisted suicide ought to be available for the 5% of dying patients who are unable to obtain pain relief despite the best pain management.

Defenders of assisted suicide often stress the findings in Oregon after the first year of enactment of the assisted suicide legislation in 1997. During that first year, 15 people ended their own lives in the state, while a few additional patients obtained the necessary medications but never committed suicide. Based on these data, providers believed that the law was not abused and, in fact, a number of people benefited from its enactment. Since that time the number of patients committing suicide under this program has stabilized at about 40 each year. However, there has been a fourfold increase in the prescription of morphine for pain in dying patients and a dramatic increase in the number of patients referred to hospice in Oregon. Thus, some supporters of assisted suicide believe that the enactment of legal assisted suicide resulted in dramatic improvements in end-of-life care to all dying patients in the state of Oregon (Lindsay, 2009).

Finally, promoters of assisted suicide will state that it allows dying people to avoid a protracted period of dependency during which they must rely on others to meet their most intimate needs. By committing suicide, these patients are not a burden to those who would otherwise be required to care for them. When dying individuals are questioned about the reasons one might commit suicide, being a burden to others is consistently near the top of the list.

Opponents of assisted suicide declare that there are limits to autonomy and no one has the right to end a human life, even his own. They seriously question whether the person requesting suicide is capable of making a rational, autonomous choice. They note that the majority of people who request assisted suicide are depressed. Depressed patients are not considered competent to make a decision about medical treatment, so opponents of assisted suicide are emphatic that depressed patients should not be allowed to make a decision about assisted suicide.

Critics of assisted suicide suggest that it would not necessarily result in a more humane death. They stress that suicide is an irreversible condition, which harms the person irrevocably by depriving him of life. For most dying patients, the last months of life can be maintained relatively symptom free and may have meaning. Most patients appear to die reasonably comfortably and peacefully, yet less predictably than if they had practiced assisted suicide. Opponents fear that if care of the dying patient is perceived as a burden by the caregivers, the dying patient would believe he must commit suicide to relieve the caregivers of the burden.

Harvath et al. (2006) explored the dilemmas encountered by hospice nurses in Oregon when their patients wished to hasten death. "The biggest dilemma arises from the conflict between important hospice values: honoring patient autonomy versus promoting a death experience in which personal and spiritual transformation are possible" (p. 200). Many nurses indicated that they tried to uncover their patient's reason for requesting assisted suicide and then tried to alleviate the patient's concern. Nurses also noted that patients' and loved ones' growth and spiritual transformation were often tied to the caregiving provided as death approached. As one nurse said, "I think the dying process has a lot to give. . . .

There's a lot of healing that occurs at the end. So, I'm saddened when people want to short circuit that" (p. 204).

The American Nurses Association (ANA, 1994) has taken a stand in opposition to assisted suicide. The ANA's opposition to assisted suicide is based on several points:

- The profession of nursing is built upon the Hippocratic tradition "do no harm" and an ethic of moral opposition to killing another human being.
- Nursing has a social contract with society that is based on trust, and therefore patients must be able to trust that nurses will not actively take a human life.
- While there may be individual cases that are compelling, there is a high potential for abuse with assisted suicide, particularly with vulnerable populations, such as the elderly, poor, and disabled. These abuses are even more probable in a time of declining resources.

Voluntary Active Euthanasia

When a patient requests that an action be taken by another to directly end her life, it is termed voluntary active euthanasia. In the Netherlands, physicians who commit voluntary active euthanasia are not prosecuted if they follow specific guidelines. They must assure that the patient is suffering unbearably, all other alternatives have been tried, and no one else will be harmed by the death. In addition, a proper consultation and appropriate reporting to authorities have to be documented.

Most Dutch citizens and physicians support the continued use of active euthanasia in these selected circumstances. However, there are grave concerns about the Dutch experience. During the more than 20 years that voluntary euthanasia has been permitted, the guidelines for euthanasia have been steadily broadening from unbearable pain to psychic disfigurement. Although the Dutch government notes that two thirds of the requests for euthanasia are refused, most studies indicate that only about 40% of the cases are reported to the local authorities as required. So the procedures are not all open to scrutiny by outside authorities, as was the original intent.

Verpoort surveyed nurses' responses to euthanasia in the Netherlands and Belgium. Verpoort et al. (2004a) found that most of the nurses believed euthanasia would be acceptable for patients who were suffering unbearably and whose suffering (whether physical or emotional) could not be relieved. In a meta-analysis,

Verpoort et al. (2004b) noted that in all the studies they reviewed, more nurses said that they could accept and understand the reasons for euthanasia than would be willing to perform or deliver care to a patient undergoing euthanasia. In a subsequent study, Gastmans et al. (2006) reviewed institutional policies related to conscientious refusal by nurses to care for patients who had requested euthanasia. Although the majority of institutions had policies that advised nurses who had conscientious objections to excuse themselves from assisting in the act of euthanasia, few institutions advised such nurses to stop caring for patients requesting euthanasia. Therefore, any nurse caring for a patient requesting euthanasia in a country where it has been decriminalized will likely face a series of dilemmas.

Perhaps the most persistent worry about the Dutch experience with euthanasia is that the Dutch may be sliding down the slippery slope to involuntary active euthanasia, purposefully ending a patient's life without the patient's consent. Researchers estimate that 3500 instances of euthanasia occurred in the Netherlands in 2001, accounting for 2.4% of deaths. Approximately 1000 deaths per year have been described in government reports as occurring from life-terminating choices not technically called euthanasia. These deaths have been interpreted by some critics of Dutch policy as deaths due to involuntary active euthanasia.

Involuntary Active Euthanasia

Involuntary active euthanasia, purposefully ending a patient's life without her consent, is usually a private, hidden act because it is illegal. Thus, it is difficult to gain a clear perspective on the extent to which healthcare providers engage in it. In a study by Asch (1996), it appeared that 16% of critical care nurses had performed active euthanasia, either voluntary or involuntary. The nurses in Asch's study most often provided large doses of narcotics to patients in pain prior to the patient's death. Because of defects in the study, it is unclear whether the nurses' intent was to relieve their patients' pain or solely to cause the patients' death. A well-controlled study by Emanuel and colleagues published the same year suggests that approximately 12% of oncologists have engaged in active euthanasia but does not identify whether it was voluntary or involuntary.

Most healthcare providers who commit involuntary euthanasia state that they are acting out of compassion. They argue that the patient's life was no longer worth living and that the burdens of the life far outweighed the benefits. They cite such reasons as the patient was suffering unbearably or the family and healthcare team were unable to reach a decision to withdraw futile, life-sustaining treatment so the patient was forced to suffer needlessly. They may also declare that the patient would never have wanted to live in her current condition and would have requested interventions to be halted if she had had a voice. Involuntary euthanasia is the judgment by another person, in this case a healthcare provider, that the patient's life is no longer worth living, followed by an action that ends the patient's life without the patient's consent.

Although according to Blendon, Szalay, and Knox (1992) the public supports the general concept of active euthanasia by physicians, oncology patients in pain usually do not (Emanuel et al., 1996). Perhaps it is telling that people who are dying, whose quality of life may appear limited to others, do not want to have healthcare providers empowered to determine whether their lives are worth living. In fact, only 3% of Americans would want their healthcare providers to make a decision and commit involuntary euthanasia on their behalf if they were not conscious and could not express their wishes (Blendon et al., 1992). Thus, there is little support for those healthcare providers who contend that in committing involuntary euthanasia they are acting in accordance with their patients' unstated wishes.

There are numerous other arguments against the use of active euthanasia. First, most medical and nursing professional organizations state that their members have a primary duty not to harm, which prohibits them from intentionally causing a patient's death. Many religious groups profess that human life should be respected and healthcare providers should never intentionally cause their patients' death. Hospice nurses have expressed concerns that palliative care might not receive adequate funding and referrals, or that patients might experience pressures to die quickly and stop being a burden if active euthanasia were available. Caring for a deteriorating or dying person takes time, a scarce commodity in our society.

Summary

Numerous ethical issues surround care of patients who are perceived to be suffering. It is imperative that nurses identify dilemmas when they encounter them and carefully consider how to intervene. Nurses can do a great deal to prevent the development of ethical dilemmas surrounding a patient's illness and to alleviate suffering even near death. They can advocate the appropriate use of technology and the withdrawal of ineffective or burdensome therapies. Nurses can ensure that their patients receive quality symptom management, that the families are educated about the experience of serious illness accompanied by suffering, and that patients receive human contact, comfort, and support even when death appears to be inevitable.

Key Points

1. Virtues that have been described as essential for palliative care nurses to possess include respect for human dignity, veracity, beneficence/nonmaleficence, fidelity, and courage.
2. Nurses can identify a moral dilemma when they encounter a situation that makes them ask themselves the question, "What should be done?"
3. Excellent pain and symptom management and alleviation of suffering are essential in serious illness.
4. Most ethicists support the withholding or withdrawal of invasive interventions when the patient has weighed the benefits and burdens and believes the interventions are too burdensome.
5. Many patients at the end of life do not experience hunger or thirst and may benefit from eating or drinking only what makes them comfortable.
6. Unlike passive euthanasia, which involves the removal of an intervention that is more burdensome than beneficial, active euthanasia is directly intervening to cause the death of a person. It is illegal in most places in the world even when the person is actively dying.

Role-Playing Exercise

Making a decision about how one ought to proceed in an ethical dilemma is difficult for any one person. However, in health care, there are usually multiple people involved in the discussion and the decision making. This exercise provides an opportunity to consider the most appropriate responses to several situations with ethical overtones and to practice ways to engage in discussions with other members of the healthcare team, patients, and families concerning what ought to be done. For each of the following situations, a different person should role-play each role, adopting the viewpoint identified for that role.

Situation 1

Roles

Leslie Evers: patient whose viewpoint is described in the dilemma.

John Evers: Leslie's husband who wants her to live but realizes she is dying. He just wants her to be comfortable.

Amy Green, RN: the nurse who has been caring for Leslie for the past few days. She is convinced she is torturing Leslie and Leslie will die the next time she is turned. She does not want to do CPR on Leslie and believes Leslie should be receiving palliative care.

Alan Walden, MD: Leslie's pulmonologist. He believes CPR would not offer any benefit, does not have any other treatment options he can provide for her, and would prefer Leslie were referred to the palliative care service.

Description of Dilemma

Leslie Evers, a 32-year-old woman with cystic fibrosis, wants to live no matter the cost. She has been married less than 5 years and has a devoted husband and caring family. Leslie is ventilator dependent and had been transferred to the ICU of a community hospital after developing pneumonia. Although she was insistent that she was on the heart-lung transplant list of two centers, both institutions declared she no longer met transplant criteria. They had informed both Leslie and her family that she was no longer on their transplant lists and they refused to have her transferred to them saying there was nothing more they could do for her. Leslie is determined to survive. Every possible therapy and intervention has been tried and her ventilator is set at the maximum settings, but still she became increasingly hypoxic. Any slight sound startles Leslie, and she awakens terrified, hypoxic, and diaphoretic. Attempts to suction or turn her result in such severe hypoxia that her heart rate drops to the low 40s. Only when she is in a quiet, darkened room with her husband holding her hand does she seem to get any rest. This, however, is not what Leslie wants; she wants to get better and live. Thus, she has asked to be turned, suctioned, and percussed despite her hypoxia and terror.

Role-Play

Role-play a meeting in Leslie's room when all four people are present. The intent of the meeting is to set goals for Leslie's care. Both the physician and nurse would like a DNR order and palliative care to be discussed.

Situation 2

Roles

Mrs. Eva Boucher: the patient whose condition is described in the dilemma. She eats what is offered to her but has not expressed an opinion about other means of nourishment when she has been asked in the past.

Mrs. Jeanne Williams: Mrs. Boucher's daughter. Her concerns are detailed in the dilemma.

Ms. Helen Redding: the day charge nurse in the long-term care facility. She has known Mrs. Boucher for many years as they lived in the same neighborhood. She believes Mrs. Boucher has already made up her own mind.

Ms. Nel Allen: a speech therapist who noted that Mrs. Boucher's mother was swallowing, not aspirating, as long as she was fed gently and not force-fed.

Description of Dilemma

Mrs. Eva Boucher is an 89-year-old widow who has had resided for 2 years in a long-term care facility. During those years, she has had recurrent strokes. Her left side has become progressively weaker, and she can barely move her arm. She has a pronounced left-sided facial droop and requires careful feeding and observation so that she does not pocket or aspirate her food. She rarely speaks and is often incontinent of urine. Her deterioration from an active, talkative 87-year-old was pronounced, and her family mourned the vivacious woman she had been.

Mrs. Boucher's daughter is concerned because her mother is eating less each week and has lost 10 pounds, a significant amount for a 4-foot, 9-inch woman. One afternoon, the daughter had finished feeding her mother lunch and was considering whether she ought to request that her mother be started on tube feedings or allow her mother to eat what she desired and perhaps slowly fade away. Mrs. Boucher was napping peacefully while her daughter sat beside her, fingering rosary beads. The daughter was remembering years earlier when she had also sat peacefully in the sun saying the rosary as her grandmother lay dying. Without warning, Mrs. Boucher's loud, clear voice interrupted her thoughts.

"What do you think you're doing? I'm NOT dying yet."

Role-Play

Role-play the discussion among the four people concerning whether Mrs. Boucher should have a feeding tube inserted.

Situation 3

Roles

Mrs. Brown's daughter: the family member whose position is described in the dilemma below.

Ms June Winning: the nurse who admitted Mrs. Brown and has just begun to take care of her.

Description of Dilemma

Mrs. Brown, a 77-year-old woman, was admitted to a medical unit of an acute care hospital. She underwent extensive surgery for colon cancer several months earlier and was in considerable pain and dehydrated at the time of admission. On admission, Mrs. Brown was barely responsive and was accompanied by a daughter, who announced she would be the medical care decision maker because she had durable power of attorney for healthcare purposes. The daughter stated that she understood her mother was dying and she did not want any measures to prolong her mother's life but would like aggressive management of her mother's pain.

Mrs. Brown was started on IV hydration and a morphine infusion with intermittent morphine boluses for severe pain. As her pain was controlled and she was rehydrated, Mrs. Brown's vital signs stabilized and she appeared quite comfortable, but she was still either unable or unwilling to communicate. Mrs. Brown's daughter cornered her mother's nurse and proclaimed, "I told you I only wanted you to control my mother's pain. I don't want her life prolonged." The nurse reassured the daughter that her mother was responding favorably to the pain medication and hydration and nothing else was being done for her. "Then," said the daughter, "I want you to give her enough pain medication to end it now. This has been going on for too long and I need it to be over."

Role-Play

Begin the role-play with the daughter's last statement and continue with the nurse's response. Also, consider what ought to be done following the interaction between the daughter and the nurse.

Questions for Reflection and Journaling

People often compare having an ethical dilemma to being on the horns of a dilemma. Do you agree with that comparison? Why or why not? Do you think it would be more appropriate to compare having an ethical dilemma to being on a winding road? How about comparing it to being caught in a maze? Which comparison do you believe is most appropriate? Why? Can you imagine another image for an ethical dilemma? If so, explain it.

When were you most recently involved in an ethical dilemma? What was your role in the situation? How was the decision made about how to resolve the dilemma? Do you believe the appropriate decision was made? Why or why not?

Have you experienced moral distress? What happened? Why was the decision that you believed was most appropriate not enacted? What, if anything, could have changed the outcome?

Do you always tell your patients and their families the whole truth? Why or why not? Describe the last time that you encountered a situation where you thought about whether you should tell someone the whole truth.

Case Study 4–2

My patient was a woman who had been diagnosed with breast cancer that had metastasized to her lungs. Her prognosis was grim and she had only a few months left to live. One dilemma the woman was having concerned eating. When I brought her breakfast, she was happy. She seemed to be joyful that there was at least one thing that she was able to do on her own—feed herself. But even that proved to be challenging. She simply did not have the strength to eat. She kept falling asleep. When my instructor explained to her that it was natural for her appetite to decrease, she broke down. She told us that her family was concerned about her eating and were insisting that she eat more. However, she simply was not able to eat much. We also spoke with her about going home and who was able to help her during the day. She was unsure if someone was able to come everyday to care for her. This was concerning because of her family; like their insistence that they wanted her to eat more, they wanted her to be at home and not to go to a hospice house. This woman had a tremendous burden on her shoulders. How would she ever die in peace if these conflicts were present? I could tell this was wearing her down.

I saw this patient again when I had my experience in a hospice house later in the semester. There, when I observed the interaction she had with her husband, I could tell he had come to terms with her prognosis. He was still very controlling and wanted to know everything that was going on with her, but he was not nearly as overbearing as before. The burden seemed to have lifted from her. She was much more cheerful and I could tell that she was cherishing the final days that she had on this earth.

Questions for Case Study 4–2

1. What ethical concerns can you identify in this case study?
2. Does the student recognize any ethical issues? What are they?
3. How are issues about continuing food at the end of life different from issues about continuing invasive measures like the ventilator described in the first case study? In what ways are they similar?
4. Who should be involved in making the decisions about food and placement after discharge from the hospital? Why?
5. What, if any, ethical responsibilities do the healthcare providers have in this situation?

Source: Courtesy of Megan Jacques, student nurse, 2010.

References

American Nurses Association. (1994). *Position statement on assisted suicide.* Washington, DC: Author.

Arman, M. (2007). Bearing witness: An existential position in caring. *Contemporary Nurse, 27*(1), 84–94.

Armstrong, A. (2006). *Towards a strong virtue ethics for nursing practice. Nursing Philosophy, 7,* 110–124.

Asch, D. A. (1996). The role of critical care nurses in euthanasia and assisted suicide. *New England Journal of Medicine, 334,* 1374–1379.

Benjamin, M., & Curtis, J. (1992). *Ethics in nursing* (3rd ed.). New York, NY: Oxford University Press.

Bergdahl, E., Wikstrom, B., & Andershed, B. (2007). Esthetic abilities: A way to describe abilities of expert nurses in palliative care. *Journal of Clinical Nursing 16,* 752–560.

Blendon, R. J., Szalay, U. S., & Knox, R. A. (1992). Should physicians aid their patients in dying? The public perspective. *Journal of the American Medical Association, 267,* 2658–2662.

Brunnhuber, K., Nash S., Meier, D., Weissman, D. E., & Woodcock, J. (2008, Spring). *Putting evidence into practice: Palliative care.* Minneapolis, MN: BMJ Publishing.

Byock, I. (1997). *Dying well: Peace and possibilities at the end of life.* New York, NY: Riverhead Books.

Carr, M. F., & Mohr, G. J. (2008). "Palliative sedation as part of a continuum of palliative care." *Journal of Palliative Medicine, 11*(1), 76–81.

Clayton, J., Hancock, K., Parker, S., Butow, P., Walder, S., Carrick, S., Currow, D., Ghersi, D., Glare, P., Hagerty, R., Olver, I., & Tattersall, M. (2008). Sustaining hope when communicating with terminally ill patients and their families: A systematic review. *Psycho-Oncology, 17,* 641–659.

Cody, W. (2001). The ethics of bearing witness in health care: A beginning exploration. *Nursing Science Quarterly, 14*(4), 288–296.

Cody, W. (2007). Bearing witness to suffering: Participating in cotranscendence. *International Journal for Human Caring, 11*(2), 17–21.

Daugherty, C. (2004). Examining ethical dilemmas as obstacles to hospice and palliative care for advanced cancer patients. *Bioethics, 22*(1), 123–131.

Emanuel, E., Fairclough, D. L., Daniels, E. R., & Clarridge, B. R. (1996). Euthanasia and physician assisted suicide: Attitudes and experiences of oncology patients, oncologists, and the public. *Lancet, 347,*1805–1810.

Emanuel, E. J. (1998). The promise of a good death. *Lancet, 351*(Suppl. Cancer), S112.

Erichsen, E., Danielsson, E., & Friedrichsen, M. (2010). A phenomenological study of nurses' understanding of honesty in palliative care. *Nursing Ethics, 17*(1), 39–50.

Gastmans, C., Lemiengre, J., & Dierckx de Casterle, B. (2006). Role of nurses in institutional ethics policies on euthanasia. *Journal of Advanced Nursing, 54,* 53–60.

Georges, J-J., & Grypdonck, M. (2002). Moral problems experienced by nurses when caring for terminally ill people: A literature review. *Nursing Ethics, 9*(2), 155–177.

Gillick, M. (2005). Rethinking the central dogma of palliative care. *Journal of Palliative Medicine, 8*(5), 909–913.

Gillick, M. (2009). Decision making near life's end: A prescription for change. *Journal of Palliative Medicine, 12*(2), 121–125.

Good, P., Cavenagh, J., Mather, M., & Ravenscroft, P. (2008). Medically assisted hydration for adult palliative care patients. *Cochrane Database Systematic Reviews, April 16* 2:CD006273.

Gran, S., & Miller, J. (2008). Norweigian nurses' thoughts and feelings regarding the ethics of palliative sedation. *International Journal of Palliative Nursing, 14*(11), 532–538.

Harvath, T. A., Miller, L. L., Smith, K. A., Clark, L. D., Jackson, M. B., & Ganzini, L. (2006). Dilemmas encountered by hospice workers when patients wish to hasten death. *Journal of Hospice and Palliative Care Nursing, 8,* 200–209.

Hebert, P. C., Hoffmaster, B., Glass, K. C., & Singer, P. A. (1997). Bioethics for clinicians: 7. Truth telling. *Canadian Medical Association Journal, 156,* 225–228.

Hermsen, M., & Have, H. (2001). Moral problems in palliative care journals. *Palliative Medicine, 15*, 425–431.

Hodkinson, K. (2008). How should a nurse approach truth-telling? A virtue ethics approach. *Nursing Philosophy, 9*(4), 248–256.

Hospice and Palliative Nurses Association. (2003). *Position statement: Palliative sedation at end of life*. Pittsburgh, PA: Hospice and Palliative Nurses Association. Retrieved from http://www.hpna.org/pdf/positionstatement_palliativesedation.pdf

Hurst, S., & Mauron, A. (2006). The ethics of palliative care and euthanasia: Exploring common values. *Palliative Medicine, 20*, 107–112.

Jakobsson, E., Bergh, I., Gaston-Johansson, F., Stout, C., & Ohlen, J. (2006). The turning point: Clinical identification of dying and reorientation of care. *Journal of Palliative Medicine, 9*(6), 1348–1358.

Jameton, A. (1984). *Nursing practice: The ethical issues*. Englewood Cliffs, NJ: Prentice Hall.

Kirk, T., & Mahon, M. (2010). National Hospice and Palliative Care Organization (NHPCO) position and commentary on the use of palliative sedation in imminently dying, terminally ill patients. *Journal of Pain and Symptom Management, 39*(5), 914–923.

Kuhse, H. (1997). *Caring: Nurses, women, and ethics*. Oxford, UK: Blackwell.

Lindsay, R. (2009). Oregon's experience: Evaluating the record. *American Journal of Bioethics, 9*(3), 19–27.

Magnusson, R, (2006, Fall). The devil's choice: Rethinking law, ethics, and symptom relief in palliative care. *Journal of Law, Medicine, and Ethics*, 559–569.

Mahon, M., & Sorrell, J. (2008). Palliative care for people with Alzheimer's disease. *Philosophy and Palliative Care, 9*, 110–120.

Mak, Y., & Elwyn, G. (2005). Voices of the terminally ill: Uncovering the meaning of desire for euthanasia. *Palliative Medicine, 19*, 343–350.

Monteverde, S. (2009). The importance of time in ethical decision making. *Nursing Ethics, 16*(5), 613–624.

Oken, D. (1961). What to tell cancer patients: A study of medical attitudes. *Journal of the American Medical Association, 175*, 1120–1128.

Rees, J., King, L., & Schmitz, K. (2009). Nurses' perceptions of ethical issues in the care of older people. *Nursing Ethics, 16*(4), 436–452.

Seo, M., Tamura, K., Shijo, H., Morioka, E., Ikegame, C., & Hirasako, K. (2000). Telling the diagnosis to cancer patients in Japan: Attitude and perception of patients, physicians, and nurses. *Palliative Medicine, 14*, 105–111.

Smith, C. & O' Neill, L. (2008). Doe not resuscitate does not mean do not treat: How palliative care and other modalities can help facilitate communication about goals of care in advanced illness. *Mount Sinai Journal of Medicine, 75*, 460–465.

Tuckett, A. G. (2004). Truth telling in clinical practice. *Nursing Ethics, 11*, 501–512.

Van der Riet, P., Good, P., Higgins, I., & Sneesby, L. (2008). Palliative care professionals' perceptions of nutrition and hydration at the end of life. *International Journal of Palliative Nursing, 14*(3), 145–151.

Varcoe, C., Doane, G., Pauly, B., Rodney, P., Storch, J., Mahoney, K. . . . Starzomski, R. (2004). Ethical practice in nursing: Working the in-betweens. *Journal of Advanced Nursing, 45*, 316–325.

Verpoort, C., Gastmans, C., & Dierckx de Casterle, B. (2004a). Palliative care nurses' views on euthanasia. *Journal of Advanced Nursing, 47*, 592–600.

Verpoort, C., Gastmans, C., De Bal, N., & Dierckx de Casterle, B. (2004b). Nurses' attitudes to euthanasia: A review of the literature. *Nursing Ethics, 11*, 349–364.

Weissman, D. (2009). Moral distress in palliative care. *Journal of Palliative Care, 12*(10), 865–866.

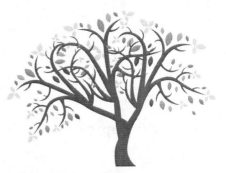

FIVE

Suffering and Palliative Care at the End of Life

■ Mary K. Kazanowski

Objectives

1. Explain different types of suffering that occur near the end of life.
2. Identify indicators of patient and family suffering near the end of life.
3. Describe interventions to optimally relieve the various types of suffering near the end of life.
4. Discuss barriers to treatment of suffering at the end of life.
5. Describe communication skills recommended to assist patients and families dealing with end-of-life issues.

Student Project

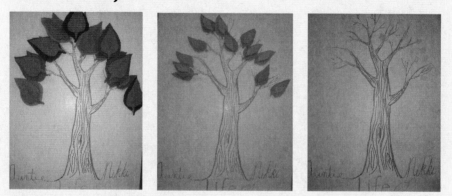

Each leaf on the tree represents one thing that the patient gave up as she weakened and eventually died.

Source: Courtesy of Kristina Michaud, student nurse, 2010.

Case Study 5–1

Linda had been diagnosed with stage IV ovarian cancer in May 2005. In September 2008, CT scans indicated that her cancer had metastasized throughout her gastrointestinal track and abdominal cavity. Surgical procedures had left her with a colostomy, a percutaneous gastrostomy tube, and a peritoneal tube that draining the ascites from her grossly distended abdomen. With the cancer progressing, she became extremely weak and experienced an increase in abdominal pain.

When I first met Linda, she was a beautiful woman who just seemed to light up a drab room. But all that changed; after her first week in the hospital, Linda took a fall and was bedridden after that. Hospital gowns hide everything when the sheets are pulled up to a person's chin. After the fall, she began to bathe at the side of her bed. I couldn't help but stare at every vertebra that stuck out prominently from her back; she was much more frail than I would choose to admit. I came to classify hers as a "cancer body" with a disproportionately thin upper frame and twig arms, but noticeable ascites and fat calves.

Linda endured much physical suffering related to the pain of having most of her abdominal cavity organs removed and enduring the scars, the ascites, the gastrostomy tube; coping with such a distortion of the body is no small feat. She had lost so much weight that her son's best friends could barely recognize Linda, with her frail frame and fat heavy legs. I spent hours with her after the visit, consoling her because she was so disgusted by the boys' shocked expression when they entered the room. Each day she grew more and more anxious, filled with fear and in a constant state of denial that she was dying. Though stoic in front of her, her husband, brother, father, and son would sob when they left the room.

Questions on the Case Study
1. In what ways might Linda be suffering?
2. How would you assess for each type of suffering?
3. What exactly would you say?
4. In what ways might the family be suffering?
5. How would you prioritize the greatest needs?
6. How would you intervene with each of the identified needs?

Source: Courtesy of Meghan McMahon, student nurse, 2007.

Introduction

People often associate dying with suffering, and for many, this may be the case. Although the dying experience may be very difficult, it need not be plagued by unrelenting suffering for patients and families. Access to healthcare providers who are knowledgeable about palliative care can do a great deal to prevent or alleviate suffering at the end of life.

Sources of Suffering at the End of Life

Types of suffering at the end of life include those experienced by the dying person and those experienced by the family. The dying person may experience physical, emotional, and spiritual suffering (see Table 5–1). The suffering of the family,

Table 5–1   Types of Suffering at the End of Life

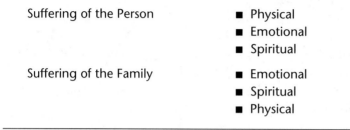

Suffering of the Person	■ Physical
	■ Emotional
	■ Spiritual
Suffering of the Family	■ Emotional
	■ Spiritual
	■ Physical

which may be emotional, spiritual, or physical, also plays a role in one's dying experience, and therefore needs attention.

Sensitivity to the pain and suffering of patients and their families is essential to developing trust and facilitating the identification of sources of suffering. Assessments of the patient's and family's perception of their greatest concerns and suffering take time and are often limited by patients' and families' reluctance and aversion to discussing end of life concerns. In conducting an assessment, it is helpful for healthcare providers to separate out the various types of suffering that commonly occur with the dying experience. Interventions for these vary, but relief of pain and suffering in one domain may bring relief in another. For example, the relief and prevention of pain, dyspnea, or other symptoms of distress in the patient often bring relief to the family witnessing the suffering of their loved one. Relief of physical symptoms also allows the patient the time and energy to address and learn how to cope with concerns that evoke emotional or spiritual suffering.

Physical Suffering of the Person

Reviews of the literature demonstrate that there are common symptoms of distress that occur near death for patients with cancer and non cancer diagnoses (Brunnhuber, Nash, Meier, Weissman, & Woodcock, 2008). Pain has been reported in 34% to 96% of patients, with fatigue being present in 32% to 90%. Breathlessness is also common near the end of life, but most common in patients with chronic obstructive pulmonary disease (90% to 95%) and heart disease (60%–88%). Other symptoms of distress may include nausea, vomiting, restlessness/agitation, and urinary problems.

Emotional Suffering of the Person

Fear of dying in pain is a major cause of suffering in individuals near the end of life. Fear of the unknown, uncertainty, and regrets for actions or relationship failures can also plague patients. It is helpful for nurses working with people near the end of their lives to recognize that physical symptoms of distress need to be addressed and treated, often before emotional suffering can be altered. Patients who are plagued by physical pain or dyspnea are unable to discuss emotional concerns, let alone analyze and work to alleviate their impact. Once physical symptoms are controlled, more efforts can be made to address emotional needs.

Patients who are physically declining are often reluctant to report signs and symptoms of decline or accept services or advice from healthcare providers. Acknowledging symptoms of decline is often difficult, and postponing dealing with the decline is often preferred. Patients becoming weak due to a chronic illness often refuse to give up their driving privileges and refuse offers of a walker, hospital bed, or commode, which to them indicate "the end." Hospice services and medications such as morphine are often declined in an effort to delay dealing with the possibility that their disease is worsening. Patients in this frame of mind often say things like "I don't need it yet," "I'm not there yet," "later," or "not now" when services or equipment are recommended. Patient refusal to accept help is particularly difficult for families who recognize that the patient is declining. Families are often fearful that the patient will fall and hurt herself, and afraid that they will not know what to do. This is particularly stressful for adult children of patients, who must now reverse their roles to take on the role of the caregiver and decision maker for their parent.

Nurses and other healthcare providers should be mindful of individual or family fears regarding the use of certain terms such as "hospice" and "morphine." Additionally, healthcare providers should avoid saying things such as "there is nothing more that we can do," which patients and families often misconstrue as an indicator that the provider will abandon them (Ngo-Metzer, August, Srinivasan, Liao, & Meyskens, 2008). Although it is important to convey the information that treatment of a disease is no longer effective, one should not focus on the limitations of care at the end of life. Instead, focus on what is available for care (e.g., symptom management, psychosocial and spiritual support), and assist individuals in identifying their goals for end-of-life care. The goals of care for an individual near the end of life may include achieving

- good quality of life;
- control of symptoms of distress;
- meaningful interactions with family and friends;
- living at home;
- avoidance of medical treatments; and
- facilitation of a peaceful death.

Talking with patients who are faced with life-limiting illnesses often includes discussion of prognosis, which initially should come from the physician. Prognostic guidelines are available for many illnesses including heart disease, pulmonary disease, HIV, liver disease, Alzheimer's disease, stroke with coma, and malignancies. However, there is variability among individuals and a certain amount of uncertainty with regard to the amount of time people may live with a poor prognosis. This variability and uncertainty often adds to the stress that patients and families experience at this time. Experts in palliative and end-of-life care suggest that discussions about prognoses be guided by patient values and goals for living. Questions to help elicit information related to values and goals include these:

- What is most important to you?
- What worries you the most?
- What is the most difficult part of your illness?
- Who is your greatest source of support?

The answers to these questions should guide the physician in his recommendations for treatment.

Depending on their values, life experiences, cognitive function, and comfort, patients and families may react to these discussions in a variety of ways, including anger, shock, and/or disbelief. These reactions will also impact how the patient reacts to the physician's recommendation for treatment. Acceptance of recommendations for treatment will likely be dependent on the person's and family's

- value of life extension over burden of treatment;
- trust in the healthcare system;
- willingness to confront the possibility of dying; and
- fear of the unknown and financial needs.

When faced with the news of a poor prognosis, many patients and families respond by saying they want "everything" done, including treatments that are unlikely to help (Quill, Arnold, & Back, 2009). After exploring patient/family values, healthcare providers should have ongoing discussions with patients and families to support their responses to the patients' prognosis, identify symptom management goals, negotiate disagreements about treatment plans, and continue to assist patients/families in goal clarification.

Spiritual Suffering of the Person

According to Lorraine Wright (2005), suffering and spirituality are connected because when you discuss suffering, issues related to spirituality often arise. Wright describes suffering as the person's perception of the meaning of the suffering and the effect of suffering on relationships. Individuals who are suffering spiritually often feel abandoned by God, saying things like "How could God do this to me? How could God let this happen? Where is God?"

Depending on the person's beliefs, life experiences, and resources to cope with suffering, individuals may remain stuck in their suffering experience. Some, however, may also grow to a point where they affirm, discover, or create interpretations of events that are comforting (Reed, 2003). The nurse should promote this spiritual growth.

When caring for patients at the end of life, nurses need to know how to initiate a discourse around spiritual issues and how to keep it open (Wright, 2005). Wright states that the "suffering experience must be acknowledged, in order for healing to occur" (p. 121). See Chapter 7 for more interventions for suffering related to faith and spirituality.

Emotional Suffering of the Family

Family members of patients near death often suffer from anticipating the loss they will experience when the patient dies. Suffering also occurs as they witness the patient's decline, which is characterized by the loss of the patient's ability to ambulate, communicate, and eat, and/or they perceive the patient to be in distress. Research has demonstrated that family members who perceive their loved one as being comfortable are less likely to suffer emotional distress than those who believe their loved one to be in pain or distress (Kazanowski, 1998).

Another emotional burden that family members experience as their loved ones decline is the problem of getting past rifts and anger that burden relationships. Recognition that individuals within a family often disagree and make mistakes and that reconciliation may help both parties move on is helpful. Although exploration of past problems may not always be possible, people's ability to forgive often impacts their ability to say goodbye. In *The Four Things that Matter Most: A Book About Living* (2004), Dr. Ira Byock advises patients and family members to consider saying "I love you," "Please forgive me," "I forgive you," and "Thank you" during this sacred time (p. 1).

Physical Suffering of Family

Family members, often the patient's spouse, play a major role in the care of patients with cancer, dementia, cerebrovascular accidents, and acquired immune deficiency syndrome (AIDS), particularly in advanced stages (Burridge, Winch, & Clavarino, 2007). Research shows that family members in the caregiver role for a loved one with a chronic disease have higher levels of physical stress and mortality (Schultz & Beach, 1999). Because much of their time is committed to caregiving tasks, family caregivers tend to ignore their own healthcare needs. Hypervigilance, which impacts a person's ability to relax, sleep, and rejuvenate, is often mentioned as the most difficult part of caregiving.

Efforts should be make to decrease the workload of family caregivers by allowing them time to rest and address their personal needs. This often takes the form of providing nurse aides to provide personal care, and volunteers who can sit with the individual for longer periods of time. Medical social workers, chaplains, and the nurse need to be available to assess family caregivers for physical and emotional stress on an ongoing basis, intervening as needed.

Interventions to Assist with Persons Suffering at End of Life

Identification of the source of suffering near the end of life can often be difficult. Reed (2003) states that many patients fear the agent that potentiates suffering. Because of this relationship of fear and suffering, Reed suggests that healthcare providers ask patients at risk for suffering, "What to you is most frightening about this situation?" The answer often reveals the major source of suffering for the patient.

Therapeutic responses to patients who are suffering at the end of life are dependent on the particular person's needs and preferences, which are often based on their lifelong experiences. Assessing them for their needs will guide the nurse in her or his comments and response to questions. Table 5–2 provides examples of therapeutic comments the nurse could make, along with responses to commonly asked questions surrounding end of life issues. Although these are helpful, the nurse should remember that listening to the patient, facilitating the opportunity for them to frame their thoughts and concerns, and acceptance of what patients have to say, are the first steps toward addressing patient concerns.

Table 5–2   Therapeutic Responses at End of Life

How to respond to patients when they ask if they're going to die.	■ "From what I know, you are very sick." (Pause, and see how they respond.) ■ "What has your doctor told you?" ■ "Do you think you may be dying?" ■ Provide support; listen; validate patient perceptions if appropriate. ■ Ask what you can do for them. ("Is there someone you need to speak to? Can I call someone for you?")
Comforting words you can say to a person near death.	■ "You are loved very much by your family here" (if appropriate). ■ "You have many things to show for your hard work here (on earth)." ■ "Your children are very kind—that says a lot about you and how they feel about you" (if appropriate).
Encourage people to say the obvious to their loved ones such as	■ "I love you." ■ "Please forgive me." ■ "I forgive you." ■ "Thank you."

Source: Byock, I. (2004). *The Four Things That Matter Most: A Book About Living.* New York, NY: Free Press.

When assisting with the care of a patient near the end of life, it is also important for the nurse to be familiar with the patient's preferences with regard to what type of care she wants. To elicit this information, the nurse could ask the following:

- What would you want to happen if you were to become sicker?
- Would you want to be in the hospital?
- Would you want to be on machines?
- Would you want to be at home?

Patient preferences should be conveyed to the family and healthcare providers, and described in advance directives. If the patient has not drawn up an advance directive, the nurse should educate the patient about the advantages of having one in place and facilitate its development. The purpose of an advance directive is to provide guidance, especially to healthcare professionals, regarding how to proceed with decision making about life-sustaining treatment for a patient with diminished capacity. When patients lack decision-making capacity, confusion can arise as to how healthcare decisions are to be made, who has the authority to make them, and what the treatment should be (Perrin, 2010). Advance directives are described as written documents prepared by individuals to specify the type of health care they would want should they lack decision-making capacity when a medical decision needs to be made. There are two general types of advance directives. The first is the instructional directive that gives guidance regarding the type and amount of care people would want if they were to become incapacitated. Living wills and medical directives such as a do not resuscitate order or do not intubate are examples of instructional directives (Perrin, 2010). The second type of advance directive is the durable power of attorney for health care (DPOAHC). The DPOAHC is a legal document in which a person appoints someone else (e.g., healthcare proxy) to make his or her healthcare decisions in the event he or she loses decision-making capacity. Advance directives vary from state to state, but are readily available through Caring Connections, an online program of the National Hospice and Palliative Care Organization (2007).

Most Americans do not have advance directives in place (Larson & Tobin, 2000), and many physicians do not talk to patients about their wishes for end-of-life care (Emanuel, Barry, & Stoeckle, 1991; O'Brien, Grisso, & Maislin, 1995). However, recent data suggest that most elderly patients would actually welcome discussions about end-of-life care (Gillick, 2010). It has also been shown that many older Americans needed decision making near the end of life, at a time when they lacked decision-making capacity, and that individuals who had prepared advance directives received care that was most closely associated with their preferences (Silveira, Kim, & Langa, 2010). Teno et al. (2007) also found a benefit of advance directives. Bereaved family members of patients with advance directives reported fewer concerns when they had communication with healthcare providers about treatment decisions and the family members believed that the directives facilitated the process.

Because of their close proximity to patients, nurses are often in the position of initiating discussions with individuals about their wishes regarding end-of-life care, especially when the person's condition starts to decline. Although the discussions may be difficult, research indicates that end-of-life discussions are not associated with patients having negative emotional states or mental health diagnoses (Wright et al., 2008). It is imperative that the nurse both verbally communicate and document patient preferences to ensure that they are honored.

Preference for where a person wants to die should be considered when planning care for individuals near death. Surveys indicate that a large percentage of Americans would prefer to die at home (Byock, 2008). Despite this, approximately 75% of Americans with chronic illnesses die in a hospital or nursing home (Gruneir & Mor, 2007) . However, there are large regional differences. Although there are exceptions, being surrounded by familiar people and things, having ready access to friends and relatives, and being free from institutional restrictions make the home setting more comfortable and give the patient and family more control. People who are unable to stay at home until death may experience a homelike environment in a hospice house. Hospice houses are generally staffed by nurses who provide direct care, but families are allowed to stay on the premises, eating their meals and sleeping with their loved ones.

Quality end-of-life care may be accessed in the hospital, nursing home, or the community, often through palliative care or hospice programs. Hospice services differ from palliative care services in that hospice has eligibility criteria which requires

- written certification of a 6-month or less prognosis by two physicians;
- a life-limiting condition or combination of diseases such as
  - cancer—metastatic or locally advanced with progression;
  - dementia— advanced;
  - end stage cardiac disease;

- end stage pulmonary disease;
- end stage liver disease;
- end stage renal disease;
- end stage human immunodeficiency virus (HIV);
- stroke coma;
- amyotrophic lateral sclerosis (ALS);
- Parkinson's disease—advanced;
- debility, with unexplained weight loss, and decline in functional status;
- patient/family goals directed toward relief of symptoms rather than cure of underlying disease (Centers for Medicare and Medicaid Services Hospice Center, 2008).

The Palliative Performance Scale (PPS), adapted from the Karnofsky Performance Scale (1996), is useful in determining when individuals are hospice appropriate. Individuals with a PPS of 50% or less may be eligible for hospice services (see Table 5–3).

Both hospice and palliative care services are based on similar fundamental philosophies as shown in Table 5–4. However, they differ in where they are placed in the course of illness (see Figure 5–1). Both provide interdisciplinary care that aims to relieve physical, emotional, and spiritual suffering, with the goal of improving quality of life for patients with advanced illness and their families. However, unlike hospice care, palliative care is offered simultaneously with other all other medical treatment.

Figure 5–1

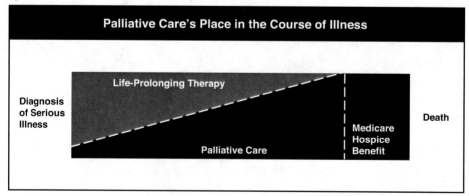

Source: National Consensus Project for Quality Palliative Care. (2009). *Clinical Practice Guidelines for Quality Palliative Care* (2nd ed., p. 6). Pittsburgh, PA: Author. Used with permission.

Table 5–3   Palliative Performance Scale (PPS)

%	Ambulation	Activity and Evidence of Disease	Self-care	Intake	Conscious Level
100	Full	Normal Activity No Evidence of Disease		Normal	Full
90	Full	Normal Activity Some Evidence of Disease	Full	Normal	Full
80	Full	Normal Activity with Effort Some Evidence of Disease	Full	Normal or Reduced	Full
70	Reduced	Unable Normal Job/Work Some Evidence of Disease	Full	Normal or Reduced	Full
60	Reduced	Unable Hobby/House Work Significant Disease	Occasional Assistance Necessary	Normal or Reduced	Full or Confusion
50	Mainly Sit/Lie	Unable to Do Any Work Extensive Disease	Considerable Assistance Necessary	Normal or Reduced	Full or Confusion
40	Mainly in Bed	As Above	Mainly Assistance	Normal or Reduced	Full or Drowsy or Confusion
30	Totally Bed Bound	As Above	Total Care	Reduced	Full or Drowsy or Confusion
20	As Above	As Above	Total Care	Minimal Sips	Full or Drowsy or Confusion
10	As Above	As Above	Total Care	Mouth Care Only	Drowsy or Coma
0	Death				

Source: Adapted with permission from Karnofsky Performance Scale; Anderson, F. et al. (1996). Palliative Performance Scale (PPS). *Journal of Palliative Care 12*, 5–11.

Table 5–4 Fundamental Elements of Hospice and Palliative Care

- Pain and symptom control, psychosocial distress, and spiritual issues are systematically addressed and treated based upon current evidence.

- Patients/families acquire ongoing information in a culturally sensitive, appropriate, and understandable manner to facilitate comprehension and realistic potential of treatment options.

- Genuine coordination of care across settings is ensured through regular and high-quality communication.

- Patient and family, however defined, are appropriately prepared for the dying process and for death when it is anticipated.

Source: Courtesy of the National Consensus Project for Quality Palliative Care Task Force (2009). *Clinical Practice Guidelines for Quality Palliative Care* (2nd ed.). Pittsburgh, PA: Author.

Despite growing acceptance of palliative care, barriers to its use continue, increasing the potential for suffering for individuals without access to this quality service. Barriers to palliative care include the following:

- U.S. health system focus on acute care model versus chronic care;
- technological advances leading to the assumption that they are appropriate in all situations;
- limited availability of palliative care services, especially in rural settings;
- lack of training in palliative care;
- lack of understanding of palliative/hospice services with regard to their availability and their relevance for patients with advanced disease;
- inaccurate media portrayal of palliative consultations and end–of-life care;
- reimbursement climate with its emphasis on increasing patient encounters, thus decreasing the amount of time caregivers spend with patients with complex needs;
- rules and regulations related to prescriptions for controlled drugs;
- misinterpretation of rules and regulations related to prescriptions for controlled drugs;
- limited access to palliative medications;
- fragmented insurance coverage for patients with advanced disease;
- complex reimbursement issues for palliative services.

Significant efforts, however, are being made by several palliative care experts to increase palliative care research, education, and practice to minimize and one day eliminate the effect these barriers can have on the care provided to those with palliative needs.

Prevalence of Symptoms at the End of Life

Several studies have defined the most common symptoms experienced by patients dying of a variety of disorders, including malignancy, dementia, heart failure, end stage renal disease, end stage hepatic disease, multiple sclerosis, ALS, AIDS, and chronic pulmonary disease (Lipman, 2009). One of the most comprehensive reports of symptom prevalence in patients receiving palliative care was from a multicenter study conducted in Spain in 1994 (Conill et al., 1997). It included 176 patients (mean age 67.7 years), who were evaluated at the time of admission to hospital, home care, or hospice, and again within the last week of life. Two-thirds of the patients had metastatic cancer. Symptom Prevalence One week before death was reported as follows

Symptom	n (%)
■ Asthenia	144 (81.8)
■ Anorexia	141 (80)
■ Dry Mouth	123 (69.9)
■ Confusion	120 (68.2)
■ Constipation	97 (55.1)
■ Dyspnea	82 (46.6)
■ Dysphagia	81 (46)
■ Anxiety	80 (45.5)
■ Depression	68 (38.6)
■ Paralysis	57 (32.4)
■ Pain	53 (30.1)
■ Sleep Disturbance	50 (28.8)
■ Cough	31 (17.6)
■ Nausea	23 (13.1)
■ Hemorrhage	21 (11.8)
■ Vomiting	18 (10.2)
■ Diarrhea	12 (6.8)
■ Dysuria	12 (6.8)

There are many interventions to alleviate physical suffering near the end of life, which include repositioning, altering the environment, and providing medications to diminish the intensity of the symptom. Interventions to alleviate specific physical symptoms of distress are discussed next.

Pain

The literature indicates that pain is one of the most feared and debilitating symptoms in patients with advanced disease (Brunnhuber et al., 2008). Most of what is known about symptoms in individuals near death has been derived from studies of patients with cancer. However, many individuals die from other chronic diseases that are also capable of causing pain and discomfort. Causes of pain in individuals near death include pain resulting from headaches, osteoarthritis, muscle spasms, stiff joints, ischemia of a limb or organ, and malignant pain, which is a result of tumor cells infiltrating organs, nerves and bone.

Assessment of Pain at the End of Life

Assessment of the pain must be performed at least daily, using a valid measurement tool (e.g., Brief Pain Inventory) that identifies the location of pain, the intensity, temporal pattern, relieving factors, and multidimensional aspects of the experience such as insomnia, depression, or anxiety. Ongoing assessments often can be as simple as a numeric rating scale of 0–10, with 0 being no pain, and 10 being the worst pain possible. Adjustments in medication are made if the intensity pattern or location of pain changes. As death nears, however, patients often lose the ability to communicate their pain because of the lethargy, decreased level of consciousness, or cognitive impairment that often accompanies the dying process. If this occurs, alternative methods of assessing pain are utilized to identify distress. Nonverbal pain behaviors include these:

- Tense body language
  - grimacing of facial muscles
  - clenched fists, knees pulled up tightly
- Frightened facial expression
  - alarmed appearance with open eyes and pleading

- Noise or speech with negative quality
  - moaning or groaning
- Restless behavior
  - constant jittery movement or squirming
  - rubbing of body parts, forceful touching, or trying to get away from hurt area (Feldt, 2000)

Pharmacologic Relief of Pain at the End of Life

At the end of life, the goal for management of pain is to control it at a level acceptable to the patient and/or to prevent it from recurring. Control/prevention of pain is considered essential for allowing patients quality time to engage in whatever conversations and activities they would like. How the patient wants the pain treated should ideally guide its treatment. However, patients and families often welcome the expertise of palliative health providers in addressing this problem.

Palliative care health providers generally recommend that patients take analgesics to control pain. Some patients, however, may prefer to avoid taking medications—to avoid side effects (e.g., sedation), out of the need to remain in full control, or because of fear of addiction (even though this should not be a concern at this time). On occasion, family members may also be averse to patients taking medications because they want the person to remain "as they know her to be" and/or awake to converse. With their understanding of issues surrounding grief and loss, palliative care health providers can be very helpful in guiding patients and families in negotiating these sensitive issues and facilitating alleviation/prevention of patient suffering.

The oral route is considered to be the best way to administer analgesics because of consistent absorption, ease of obtaining the medication, and ease of administration. However, most important is the ability and comfort of the person in swallowing medication at the end of life, when dysphagia often becomes a problem, and this takes precedence in the decision of what medications are used. For example, analgesics in liquid form (e.g., acetaminophen suspension, morphine sulfate concentrate elixir) are often well tolerated by patients with dysphagia. Patients who lose the ability to swallow safely (and avoid chewing) long-acting analgesics (e.g., morphine sulfate controlled release or oxycodone often benefit from changing to the transdermal route with fentanyl at an equianalgesic level.

Ability and convenience for caregivers administering medications is also a consideration. Elixirs for short-acting analgesics and transdermal patches for long-acting analgesia often ease the caregiver burden in administration of medications. If administration by the oral or transdermal route is problematic for caregivers, medications such as morphine sulfate may be administered by pump, either subcutaneously or intravenously. Intramuscular administration of medications near the end of life is avoided because of the pain associated with injections and the cachetic nature of many individuals near death.

Nonopioid Analgesics

Nonopioid analgesics include acetaminophen and nonsteroidal anti-inflammatory drugs (NSAIDs) such as aspirin and ibuprofen. Although often effective for mild to moderate pain of somatic or visceral origin, these drugs have a ceiling effect that limits the amount of the drug that can be administered safely. The NSAIDs may also cause adverse effects such as gastrointestinal upset and bleeding. Although individuals with rheumatoid arthritis or bone pain often benefit from NSAIDs, histories of gastrointestinal hemorrhage, a low platelet count, or renal insufficiency may make these drugs a poor choice. A thorough assessment of the client's past experiences with pain and analgesics and their side effects is essential to optimal pain management. The experience of pain is somewhat individual, and using analgesics that have been effective for past pain experiences is recommended.

With some exceptions, nonnarcotics such as acetaminophen or NSAIDs are the first line of treatment for mild to moderate pain. However, acetaminophen is contraindicated in liver disease; NSAIDs are contraindicated in the elderly or people with renal failure or gastrointestinal bleeding. When pain persists or increases, an opioid such as codeine or hydrocodone is added, often in the form of a combination drug (e.g., oxycodone and acetaminophen). Although combination medications are often effective in controlling mild to moderate pain, their use is limited by the content of acetaminophen or NSAID in the medication. For example, 4 grams of acetaminophen is the 24-hour limit for adults. Toxicity could occur with doses exceeding this.

Opioid (Narcotic) Analgesics

Persistent pain or pain that is moderate to severe in intensity should be treated with opioids. Unfortunately, many patients, family members, and even healthcare providers fear that the administration of uploads will hasten death. Experts in palliative care, however, state that with proper dosing, death should not occur prematurely (Portenoy, et al., 2006). Pure opioid agonists such as morphine, oxycodone, and hydromorphone are the drugs of choice for patients with moderate to severe pain because they do not have a ceiling effect (i.e., limited dose requirement). Because of this, they can be increased as needed. These pure agonists are also available in extended-release formulas to ease administration and prolong pain relief. Prevention of recurrent pain often requires administering medication in scheduled around-the-clock dosing to maintain an adequate level of analgesia. Medications without a ceiling effect in long-acting formulas include extended-release morphine (e.g., MS Contin; Oramorph) and controlled or sustained-release oxycodone (e.g., Oxycontin SR). Transdermal fentanyl (Duragesic) also provides sustained control of pain, but because of its potency, it should be used only in opioid tolerant patients. Transdermal fentanyl should also be limited to patients with stable pain, as it is not suitable for rapid dose titration and does not reach peak effect for 12 to 17 hours after it is first initiated. Another limiting factor for use of transdermal fentanyl is the decreased blood flow to the skin that often occurs in a person near death. This may impede absorption of the drug. For this reason, patients who are not candidates for transdermal fentanyl may need to be started on continuous opioid infusions given via subcutaneous or intravenous routes.

Changing a patient from the oral route to subcutaneous or intravenous infusion requires calculation of the 24-hour dose of oral analgesia (controlled release and immediate release) and calculation of the equianalgesic dose for the parenteral route. An hourly rate is calculated by dividing the 24-hour total parenteral equianalgesic dose of drug by 24 and dividing that number by 2. Division by 2 is done when first making the change from oral to parenteral to ensure that the dose is not too potent. Once the parenteral infusion is initiated, the dose can be titrated up as needed to control the pain. Because treatment of pain is often complex, specialists in palliative care may be needed to achieve optimal comfort.

Limitations of Opioids for Pain at End of Life

Patients at times may require such high doses of analgesia that sedation occurs as a side effect. Although sedation is not ideal, its occurrence as a side effect of treatment for symptoms of distress at the end of life may be acceptable if there is no alternative for comfort. It is important that both healthcare providers and the public understand that adequate symptom management may at times result in sedation. The sedation that occurs is a side effect of treatment—it is not a treatment goal or an effect meant to hasten death.

The administration of medications for symptoms of distress at the end of life is guided by protocols using doses of medications that are considered safe. These guidelines and protocols are used with the intention of alleviating suffering, not hastening death. While it is true that individuals are more likely to receive higher doses of both opioids and sedatives as they get closer to death, there is no evidence that initiation of treatment or increases in dose of opioids or sedatives is associated with precipitation of death (Sykes & Thorns, 2003). Despite this, some healthcare providers may continue to express concern that opioids or benzodiazepines will hasten death. Healthcare providers with this concern should be reminded that an increased risk of earlier death counts little against the benefit of pain relief and painless death in a person who faces imminent death from progression of a primary disease (Guideline Panel for Management of Cancer Pain, 1994). The ethical duty of healthcare providers in caring for clients near death is to follow guidelines in the medication management of symptoms and to facilitate prompt and effective symptom management.

The occurrence of myoclonus, (i.e., uncontrolled jerking movements of the patient's limbs or torso) can occur as a neurotoxic side effect of opioid therapy. This is more likely to occur when doses of opioids are increased quickly and/or they accumulate. It is essential that healthcare providers recognize myoclonus as a possible dose-related effect of opioid therapy and rotate (i.e., change) to another narcotic. A benzodiazepine such as clonazepam may also be ordered to ease the twitching (Furst & Doyle, 2004).

Adjuvant Medications for Pain

In addition to opioids, patients with severe pain may require medications with other pharmacologic properties to achieve pain relief. Corticosteroids such as dexamethasone are often given for pain secondary to swelling or nerve compression, as seen in malignant disease. Neuropathic pain is often treated with antidepressants such as amitriptyline or anticonvulsants such as gabapentin. Antidepressants and anticonvulsants, however, are not routinely initiated when death is imminent because they take days before they show effect.

Poor Analgesic Response

Individuals who not obtain an acceptable level of pain control should have consultations with experts in palliative care. Poor analgesic response to pain in palliative care patients occurs in 10% to 30% of patients (Brunnhuber et al., 2008). A change in the opiate, referred to as rotation, is often done in an attempt to better control the pain. In one prospective study of patients requiring rotation, 20% required two or more changes in opioids to obtain adequate analgesia. Concomitant use of anxiolytics, corticosteroids, and local anesthetics should also be considered.

Despite optimal treatment of pain at the end of life, a small percentage of individuals may continue to suffer. Pain despite exhaustive treatment is defined as intractable or refractory. Palliative sedation for patients with intractable or refractory symptoms of distress is gaining acceptance in the hospice and palliative care community as a therapy of last resort (Kirk, Coyle, Poppito, & Bigoney, 2010). The National Hospice and Palliative Care Organization (NHPCO; 2010) defines palliative sedation as "the lowering of patient consciousness using medications for the express purpose of limiting patient awareness of suffering that is intractable and intolerable" (p. 21). NHPCO states that palliative sedation should be considered for "the limited number of imminently dying patients who have pain and suffering that is (a) unresponsive to other palliative interventions less suppressive of consciousness and (b) intolerable to the patient" (*www.jpsmjournal.com*). The goal of palliative sedation is to control symptoms of distress, not hasten the patient's death (Blinderman & Fowler, 2010). The intent to promote comfort, and not hasten death, differentiates it from euthanasia.

Pharmacotherapy in Palliative Sedation
Medications used to provide palliative sedation include opioids, benzodiazepines, neuroleptics, barbiturates, or anesthetic agents. The choice of the agent is dependent on what other medications have been used to treat symptoms, available route of administration, the setting, and cost. Many patients receiving palliative sedation are already on opioids for pain. Opioid escalation can be inadequate or it can lead to adverse effects such as myoclonus, agitation, or delirium (Blinderman & Fowler, 2010). In these cases, a benzodiazepine such as lorazepam or midazolam is often used. Barbiturates used include phenobarbital or pentobarbital. Propofol (Diprivan) is a sedative anesthetic that may be used in some settings.

For a summary of the types of medications available for pain management at the end of life, see Table 5–5.

Integrative Therapy for Pain at the End of Life

Massage has been shown to decrease pain in individuals with cancer (Cassileth & Vickers, 2004) and it is one of the most popular complementary services being offered to patients at the end of life (Demmer, 2004). Patients who are frail may

Table 5–5   Pharmacologic Interventions for Pain at End of Life

Type of Pain	Medication	Dose	Advantages	Limitations
Mild–Moderate	Aceta-minophen	325–650 mg PO/PR every 4–6 hrs. Not to exceed 4 gm/24 hrs	Readily available in multiple forms	Ceiling effect risk for hepatotoxicity
	(NSAIDS) Ibuprofen	400–600 mg PO every 6 hrs.	Effective for bone pain	Ceiling effect risk for GI bleeding; risk for renal toxicity
Persistent Pain Moderate–Severe	(Opioids) Morphine Sulfate Oxycodone	5 mg every 2–4 hrs. prn or increase existing dose by 25–50%	No ceiling effect Multiple forms	Sedation
Adjuvants for Pain	(Cortico-steroids) Dexametha-sone	4 mg PO/IV/SC 1–2 times per day	Indicated for swelling or nerve compression	GI Upset Insomnia

not tolerate an extensive treatment but may benefit from a short treatment to sites of their choice. In working with patients with cancer, light pressure is best, and deep or intense pressure should be avoided (Berenson, 2005; Deng et al., 2004). Massage is contraindicated over the site of tissue damage (i.e., open wounds or tissue undergoing radiation therapy), in patients with bleeding disorders, and in patients who are uncomfortable with touch (Layman-Goldstein & Coyle, 2006).

Music therapy has also been shown to decrease pain in patients near death (Layman-Goldstein & Coyle, 2006). Therapeutic touch, which involves moving one's hands through the person's energy field, has also been shown to relieve pain (Newshan & Schuller-Citella, 2003) and should be offered to patients with pain near the end of life. Aromatherapy can be used with other treatments. Lavender, capsicum, bergamot, chamomile, rose, ginger, rosemary, lemongrass, sage, and camphor have been recommended for use in palliative care (Mariano, 2006).

Breathlessness or Dyspnea

Dyspnea is a subjective experience during which the person experiences an uncomfortable feeling of breathlessness, which is often described as terrifying. It can manifest itself as air hunger, copious secretions, cough, chest pain, or fatigue. It is a common symptom in advanced cancer, chronic obstructive pulmonary disease (COPD), and heart failure, and tends to increase in individuals approaching death (Booth et al., 2004). Many patients, family members, and healthcare providers consider this to be the worst symptom of distress near death.

Causes of dyspnea can be

- directly related to the patient's primary diagnosis (e.g., lung cancer, breast cancer, or coronary artery disease);
- secondary to the primary diagnosis (e.g., pleural effusion, metastasis to the lung or pleura);
- related to treatment of the primary disease (e.g., heart failure caused by chemotherapy, constrictive pericarditis due to radiation therapy, anemia related to chemotherapy);
- related to an etiology unrelated to the primary disease (e.g., pneumonia).

Depending on the cause, the pathophysiology of dyspnea can involve the following:

- obstructive, restrictive, or vascular disturbances in the airways with tumor or nodal involvement;
- pulmonary congestion secondary to fluid overload and/or cardiac dysfunction;
- bronchoconstriction and bronchospasm as seen with respiratory infection;
- COPD, or airway blockage by a tumor;
- a decreased hemoglobin-carrying capacity, as with anemia;
- hyperventilation secondary to neuromuscular disease, with limited movement of the diaphragm.

Diagnostic testing to identify the cause of dyspnea is usually not done on patients at the end of life. Management is based on physical assessment and knowledge of the underlying condition.

Pharmacologic Interventions for Dyspnea

Treatment of dyspnea near the end of life should initially be aimed at reversing treatable causes such as bronchospasm or fluid overload. Individuals with chronic pulmonary disease often have bronchodilators available, such as albuterol or ipratropium bromide. Corticosteroids such as prednisone or dexamethasone may also be given for bronchospasm and inflammatory problems within and exterior to the lung. Patients with manifestations of heart failure may benefit from maintenance of their diuretic therapy and/or an increase in dosage even if their other oral medications are being discontinued.

Oxygen has been shown to be helpful for individuals with chronic respiratory disease and may be helpful for other conditions causing dyspnea near death, regardless of the presence or absence of hypoxia. Oxygen has not, however, been established as a standard of care for all individuals with dyspnea. Individuals with dyspnea that cannot be controlled by other pharmacologic or nonpharmacologic interventions may be provided with 2 to 6 liters of oxygen by nasal cannula to assess its effect. Ideally, it is provided by nasal cannula, because masks can be frightening to the patient.

For dyspnea refractory to an individual's usual medications and/or other causes of dyspnea, opioids such as morphine and fentanyl are the mainstay of pharmacologic treatment. Opioids in this situation work by (1) altering the perception of air hunger, reducing anxiety and associated oxygen consumption; and (2) reducing pulmonary congestion by dilating pulmonary blood vessels. Patients who have not been receiving opioids are given starting doses of 2.5 mg to 5 mg orally, which may be repeated as needed. Individuals who have been taking morphine or other opioids for pain may need higher doses of morphine (up to 50% of their usual dose) for relief of dyspnea.

Fear and anxiety may be components of respiratory distress at the end of life. For this reason, benzodiazepines are commonly given when morphine does not fully control the person's dyspnea. Low dose lorazepam (Ativan) (e.g., 0.25 mg to 0.5 mg) is administered orally, sublingually, or intravenously every 4 hours PRN or around the clock.

Antibiotics may be indicated in clients with dyspnea secondary to a respiratory infection. A thorough workup for a respiratory infection, however, is not appropriate when death is imminent. If signs or symptoms of a respiratory infection are present (i.e., fever, adventitious breath sounds, congested cough) along with the dyspnea, a trial of an appropriate antibiotic may be considered. For a summary of the pharmacologic management of dyspnea at the end of life see Table 5–6.

Table 5–6   Pharmacologic Interventions for Dyspnea at End of Life

Cause of Dyspnea	Medication	Dose	Advantages	Limitations
Bronchospasm	(Bronchodilators) Albuterol	2 puffs every 4–6 hrs. PRN or 1 unit dose solution every 6–8 hrs.	Prompt action	Requires patient synchronized breathing
	(Corticosteriods) Prednisone	20–40 mg every day	Readily available in patient with h/o bronchospasm	Insomnia Agitation
Fluid Overload	(Diuretics) Furosemide	40 mg PO/IV/IM daily and prn	Prompt action Readily available in patient with h/o fluid overload	Diuresis will cause need to void
Anxiety/Fear	(Benzodiazepines) Lorazepam	0.25–0.5 mg PO/IV every 4 hrs prn	Prompt action	Sedation
Any Cause	Oxygen	2 liters—increase as ordered	Prompt action	Patient may dislike nasal prongs or mask
	Morphine Immediate Release	5 mg PO every 30 minutes until relief. Give effective dose every 2–4 hrs. prn. Increase dose of current opioid by 25–50% and give every 2–4 hrs. prn	Prompt action	Sedation

Nonpharmacologic Interventions for Dyspnea

Pharmacologic interventions should be initiated early in the course of dyspnea near the end of life. Nonpharmacologic interventions can be used in conjunction with, but should not be used in place of, medications. Nonpharmacologic interventions include the following:

- altering the environment to facilitate the circulation of cool or cold air (e.g., via air-conditioner and fan);
- applying wet cloths to the patient's face;
- positioning the patient to facilitate chest expansion;
- intervening to conserve patient's energy through frequent rest periods;
- encouraging imagery and deep breathing.

Upright positioning with arms elevated and supported by pillows facilitates diaphragmatic excursion and an optimal lung capacity. Insertion of a Foley catheter to avoid the need for exertion with voiding may be considered if the individual agrees.

Management of Dyspnea from Oral Secretions

Secretions in the upper airways and oral cavity may contribute to a person's dyspnea near death. Generally, however, these secretions are heard when the patient is unconscious, and it is believed they do not cause distress. These loud, wet respirations (referred to as death rattle) may be disturbing to family even when they do not seem to cause dyspnea or respiratory distress. Patients with loud secretions should be repositioned, usually on their sides. Anticholinergics such as hyoscyamine (Levsin) are commonly given orally or sublingually to dry up secretions. Transdermal scopolamine can also be used to reduce secretion production. Oropharyngeal suctioning is not recommended for loud secretions in the bronchi or oropharnyx because it is frequently ineffective and may only stimulate the individual. For a summary of the types of medications available for management of oropharyngeal secretions at the end of life, see Table 5–7.

Anxiety/Restlessness

Anxiety and restlessness at the end of life require assessment for pain, urinary retention, constipation, fear, or another potentially reversible cause. Administration of an opioid can be helpful in treating agitation related to pain, and insertion of an

Table 5–7   Pharmacologic Interventions for Oropharyngeal Secretions at End of Life

Medication	Dose	Advantages	Limitations
Atropine Ophthalmic Solution 1%	1–2 gtts PO/SL every 4–6 hrs ATC or prn	Ease of administration in unconscious patient	Risk for tachycardia
Hyoscyamine	0.125 mg–.25 mg PO/SL every 4–6 hrs. ATC or prn	Readily available	Tablets need to be crushed and mixed with small amounts of water
Scopolamine Transdermal Patch	1–3 patches every 3 days	Ease of administration	Delayed effect

indwelling urinary catheter is appropriate if urinary retention is suspected. Eliciting what is causing fear and providing reassurance that the patient will receive the help she needs may be all that is needed to alleviate patient distress. Consultation with a spiritual and/or bereavement counselor should also be considered to assess for unfinished business or spiritual distress as a cause of the anxiety.

In a patient with anxiety without signs of delirium, a benzodiazepiene such as lorazepam may be tried. When delirium is present, however, benzodiazipines are not the drugs of choice. Delirium is defined as a neuropsychiatric syndrome composed of disturbances of consciousness, attention, and cognition, with abrupt onset and a fluctuating course (APA, 2000). It is common in the last weeks of life, occurring in up to 85% of patients (Breitbart & Alici, 2008).

There are two types of delirium: agitated and hypoactive. Hypoactive delirium is probably not uncomfortable for patients. Agitated delirium can be uncomfortable, especially for the family. Although a diagnostic workup is not appropriate when either type of delirium develops near end of life, healthcare providers should consider possible causes such as the adverse effects of opioids, benzodiazepines, anticholinergics, or steroids. A decrease or discontinuation of these agents should be considered, particularly if they were recently started. Low doses of the antipsychotic haloperidol (Haldol) is the first-line therapy for terminal delirium manifested by agitation, paranoia, hallucinations, and altered sensorium. Other antipsychotics used include chlorpromazine, olanzapine, risperidone, or quentiapine. Use of more

Table 5–8   Pharmacologic Interventions for Delirium at End of Life

Medication	Dose	Advantages	Limitations
Haloperidol	0.5–2 mg PO/SL/SC/IM every 2–8 hrs. ATC or prn	Nonsedating	Risk of extrapyramidal side effects in elderly. Not allowed at some facilities.
Chlorpromazine	12.5 mg–50 mg PO q 4–12 hr ATC or prn	Readily available	Sedation. Risk of extrapyramidal side effects in elderly.
Olanzapine	2.5 mg ODT	Tolerated well	Sedation
Risperidone	0.25 mg–1 mg PO 1–2 times day	Tolerated well	May not provide rapid effect

than one neuroleptic at a time is strongly discouraged because of the risk of adverse reactions.

Although antipsychotic medications are considered the drug of choice for anxiety related to delirium, patients with a known history of anxiety may be tried on a benzodiazepine such as lorazepam (Watson, Lucas, Hoy, & Wells, 2009). Development of increased agitation in this situation would represent a paradoxical reaction and indicate that the benzodiazepine be tapered or discontinued. For a summary of the types of medications available for management of delirium at the end of life, see Table 5–8.

Nausea and Vomiting

Although not as common a problem as pain or dyspnea, nausea, and vomiting are thought to occur in about 40% of terminally ill individuals during the last week of life. It is particularly prevalent in individuals with (AIDS) or breast, stomach, or gynecologic cancers. Common causes of nausea and vomiting at the end of life include

- uremia;
- hypercalcemia;
- increased intracranial pressure secondary to brain metastasis;
- vagal stimulation secondary to oral candida;
- stretching of the hepatic capsule;
- constipation or impaction; and
- bowel obstruction.

If constipation is identified as the cause, a biphosphate enema is administered to release stool quickly. If stool in the rectum cannot be evacuated, a mineral oil enema followed by disimpaction may be required to relieve the person's distress. Nausea and vomiting related to other causes can generally be controlled by one or more antiemetic agents. Combinations of antiemetics as rectal suppositories, gels, or oral troches can be tried and individualized for maximal relief and control. Aromatherapy using peppermint and rosewood has been found to be helpful in relieving nausea. Aromatherapy using chamomile, camphor, fennel, lavender, peppermint, and rose has been shown to relieve vomiting (Duke, 1997). For a summary of the types of medications available for management of nausea and vomiting at the end of life, see Table 5–9.

Urinary Discomfort

Urinary discomfort near the end of life can occur secondary to urinary retention, urine incontinence, urinary tract infections, or bladder spasms (usually with indwelling catheter in place). Retention and incontinence are often resolved with insertion of an indwelling catheter. Bladder spasms in a person with an indwelling catheter may decrease by removing water from the balloon or with oxybutynin given orally. Treatment with antibiotics is appropriate for a presumed urinary tract infection causing symptoms of distress.

Fatigue

Fatigue is one of the most prevalent and troublesome symptoms experienced by individuals receiving palliative care (Del Fabbro, Dalal, & Bruera, 2006). As death approaches, weakness and fatigue usually increase. Interventions such as physical activity, hematopoietic growth factors, or psychostimulants may be appropriate at points in the illness trajectory. At the end of life, however, fatigue may provide

Table 5–9   Pharmacologic Interventions for Nausea/Vomiting at End of Life

Medication	Dose	Advantages	Limitations
Prochlorperazine	10 mg PO every 6 hrs. prn or 25 mg PR every 12 hrs. prn	Readily available	Sedation Risk of extrapyramidal side effects
Haloperidol	0.5–2 mg PO/IM every 6 hrs. prn	Nonsedating	Risk of extrapyramidal side effects
Dexamethasone	4 mg. PO/IV/SC/IM twice a day	Effective with increased intracranial pressure	Agitation/ insomnia
Metochlopramide	10–20 mg PO/gel every 6 hrs. prn	Effective with gastric stasis	Risk of extrapyramidal side effects

Compounds of the above medications are often available for N/V that is refractory to treatment with one or two anti-emetics.

protection from suffering as it will facilitate rest; this, in turn, could decrease pain and dyspnea related to movement. Thus, treatment of fatigue near the end of life is not generally appropriate. It is, however, important for healthcare providers to acknowledge the distress that fatigue can cause the patient and family so as to alleviate emotional suffering. Healthcare providers play a role in identifying the point at which treatment of fatigue is no longer indicated or beneficial.

Interventions to Assist the Family of a Person Near the End of Life

Although emotionally challenging, witnessing the death of a loved one may actually facilitate the family's acceptance of the death. Witnessing a patient's decline makes the event real and enhances an understanding of how disease affects bodily function.

Family and friends who are anticipating the death of a loved one often fear that the death will be characterized by pain and suffering. Families need to be assured that many signs and symptoms that occur during the dying process do not cause discomfort and that symptoms of distress can be promptly treated. Such assurances diminish the emotional pain of suffering that families may experience. Written and verbal information about common signs and symptoms of approaching death with ways to alleviate any discomfort are provided to families at this time (see Table 5–10). Nurses should emphasize to families that the dying person often emotionally withdraws from others. This should be viewed not as an insult but as a way of saying goodbye.

Grief is the emotional feeling related to the perception of the loss. Mourning is the outward social expression of the loss. Interventions to assist individuals and families in grieving and mourning are based on the cultural beliefs, values, and practices of patients and families (see Chapter 7, Spirituality and Suffering). Interventions are aimed at providing appropriate emotional support to allow patients and families the opportunity to verbalize their fears and concerns. Nurses can assist by keeping patients/families involved in healthcare decisions, reframing the situation to emphasize the goal of keeping the individual comfortable, and ensuring that the patient will remain comfortable until death.

Nurses can also intervene with those grieving an impending death by "being with" as opposed to "being there." "Being with" implies that you are physically and psychologically with the grieving person and empathizing with their loss. Listening and acknowledging the legitimacy of the patient and/or family's pain are often more therapeutic than speaking; this concept is sometimes referred to as "presence." Nurses also facilitate the expression of grief by giving the person who is mourning permission to express this grief. One's manner and words show that these expressions of grief are acceptable and expected. Saying something such as "This must be very difficult for you" or "I'm sorry this is happening" is therapeutic.

A family member's pain of loss should not be minimized. The nurse must avoid trite assurances such as "Things will be fine. Don't cry," or "Don't be upset" or "In a year you will have forgotten." Such comments can actually be barriers to demonstrating care and concern. The nurse should accept whatever the grieving person says about the situation and remain present, ready to listen attentively and guide gently. This will help the bereaved prepare for the necessary reminiscence and integration of the loss.

Storytelling through reminiscence and life review can be an important activity for individuals who are dying, and for family. Life review is a structured process of reflecting on one's life experience. It is often facilitated by an interviewer.

Table 5–10   Interventions to Facilitate Comfort for Signs and Symptoms
of Approaching Death

Signs/Symptoms	Interventions for Comfort
Increase in weakness and fatigue	▪ Encourage person to remain in bed for comfort and safety. ▪ Assist person to move using draw sheet for turning and pulling up in bed ▪ Provide cushioning with air mattress and pillows to support joints.
Decrease in level of consciousness	▪ Talk to patients as if they were conscious. ▪ Create a familiar and pleasant environment, with music, pets, and people they love. ▪ Encourage family members to say what they need to say. ▪ Give patients permission to let go and die when they are ready. ▪ Encourage family members to say they will miss the patient but that the family will be all right.
Loss of appetite Loss of ability to swallow	▪ Offer sips of liquids or soft food as desired. Do not force the person to eat/drink. ▪ Avoid parenteral fluids that can lead to urge to void and/or third spacing.
Loss of bowel/bladder control	▪ Use Attends, Chux, and/or Foley catheter to contain body fluids. ▪ Apply barrier creams to protect skin.
Change in breathing pattern	▪ Check to see if person is struggling to take a breath. ▪ Elevate head of bed. ▪ Contact hospice nurse who will assist in determining if breathing pattern represents suffering versus expected response.
Confusion/hallucinations	▪ Gently encourage patients to share what they see and hear. ▪ Avoid arguing with person. ▪ Contact hospice nurse who will assist in determining if medication is indicated.

Signs/Symptoms	Interventions for Comfort
Oral mucosal drying	■ Moisten mouth and lips with mouth swab dipped in solution of choice. ■ Apply petroleum-based lubricant to lips (nonpetroleum if using oxygen).
Discoloration/mottling of skin	■ Ask if person is warm enough. ■ Provide blankets as needed.

REPORT ANY SIGNS/ SYMPTOMS OF PAIN (E.G., MOANING, GRIMACING), DIFFICULTY BREATHING, AGITATION, OR OTHER SIGNS OF DISCOMFORT. Your Loved One Need Not Suffer.

Reminiscence is the process of randomly reflecting on memories of events in one's life. The benefits of storytelling through either method include catharsis, the ability to attain perspective, and enhancement of meaning. Familiar objects such as photographs and favorite jewelry pieces can be used to spark ideas for stories that the person may want to tell.

After the death, "being with" family members remains important. At this time, out-of-town relatives return home, and friends and local relatives resume their own lives. Healthcare providers should consider contacting family members after the death to allow them the opportunity to voice their perceptions of the experience. Family caregivers who assumed the role of symptom manager in the home often welcome the opportunity to discuss their experience. Bereavement counselors with training in caring for individuals and families facing loss and suffering related to end-of-life issues should also be available to assist family to cope both before and after death. Medical social workers and chaplains often serve as bereavement counselors in palliative care or hospice programs.

Participation in bereavement support groups by individuals who are grieving a person's pending or past death has been shown to facilitate the grieving process. Being a part of a support group can help people to discover that others have suffered through an experience just as devastating as their own. This discovery makes them more likely to share their feelings with others and work toward some resolution of the experience.

Summary

Although physical, emotional, and spiritual suffering can occur near the end of life, access to quality palliative and end-of-life care can alleviate much suffering and facilitate an opportunity for the patient and family to experience a "good death." Consultation from a palliative care team will assist the nurse in addressing the multiple issues that often occur at this difficult, but sacred time.

The case study at the start of this chapter illustrates various types of suffering that the patient and family can experience as death nears. The nurse understands that Linda's stage 4 ovarian cancer with metastasis through her abdominal cavity is a life-threatening disease with a poor prognosis. Linda is at high risk for bowel obstruction and septicemia, either of which can cause death within days. Linda's increase in weakness, sleep, pain, and draining ascites are symptoms that support the fact that death may be near. Linda's anxiety and fear, along with her sobbing when her family leaves the room, indicate that she is suffering emotionally. She does not tell others she is suffering and does not ask for help; but much can be done to facilitate some relief.

A comprehensive assessment of Linda's concerns, with discussion of a plan to address them, is essential. However, treatment and control of the pain must be initiated before Linda will be able to explore her emotional concerns. Once the physical pain is relieved, Linda may be asked what she is afraid of. Possible responses include (1) fear of dying, (2) fear of having uncontrolled pain, (3) fear of frightening her family and friends, (4) fear of leaving her family and friends with an unattractive image of her, or (5) fear of losing control. Acknowledgment of her anguish with some suggestions of how she could deal with these fears along with a referral to spiritual and social workers on the palliative team could diminish the intensity of her suffering. A decrease in Linda's suffering would also diminish the suffering of the family.

Key Points

1. Although the dying experience may be very difficult, it need not be plagued by unrelenting suffering for patients and families.
2. Types of suffering at the end of life include those the dying person experiences, and those experienced by the family, each of which may be physical, emotional, and/or spiritual.

3. When trying to identify the source of someone's suffering near the end of life, ask "What to you is most frightening about this situation?"
4. The ethical duty of healthcare providers in caring for individuals near death is to follow guidelines in the medication management of symptoms and to facilitate prompt and effective symptom management.
5. The goals of care for an individual near the end of life may include achieving
    - good quality of life;
    - control of symptoms of distress;
    - meaningful interactions with family and friends;
    - living at home;
    - avoidance of medical treatments; and
    - facilitation of a peaceful death.

Visualization Exercise for End-of-Life Care*

Close your eyes and imagine, if you will for a moment, that you are at the last stage of your life. Let me set the scene for you.

You are at home, in your own bed, surrounded by loved ones. You have said your goodbyes; all your business is in order. Quiet surrounds you. You can smell the fresh-cut lilacs from your garden at your bedside. The air is cool and the breeze gently fans your face. You have no pain, nausea, hunger, or thirst. You are awake but drowsy and able to communicate.

Your family member holds your hand as you take your last breath. At peace. And you are gone. Now, please stay in this visualization. I would like to create an image for you that may be much different from the ideal situation you were just visualizing—a situation that one of your patients may experience. Stay with me if you will.

You are lying in bed, but it's not your own. You are in the hospital. The bed is uncomfortable and bends in the wrong place. You can feel the plastic of the mattress under the starched sheets. Noises. The beeps and bells. Doors opening and closing. It smells so sterile in here, not like home. Your family members come in to be with you and speak words from the foot of the bed. You faintly hear their voices but can not respond. Pain. Hurt. It hurts in many different places. The pain medication is wearing off. You don't have the strength or ability to cry out, to

*Courtesy of Laurie Tyer, MS, RN.

move in bed. You always sleep on your left side, but today you are positioned on your right side. Who can help?

Your family members cry, but you can't comfort them. Can someone comfort them? Can someone assure them that everything is all right? Tell them that they did everything they could but the time has come and it's okay. It is so painful to see them so sad. You want them to know how much you love them. You want them to remember you as you were before this illness: full of life and love.

Can they come close to the bed? Why are they so distant? You want them close to you. Come closer. Could someone hold your hand; moisten your dry, chapped lips? Talk soothing words to you or perhaps reminisce about our past together?

If only you could communicate. If only those around you could tell what you need.

Now, as we close this visualization, let us look forward. Let's imagine that a healthcare provider enters. Perhaps a nurse, a nursing assistant, or a hospice worker. They understand. They acknowledge you and your family. They provide support, empathy, and knowledge. They bridge the disconnection and help everyone be present, respectful, and embrace the moment.

Thank you for participating in this visualization exercise. You may open your eyes. And now, to reflect.

At how many moments during this visualization did you think about what interventions you, as a healthcare provider, could have done to make a difference? Assess pain and provide relief? Speak comforting words and share a warm touch? Reposition? Educate the family about end-of-life issues? Provide support and listen to the loved ones talk about the past? Encourage the loved ones not to shy away from the bedside? Be a part of this moment in life? What greater gift can you give than your presence, participation, and professional knowledge at this time?

Birth and death are two of the most significant times in any individual's life; and the nursing profession and healthcare providers may have the honored privilege of being present at these events. While birth is generally witnessed in a specialty unit, the ending of a life can take place in any area of the healthcare system. It is, therefore, essential that end-of-life issues are acknowledged and addressed in education so that care providers are knowledgeable about the changes that occur, the care that is needed, and the impact they can make on the experience for all those involved.

Questions for Reflection and Journaling

1. As a nurse caring for a patient near death, what would be your first priority? Why?

2. You believe your patient is suffering from pain, but the family asks you not to administer any medication. What would you do?

3. What if the patient asked you not to administer anything for pain? Would that be different? Why?

Case Study 5–1   (continued)

As Linda grew more and more anxious, she was placed on lorazepan (Ativan) scheduled around the clock, but I felt the power of touch tended to ease her apprehension. I held her cold hand when she looked at me with trepidation. Her sister was always painting her toes a shade of red or rubbing wild honey lotion on her edematous legs. I loved the smell so it was calming and therapeutic to step into the room and take her vital signs while she received a massage.

The doctors expected her to pass before the fourth of July. That weekend I prayed that she would make it through the weekend so I could say goodbye on Monday. I came into work on the fourth and she was there to greet me with a smile. That night I wheeled her up to the roof to watch the fireworks.

Days passed by with uncertainty and the family postponed several funeral dates because Linda persevered. It was hard for the family; they had been told on several occasions to make arrangements, and each time Linda had fought back. The doctors were shocked to still find her on the white board. By the end of July, the nurses and I collaborated, commenting that too much time had been wasted. Why was she still in the hospital? We all believed she should be home for her final days. That was what she wanted more than anything else and that was my promise to her, that we would work tirelessly until she was discharged home so she could enjoy her beautifully landscaped yard and stunning interior design one last time. I know better now not to make such promises Yet, going home was the one fragment of hope she had left in her life. I wanted her to go home as much as she did, and I would not take no for an answer. The nurses and I believed that once she went home, she could rest in peace and stop fighting. Till this point, she was enduring. The day she was to be discharged, Linda seemed different, as though she had given up. Until then, the problem had been that too much time had been spent on curing Linda's illness that could not be cured instead of caring for her personal needs and getting her home to enjoy the rest of her days.

At long last, the staff was able to arrange to transfer Linda to her home by ambulance. At home, her husband managed her parenteral nutrition and morphine pump in addition to diligently emptying her Foley and ostomy bag. For a few weeks, she could sit up in a chair and read a book every day, and the cancer support meetings were held in her home. I visited her at home once and she seemed so relaxed and content—in fact, she looked better than ever. But people always do get better before they decline. Within a few weeks, Linda slipped into a coma-like state and she died peacefully in her sleep at four in the morning.

Questions on the Case Study
1.   What might you have done differently in this situation?
2.   Do you think a palliative care consult may have helped in this situation? In what way?
3.   List four additional nursing interventions that could have facilitated comfort for Linda or her family.

Source: Courtesy of Meghan McMahon, student nurse, 2008.

References

Anderson, F., Downing, G., Hill, J., Cosorso, L., & Lerch, N. (1996). Palliative Performance Scale (PPS). *Journal of Palliative Care 12,* 5–11.

Berenson, S. (2005). Complementary and alternative therapies in palliative care. In B.R. Ferrell & N. Coyle (Eds.). *Textbook of palliative care nursing.* St. Louis, MO: Mosby.

Blinderman, C., & Fowler, B. C. (2010). Palliative sedation for physical, psychological, or existential distress. *Practical aspects of palliative care.* Cambridge, MA: Harvard Medical School Center for Palliative Care.

Booth, S., Wade, R., Johnson, M., Kite, S., Swannick, M., & Anderson, H. (2004). The use of oxygen in the palliation of breathlessness. A report of the expert working group of the Scientific Committee of the Association of Palliative Medicine. *Expert Working Group of the Scientific Committee of the Association of Palliative Medicine Respiratory Medicine 98,* 66–77.

Breitbart, W., & Alici, Y. (2008). Agitation and delirium at the end of life. *Journal of the American Medical Association, 300,* 2898–2910.

Brunnhuber, K., Nash S., Meier, D., Weissman, D.E., & Woodcock, J. (2008, spring). *Putting evidence into practice: Palliative care.* Minneapolis, MN: BMJ.

Burridge, L., Winch, S. & Clavarino, A. (2007). Reluctance to care: A systematic review and development of a conceptual framework. *Cancer Nursing, 30,* E9–E19.

Byock, I. (2004). *The four things that matter most: A book about living.* New York, NY: Free Press.

Byock, I. (2008). *Reclaiming the end of life.* Retrieved from http://www.ReclaimTheEnd.org

Cassileth, B.R., & Vickers, A.J. (2004). Massage therapy for symptom control: Outcome study at a major cancer center. *Journal of Pain and Symptoms Management, 28,* 244–249.

Centers for Medicare and Medicaid Services Hospice Center. (2008). Retrieved from https://www.cms .hhs.gov/center/hospice.asp

Conill, C., Verger, E., Henriquez, I., Saiz, N., Espier, M., Lugo, F., & Garrigos, A. (1997). Symptom prevalence in the last week of life. *Journal of Pain and Symptom Management, 14,* 328–331.

Del Fabbro, E., Dalal, S., & Bruera, E. (2006). Symptom control in palliative care—Part II: Cachexia/anorexia and fatigue. *Journal of Palliative Medicine 9,* 409–421.

Demmer, C. (2004). A survey of complementary therapy services provided by hospices. *Journal of Palliative Medicine, 7,* 510–516.

Deng, G., Cassileth, B.R., & Simon Yeung, K. (2004). Complementary therapies for cancer-related symptoms. *Supportive Oncology, 2,* 419–429.

Duke, J. (1997). *The green pharmacy.* New York, NY: St. Martin's Press.

Emanuel, L. L., Barry, W., & Stoeckle, J. D. (1991). Advanced directives for medical care—A case for greater use. *New England Journal of Medicine, 324,* 889–895.

Feldt, K. (2000). The checklist of nonverbal pain indicators (CNPI). *Pain management in nursing. 1*(1), 13–21.

Furst, C. J., & Doyle, D. (2004). The terminal phase. In D. Doyle, G. Hanks, N. Cherny, & K. Calman (Eds.), *Oxford textbook on palliative medicine* (3rd. ed., pp. 1117–1134). Oxford, UK: Oxford University Press.

Gillick, M. R. (2010). Reversing the code status of advance directives? *New England Journal of Medicine 362,* 1239–1240.

Grunier, A., & Mor, V. (2007). Where people die: A multilevel approach to influences on the site of death in America. *Medical Care Research Review, 64,* 351–378.

Kazanowski, M. (1998). Commitment to the end: Family caregivers' medication management of symptoms in patients with cancer near death. PhD dissertation. Graduate School of Nursing. Boston College. Chestnut Hill, MA.

Kirk, T., Coyle, N., Poppito, S., & Bigoney, R. (2010). Palliative sedation and existential suffering: A dialogue between medicine, nursing, philosophy, and psychology. *American Academy of Hospice and Palliative Medicine.* Boston, MA, Friday, March 5, 2010.

Larson, D. G., & Tobin, D. R. (2000). End-of-life conversations: Evolving practice and theory. *Journal of the American Medical Association, 284,* 1573–1578.

Layman-Goldstein, M., & Coyle, N. (2006). Nondrug pain interventions. In M. L. Matzo & D. W. Sherman (Eds.) *Palliative care nursing: Quality care to the end of life* (2nd ed). (pp. 407–442). New York, NY: Springer.

Lipman, A. G. (2009). Evidence-based palliative care. In A. G. Lipman, K. C. Jackson, & L. S. Tyler (Eds.), *Evidence-based symptom control in palliative care* (pp. 1–9). New York, NY: Informa Healthcare.

Mariano, C. (2006). Holistic integrative therapies in palliative care. In M. L. Matzo & D. W. Sherman (Eds.). *Palliative care nursing: Quality care to the end of life (*2nd ed.*)* (pp. 51–86). New York, NY: Springer.

National Consensus Project for Quality Palliative Care Task Force. (2009). *Clinical practice guidelines for quality palliative care* (2nd ed.). Pittsburgh, PA: Author.

National Hospice and Palliative Care Organization. (2007). *Caring connections: Download your state specific advance directive.* Retrieved from http://www.caringinfo.org

National Hospice and Palliative Care Organization. (2010). *NHPCO position statement and commentary on the use of palliative sedation in imminently dying terminally ill patients.* Retrieved from http://www.jpsmjournal.com

Newshan, G., & Schuller-Citella, D. (2003). Large clinical study shows value of therapeutic touch program. *Holistic Nursing Practice, 17*(4), 189–192.

Ngo-Metzer, Q., August, K., Srinivasan, M., Liao, S., & Meyskens, F. (2008). End of life care: Guidelines for patient-centered communication. *American Family Physician, 77,* 167–174.

O'Brien, L. A., Grisso, J. A., & Maislin, G. (1995). Nursing home residents' preferences for life sustaining treatments. *Journal of the American Medical Association, 274*(22), 1775–1779.

Perrin, K. (2010). Legal aspects of end-of-life decision making. In M. Matzo & D. W. Sherman (Eds.), *Palliative care nursing* (3rd ed.). New York, NY: Springer.

Portenoy, R. K., Sibirceva, U., Smout, R. , Horn, S., Connor, S., Blum, R. . . . Fine, P. (2006). Opioid use and survival at the end of life. *Journal of Pain and Symptom Management, 32,* 532–540.

Reed, C. F. (2003). *Suffering and illness: Insights for caregivers.* Philadelphia, PA: F. A. Davis.

Quill, T., Arnold, R., & Back, A. L. (2009). Discussing treatment preferences with patients who want "everything." *Annals of Internal Medicine, 151,* 345–349.

Schultz, R., & Beach, S. R. (1999). Caregiving as a risk factor for mortality: The caregiver health effects study. *Journal of the American Medical Association, 282,* 2215–2219.

Silveira, M. J., Kim, S. Y. H., & Langa, K. M. (2010). Advance directives and outcomes of surrogate decision making before death. *New England Journal of Medicine, 362,* 1211–1218.

Sykes, N. & Thorns, A. (2003). The use of opioids and sedatives at the end of life. *Lancet Oncology, 4*(5), 312–318.

Teno, J., Gruneir, A., Schwartz, Z., Nanda, A., & Wetle, T. (2007). Association between advance directives and quality of end of life care: A national survey. *Journal of the American Geriatrics Society, 55*, 189–194.

US Public Health Service, Agency for Health Care Policy and Research, US Department of Health and Human Services. (1994). *Guideline Panel for Management of Cancer Pain.* Silver Spring, MD: Author.

Watson, M., Lucas, C., Hoy, A., & Wells, J. (2009). *Oxford handbook of palliative care* (2nd ed.). Oxford, UK: Oxford University Press.

Wright, A. A., Zhang, B., Ray, A., Mack, J. W., Trice, E., Balboni, T. . . . Prigerson, H. G. (2008). Associations between end-of-life discussions, patient mental health, medical care near death, and caregiver bereavement adjustment. *Journal of the American Medical Association, 300*, 1665–1673.

Wright, L. (2005). *Spirituality, suffering, and illness: Ideas for healing.* Philadelphia, PA: F. A. Davis.

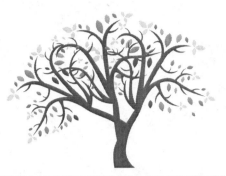

SIX

Acute and Chronic Pain as Sources of Suffering

■ Caryn A. Sheehan

Objectives

1. Compare and contrast the experience of acute and chronic pain.
2. Examine the human experience of living with chronic pain and suffering.
3. Identify nursing interventions that can be used to manage chronic pain.
4. List sources of support for people with chronic pain.

Student Project

Figure 6–1   Girl in the Pepper

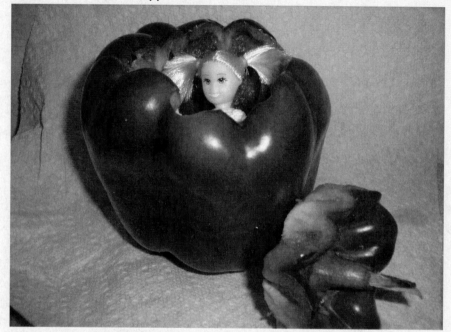

Source: Courtesy of Katie Powers, RN.

Case Study 6–1

The girl in the pepper is a student project based on the heart-wrenching story of a young woman who has spent the last 15 years in a long-term care facility in a "vegetative state." As a young teenager, she sustained a head injury in a motor vehicle accident that left her nonverbal and minimally responsive. Subsequently, she was transferred to a long-term care facility and kept alive with artificial nutrition. While the nurses there care for her and speak to her as a family member, her only responses include occasional grimacing, moaning, and slight movement of her grossly contracted arms and hands. She has frowned for so long that she has deep lines in her forehead. She appears to be in pain, though it is impossible to determine where the pain originates or how much pain she is in.

The symbolism of a young girl trapped inside a pepper represents a student nurse's ability to see beyond this patient's painful scowl and her limiting "vegetative" body, to see a young girl who was normal and healthy up until the day of her accident. To imagine that this young woman appears to suffer in pain on a daily basis can be overwhelming.

Source: Courtesy of Katie Powers, student nurse.

Questions on the Case Study
1. How does the human body respond to and endure chronic pain?
2. What are the best options for managing chronic pain?
3. Should this patient be treated for pain?
4. What would be the best nursing interventions to make her more comfortable?

Introduction—What Is Pain?

Pain is a deeply personal, yet universally common, subjective experience; pain has been described as a feeling, a symptom, a sign, or an interpretation (Kugalmann, 2003). Throughout history, mankind has viewed pain in several constructs that have ranged from a type of physical insult to a source of mystery and even a sign of evil or punishment (Matteliano, 2003). The widely accepted notion that pain serves as an indicator of dysfunction or injury still has credence, though pain can also exist where science is unable to detect any impairment. While suffering can occur with both brief acute pain and chronic pain, the consequences of pain and suffering that persist despite the lack of physical evidence can be particularly problematic and are therefore the major focus of this chapter.

Types of Pain

Pain can be differentiated based on the duration of existence, with acute pain generally referring to pain limited in scope and duration. Acute pain is common and is generally associated with some reversible impairment such as a sore throat, fractured bone, or a muscle tear. When the source of pain is known, treatment focuses not only on pain relief but also on correcting the underlying issue, such as treating with antibiotics, a cast, or rest. Acute pain has been the focus of increased awareness since The Joint Commission issued the 2001 pain management standards requiring healthcare facilities to diligently assess, treat, and document each patient's experience of pain (The Joint Commission, 2001). Many nurses are quite familiar with how to assess, treat, and evaluate patients who experience acute pain.

Cancer Pain versus Chronic Nonmalignant Pain

Chronic pain can persist beyond a few weeks or months and is associated with several debilitating consequences including insomnia, depression, and the inability to work or care for oneself (Arnstein, 2003). Chronic pain can be from a known source such as cancer or arthritis. One common cause of chronic pain is that related to malignancy. In the United States, organizations such as the Oncology Nurses Society and the Hospice and Palliative Care movement have fought to make a priority of aggressive pain management for people with cancer and for people at the end of life (Dormandy, 2006). Their efforts have advanced the acceptability of aggressively managing pain in this country.

Sometimes chronic pain lingers after the known cause is believed to be resolved. One classic example of this is phantom pain; a patient who has suffered with multiple skin and bone infections of the foot and then has the extremity amputated, only later to experience chronic pain where the foot once was. Phantom limb sensations can be the feeling of discomfort, twisting, or burning in a body part that no longer is attached to the body (Meinhart & McCaffery, 1983). For all scientific purposes, the insult to the body has been removed, yet the pain persists. These types of nonmalignant chronic pain can be among the most challenging to understand and manage.

Case Study 6–2

Thomas, age 41 (name and age changed to protect identity), is a sharp-witted adult who made a living as a truck driver before having to leave work on disability 2 years ago. During the past 30 months he had been hospitalized more than 10 times in order to manage his rapidly progressive arterial disease. As a result of the devastating effects of Burger's disease, he had severely compromised circulation in his distal extremities. Subsequently, he had endured several surgical amputations of both his fingers and his toes, leaving him with only three intact fingers and one intact thumb. His most recent hospitalization was to rule out osteomyelitis and to debride his lower leg wounds that extended from his feet to his knees bilaterally. Thomas's major concern was not his frequent surgeries or hospitalizations. He was not overly concerned about the wound packing procedures that lasted over two hours per day. His primary concern was his pain management.

The surgical nurses could scarcely comprehend how he could possibly consume 600 mg of oxycontin every 6 hours and be alert enough to watch television and talk on the phone. The nursing staff was concerned because he would occasionally "chew" his oxycontin tablets when his scheduled dose occurred during an exacerbation of pain. Thomas's medical record was filled with notes detailing how the staff advised him that chewing a long-acting opioid could lead to respiratory depression and possibly even death. Furthermore, some staff doubted him when he calmly stated his pain rating was still "10 out of 10" and hesitated to offer him the 60 mg (twelve 5 mg tablets) PRN dose of oxycodone for breakthrough pain. Thomas spoke openly about his frustration with his situation because he felt pressure to "prove" he was in legitimate pain and that he was not a drug addict.

Questions on the Case Study

1. How does the assessment differ between a patient who has acute pain, one who has chronic pain, and one who has both types of pain?
2. How can the nurse distinguish between a patient who is a drug abuser and a patient who is in legitimate pain?

Scope of the Problem of Pain

Estimates suggest more than 75 million Americans have some recurrent or persistent pain (Adams et al., 2001). The Centers for Disease Control and Prevention (CDC) estimated in 2006 that 1 in 10 Americans reported they had pain that lasted longer than 1 year in duration (National Center for Health Statistics, 2006). Low back pain, headache pain, and joint pain were the most common types of pain reported among Americans, with an estimate of nearly one quarter of adults in America reporting back pain within the past 3 months in 2007 (National Center for Health Statistics, 2009). According to Adams et al. (2001) and Lazarus and Neumann (2001), common sources of nonmalignant chronic pain include

- lumbar/low back pain;
- joint disease/arthritis;
- headache/migraine
- neck/upper back;
- neuropathic pain; and
- fibromyalgia.

Chronic pain is not only costly physically and emotionally; it also consumes an inordinate amount of healthcare resources. Low back pain alone accounts for more than eight million physician visits yearly and for 25% of worker compensation claims (Adams et al., 2001). Lost wages, physical therapy, alternative therapies, and prescription and over the counter medication costs must also be figured into the chronic pain financial equation. By definition, chronic pain exists over a long period of time or a lifetime; thus considering the duration of services required, the burden of cost for chronic pain management is immense.

Variables in Suffering with Pain

The perception of pain varies not only based on duration and type of pain but also on many other factors including age, gender, and culture. Pain assessment and management is distinctly different for children. Children and infants may not be able to describe their pain or the efficacy of treatments. Various pediatric assessment tools and prescription dosage recommendations exist for this special population. While acute pain is reportedly common in children, chronic pain is rare; one study estimated chronic pain to be present in less than 3% of people younger than age 30 (ABC News/USA Today/Stanford Medical Center Poll: Pain, 2005). To learn more about suffering in children see Chapter 2 "Suffering in Special Populations"; to learn more about chronic pain management in the pediatric population consult *Pain in Infants, Children and Adolescents* (2002) by Schechter, Berde, and Yaster. The remainder of this chapter focuses on adults with chronic pain.

Males and females also experience pain differently. Women have been observed to have a lower pain threshold and tolerance, and be more willing to report their pain (Wise, Price, Myers, Heft, & Robinson, 2002). Whether this gender disparity has biological roots or social-psychological explanation has yet to be determined. In American culture women are encouraged to share their feelings; in fact, pop culture overflows with talk shows and magazines targeting women's issues. The observation that women are more likely to talk about their pain is consistent with observations that middle-age women visit their doctors more often than men (Song, Change, Manheim, & Dunlop, 2006). Whether the reason is social or biological, gender appears to play a role in the experience of pain.

Diagnosis: Chronic Pain

Most people realize when they can no longer manage their pain, and seek help. This journey often begins at the office of their primary care provider (PCP). Most pain from acute illnesses can be managed well by the PCP. However, when usual pain interventions lack efficacy, most PCPs will send patients to a specialist for further evaluation and treatment. Herein lies the beginning of what may seem like an endless, hopeless journey for people with chronic pain. Many people with generalized or joint pain make their next visit to a rheumatologist or orthopedic surgeon. Then, between visits to physical therapy, pre-operative consultations, chiropractors, and neurologists, the patient continues to purchase several over the counter and prescription medications. Human nature directs people to seek help and look for a cure. Months and years later, even sometimes after undergoing several surgical procedures, the patient may continue to visit several providers seeking relief. Ultimately some fortunate chronic pain patients will be referred to a pain specialist. The journey with a diagnosis of chronic pain is long and frustrating, and can negatively impact the relationship between healthcare providers and patients.

Pain and Suffering Intertwine with Trust and Frustration

Issues with trust can develop between the person with chronic pain and the healthcare system. Pain is fundamentally subjective and therefore clinicians must rely on the patient's self-report. However, with the surge of false worker's compensation and disability claims and the risk of narcotic abuse and diversion, clinicians may be overly alert. These concerns can be a source of frustration for people with chronic pain who often feel as though they have to constantly "convince" healthcare providers about the legitimacy of their pain. People with chronic pain can experience frustration from many sources including the difficulty in obtaining a diagnosis, the inability of treatments to provide lasting relief from pain, doubting family members and/or healthcare providers, personal worry about burdening their families, and even frustration with the healthcare system that is purported to be so technologically advanced but cannot offer a cure (Thomas, 2000). A two-way culture of mistrust can develop when the patient in pain fears the healthcare system may not be able to help and the healthcare providers fear the patient is not truthful about the pain.

Believing the patient's report of pain is a leap of faith nurses take every day. The special assessments for chronic pain listed later in this chapter can give nurses the evidence to support their desire to believe the patient. Believing is an important step in creating rapport and can minimize the issues of mistrust that are inherent in the care of people with chronic pain.

Pain and Suffering and Functional Limitations

One of the causes of frustration and a major theme among people with chronic pain is a concomitant decline in functional ability. "The chronic pain patient dwells in the world of 'I cannot' instead of the world of 'I can'" (Thomas, 2000, p. 697). Chronic pain affects a person's ability to accomplish simple daily tasks such as making breakfast for the children, driving to work, lifting groceries, and other daily feats people without pain take for granted. Lazarus and Neumann (2001) observed that 67% of people with chronic pain say their daily lives have been altered by the pain. Some chronic pain sufferers go to great lengths to accomplish everyday activities. One woman with chronic pain described how she had learned to choose the "correct" seat to sit in when she took bus trips as to avoid the bus seats that bounced too hard from poor suspension (Peolsson, Hyden, & Larsson, 2000). The inability to care for oneself or one's family and the inability to work are significant stressors that create isolation and affect self-esteem.

Pain and Suffering and Isolation

Over time, people with chronic pain are excluded or intentionally withdraw from vocational, recreational, family, and even intimate relationships (Arnstein, 2003). The inability to work or participate in the physical demands of such relationships because of pain tends to fuel this disengagement. Some patients with chronic pain say they avoid social situations so they will not be the target of pity, because they do not want to burden or disappoint others, or simply because they have difficulty focusing on anything other than their pain (Lansbury, 2000; Thomas, 2000). Depression both contributes to and is a consequence of this social isolation.

The Emotional Burden of Pain and Suffering

One of the concepts that establishes chronic pain as such a significant source of suffering is how negatively it affects quality of life (QOL). People with chronic pain have been observed to rate their QOL lower than people with other chronic illnesses such as renal failure, multiple sclerosis, and even cancer (Gerstle, All, & Wallace, 2001). Among people who have chronic pain, factors such as high medical costs, low income, and no workman's compensation insurance have been associated with the lowest ratings of QOL (Gerstle et al., 2001). The highest QOL ratings among people with chronic pain were from people who were older and were still able to work (Gerstle et al., 2001). The effect of pain on quality of life has much more to do with how the pain affects every facet of daily living rather than just the pain experience alone. For instance, some people with chronic pain begin to shape their lives to accommodate the pain. They often have to leave or change their jobs and lose the companionship of co-workers. They may no longer be able to participate in simple family activities such as bowling or camping because of physical limitations from pain.

Eventually the life of people who have chronic unrelieved pain can become so enveloped with trying to control potential sources of pain and seeking pain relief that focusing on the pain becomes the very center of their attention. Suffering and pain become their life. Popular press has even referred to the combination of suffering, sleeplessness, and sadness associated with chronic pain as the "terrible triad." The inability to get enough pain relief to sleep at night contributes to the lack of pain tolerance and increases focus on the pain, which then can contribute to insomnia. This common cycle is self-perpetuating and undoubtedly frustrating for the patient, the family, and the caregiver. Important nursing concerns related to chronic pain are

- pain description/perception;
- functional ability/disability;
- isolation;
- depression;
- trust issues/frustration;
- insomnia.

The link between chronic pain and its ensuing emotional response is an area that nurses need to tend to (Lin et al., 2003). People with chronic pain who doubt their ability to cope or move forward (low self-efficacy) tend to report more depression and disability than others (Arnstein, Caudill, & Wells-Federmann, 2000). In fact, chronic pain has even been identified as a significant risk factor for suicide (Meeks et al., 2008). The next two sections of this chapter specifically address how the nurse can best assess and intervene to help patients manage their suffering related to chronic pain.

Assessing Chronic Pain

Traditional pain scales may not be the ideal way to assess chronic pain (Arnstein, 2003). The premise of having patients rate their pain on a scale from 0 to 10 is to capture the level of pain at a single moment in time. People with chronic pain often experience periods of exacerbation and remission of their pain that can impact the degree of pain from week to week, day to day, or even moment to moment. Therefore, an ideal pain assessment would need to capture a longer interval of time. In addition, the associated sequela of chronic pain have tremendous impact on the suffering involved. The following symptoms are essential to include in a chronic pain assessment, so they too can be addressed (Kerns, Turk, & Rudy, 1985):

- Description of pain/pain severity over a designated period of time (last week or month)
- Sleep habits and quality
- Ability to complete activities of daily living/general activity level
- Ability to work/volunteer
- Emotional well-being/mood/affective distress
- Relationships/socialization/social support
- Patient's level of satisfaction with current pain management plan

See Figure 6–2 and Figure 6–3 for examples of assessment forms appropriate for use with patients in chronic pain.

Figure 6–2   Sample Chronic Pain Assessment Flow Sheet

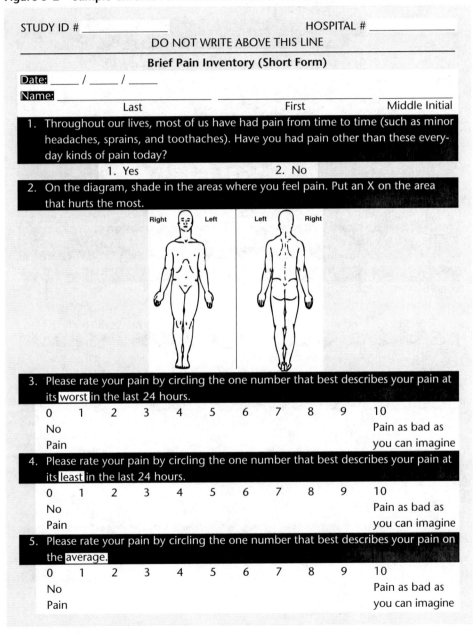

STUDY ID # _____   HOSPITAL # _____

DO NOT WRITE ABOVE THIS LINE

Brief Pain Inventory (Short Form)

Date: _____ / _____ / _____

Name: _____ _____ _____

Last   First   Middle Initial

1. Throughout our lives, most of us have had pain from time to time (such as minor headaches, sprains, and toothaches). Have you had pain other than these every-day kinds of pain today?

1. Yes   2. No

2. On the diagram, shade in the areas where you feel pain. Put an X on the area that hurts the most.

3. Please rate your pain by circling the one number that best describes your pain at its **worst** in the last 24 hours.

0   1   2   3   4   5   6   7   8   9   10

No   Pain as bad as
Pain   you can imagine

4. Please rate your pain by circling the one number that best describes your pain at its **least** in the last 24 hours.

0   1   2   3   4   5   6   7   8   9   10

No   Pain as bad as
Pain   you can imagine

5. Please rate your pain by circling the one number that best describes your pain on the **average.**

0   1   2   3   4   5   6   7   8   9   10

No   Pain as bad as
Pain   you can imagine

(continued)

Figure 6–2 (continued)

6. Please rate your pain by circling the one number that tells how much pain you have right now.

0	1	2	3	4	5	6	7	8	9	10

No
Pain

Pain as bad as
you can imagine

7. What treatments or medications are you receiving for your pain?

_____

8. In the last 24 hours, how much relief have pain treatments or medications provided? Please circle the one percentage that most shows how much relief you have received.

0%	10%	20%	30%	40%	50%	60%	70%	80%	90%	100%

No
Pain

Pain as bad as
you can imagine

9. Circle the one number that describes how, during the past 24 hours, pain has interfered with your:

A. General Activity

0	1	2	3	4	5	6	7	8	9	10

Does not
Interfere

Completely
Interferes

B. Mood

0	1	2	3	4	5	6	7	8	9	10

Does not
Interfere

Completely
Interferes

C. Walking Ability

0	1	2	3	4	5	6	7	8	9	10

Does not
Interfere

Completely
Interferes

D. Normal Work (includes both work outside the home and housework)

0	1	2	3	4	5	6	7	8	9	10

Does not
Interfere

Completely
Interferes

E. Relations with other people

0	1	2	3	4	5	6	7	8	9	10

Does not
Interfere

Completely
Interferes

Figure 6–2 (continued)

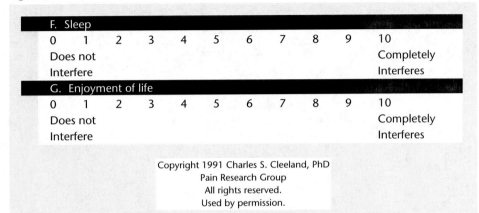

F. Sleep										
0	1	2	3	4	5	6	7	8	9	10
Does not Interfere										Completely Interferes

G. Enjoyment of life										
0	1	2	3	4	5	6	7	8	9	10
Does not Interfere										Completely Interferes

Believing the patient's report of pain and symptoms is the foundation of any pain assessment. In the case of chronic pain, this can be particularly challenging for nurses. Often nurses look for the traditional signs of pain include wincing, crying, screaming, gritting of teeth, or moaning which can also be associated with increases in blood pressure and heart rate. These typical signs of pain are largely due to the body's normal "fight or flight" response to stress (Selye, 1976). These signs are so universally recognized that most nurses respond rapidly when patients exhibit such behavior. However, the aroused physiological state and the self-preservation response can be maintained for only a limited period of time before the body becomes exhausted. Therefore, when the noxious stimulus (pain) becomes chronic, the body is unable to continue to respond in the expected manner. This may explain why patients in chronic pain may lack the typical signs and symptoms associated with the experience of pain. This also explains why so many patient reports of chronic pain are doubted by healthcare workers. The following scenario is common:

Case Study 6–3

A patient in the hospital who has chronic pain talks quietly on the phone with a family member, while lying in bed with the TV playing. When the nurse comes in to assess her pain using a pain scale, the patient states her pain is a "10" and would gladly accept a PRN dose of pain medication. The nurse does not observe any physical signs of discomfort and hesitantly prepares the medication as she worries the woman may be addicted to narcotics.

Figure 6–3   Sample of a Functional Assessment Pertinent to Chronic Pain

American Chronic Pain Association

Quality of Life Scale
A Measure of Function for People with Pain

Non-functioning

0 Stay in bed all day.
Feel hopeless and helpless about life.

1 Stay in bed at least half the day.
Have no contact with outside world.

2 Get out of bed but don't get dressed.
Stay at home all day.

3 Get dressed in the morning. Minimal activities at home.
Contact with friends via phone, email.

4 Do simple chores around the house.
Minimal activities outside of home two days a week.

5 Struggle but fulfill daily home responsibilities.
No outside activity. Not able to work/volunteer.

6 Work/volunteer limited hours.
Take part in limited social activities on weekends.

7 Work/volunteer for a few hours daily. Can be active at least five hours a day.
Can make plans to do simple activities on weekends.

8 Work/volunteer for at least six hours daily. Have energy to make
plans for one evening social activity during the week. Active on weekends.

9 Work/volunteer/be active eight hours daily. Take part in family life.
Outside social activities limited.

10 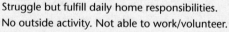 Go to work/volunteer each day. Normal daily activities each day.
Have a social life outside of work. Take an active part in family life.

Normal Quality of Life

Figure 6–3   (continued)

Quality of Life Scale
A Measure of Function for People with Pain

Pain is a highly personal experience. The degree to which pain interferes with the quality of a person's life is also highly personal.

The American Chronic Pain Association Quality of Life Scale looks at ability to function, rather than at pain alone. It can help people with pain and their healthcare team to evaluate and communicate the impact of pain on the basic activities of daily life. This information can provide a basis for more effective treatment and help to measure progress over time.

The scale is meant to help individuals measure activity levels. We recognize that homemakers, parents and retirees often don't work outside the home, but activity can still be measured in the amount of time one is able to "work" at fulfilling daily responsibilities be that in a paid job, as a volunteer, or within the home.

With a combination of sound medical treatment, good coping skills, and peer support, people with pain can lead more productive, satisfying lives. The American Chronic Pain Association can help.

For more information, contact the ACPA:

Post Office Box 850
Rocklin, CA 95677
916.632.0922
800.533.3231
Fax: 916.632.3208
E-mail: acpa@pacbell.net
Web Page: www.theacpa.org

Source: American Chronic Pain Association. Used with permission.

In reality, this patient is exhibiting the expected signs and symptoms of chronic pain: none. The only way to correctly assess the pain is to ask the patient. When patients repeatedly sense skepticism from healthcare providers, some even try to intentionally "act" in a manner that is more convincing that they are really in pain. These "acts" are usually apparent to nurses and may even cause more distrust. The situation is truly a dilemma for the patient who desperately seeks to be believed and to be treated appropriately for pain.

An important concept in assessing chronic pain is consideration of the multitude of associated symptoms that can accompany the pain and contribute to suffering. These symptoms often include depression, decreased activity, forgetfulness, anxiety/panic disorders, and difficulty concentrating (Adams et al., 2001; McCracken & Iverson, 2001). While these cognitive complaints that patients with chronic pain endure can be particularly frustrating, little is known about their exact etiology. The inability to "think correctly" may be associated with many causes including stress, sleep deprivation, medication, or even the pain itself. Recent research has demonstrated that magnetic resonance imaging (MRI) can actually detect changes in the neurons of the brain in people with chronic low back pain, and this may account for some of their depression and cognitive changes (Baliki, Geha, Apkarian, & Chialvo, 2008). Patients may take comfort in explanations that demonstrate that their concerns are valid, are common, and have some basis in physiological changes that occur in the brain with chronic pain.

Goals for People with Chronic Pain

The goal of pain management is to alleviate pain by eliminating the underlying cause of the pain; however, for many people with chronic nonmalignant pain, the cause may be neither identifiable nor easy to treat. For instance, a patient who had a traumatic shoulder injury several years ago may show resolution of the original injury on recent MRI but continue to have pain. Or a patient with a mild spinal stenosis may admit to pain that is disproportionate to the x-ray findings. Once treatment of the cause is no longer feasible, controlling the pain and maximizing quality of life become the focus of treatment.

The goals and treatment of chronic pain need to be realistic. In many circumstances complete relief of pain is not feasible and patients need to know this upfront. However, many aspects of daily life for people with chronic pain can be significantly improved, including quality of life. According to the Scoping Document for the WHO Treatment Guidelines on Chronic Non-Malignant Pain in Adults (2008), some reasonable goals for patients who have chronic pain would include these:

- Reduce pain.
- Improve quality/duration of sleep.
- Decrease feelings of depression/anxiety/isolation.
- Improve daily functioning.
- Return to or maintain employment.
- Improve sense of control over pain/increase quality of life.
- Minimize adverse effects/complications/cost associated with treatment.

Questions for Reflection and Journaling
1. Are chronic pain patients too "passive" in playing their role in obtaining pain relief?
2. At what point, if any, should patients with chronic pain be encouraged to stop seeking a miracle cure and begin to learn new ways to adapt to their life with pain?

Management of Chronic Pain and Suffering

Successful management of chronic pain and its associated suffering is a complex process that often involves a multidisciplinary approach utilizing several providers and multiple modalities. It is not uncommon to see patients with chronic pain who have consulted with many of the following healthcare specialist areas (Koestler & Myers, 2002):

- Anesthesiology
- Chiropractic
- Counseling
- Neurology
- Nursing
- Occupational therapy
- Orthopedic surgery
- Pain specialists
- Physical therapy
- Psychiatry
- Psychology
- Rheumatology

Barriers to Effective Management of Chronic Pain

Treatments can be divided into three main categories: (1) medications, (2) physical interventions, and (3) behavioral interventions. A basic overview of some of the barriers and the more common options among these treatments are included in this section.

Despite the increase in pain assessment and management awareness over the past 2 decades, some people continue to suffer in pain. Some of the most common reasons for this are that healthcare providers may (1) incompletely assess pain, (2) have inadequate knowledge about the prescription of analgesics, or (3) fear narcotic addiction (Laccetti & Kazanowski, 2009).

Although helping patients navigate through the overwhelming options for chronic pain can be exhausting for the care providers as well as the patients, Meinhart and McCaffery (1983) argue that "failure to treat pain is inhumane and constitutes professional negligence" (pp. vi).

Medications for Chronic Pain

Appropriate pharmacologic intervention can significantly reduce the suffering resulting from pain. In 1990 the World Health Organization (WHO) developed the landmark guideline for managing pain entitled *"Cancer pain relief and palliative care: report of a WHO expert committee."* While the intended population was patients with cancer, many of the principles are also applicable to people suffering with nonmalignant chronic pain. The WHO's 3 step analgesic ladder recommends beginning with nonopioid analgesics and adjuvant therapy. Many patients report significant relief with scheduled NSAIDs such as ibuprofen or naproxen. Patients who routinely use these medications should be monitored for gastrointestinal and renal complications. If pain continues, the WHO protocol calls for the addition of a weak opioid. In cases where pain persists despite all of these interventions, strong opioid medications can also be added. Some of the frequently prescribed opioids for chronic pain in primary care (and their associated percentage of use) are Percocet (31%), Morphine (19%), Tylenol #3 (15%), Vicodin (14%), and Oxycontin/Oxycodone (3–12%) (Adams et al., 2001). In a recent poll of 1200 Americans, people with pain reported that the use of prescription medications was one of the most effective pain interventions; however, among people with chronic pain, less than one third of the people polled said prescription drugs worked "very well" (ABC News, 2005).

The use of narcotics to treat nonmalignant chronic pain has been controversial because of concerns about drug abuse and addiction. Variability in treatment of chronic pain along with the low confidence and low likelihood of using opioids for nonmalignant pain has been documented in the research (Green, Wheeler, LaPorte, Marchant, & Guerrero, 2002). Providers often fear that narcotics will precipitate respiratory depression or addition. Narcotic-induced constipation is a realistic but treatable side effect of this therapy. When narcotics are prescribed appropriately and increased gradually, the risk of respiratory depression and addiction in long-term use is small.

Addiction is the psychological compulsive need for a medication or the excessive use of medication in a way that is not intended and may be harmful (*Merriam-Webster,* 2010). Unfortunately, the signs of unrelieved chronic pain can be mistaken for addiction. Patients in pain will ask for additional or higher doses of pain medication despite the lack of objective signs of acute pain (crying, guarding, moaning) that nurses are familiar with. Nurses can be uncomfortable when patients ask for medication by name or dosage at specific time intervals, thinking these are indications of addiction. Such thinking can send the message to patients that it is not acceptable to be knowledgeable about their own treatment. The irony is that this is not necessarily so in other situations: if a patient newly diagnosed with diabetes asked for insulin by name and dose, the nurse would consider this request an indication of successful patient teaching. Nurses need to balance their fear of addiction with accurate knowledge of chronic pain management. Using an "opioid contract," a signed, formal agreement to the safe use and storage of prescribed narcotics, can also alleviate provider fears of diversion of these medications. The overall efficacy and effect of narcotics in chronic pain is very individualized. As one person with chronic pain suggested, "I've taken all the medication they tell you to. For a while they're like magic and then they don't work anymore" (Davis, Hiemenz, & White, 2002, pp. 124). While debate over proper use of opioids in chronic pain persists, some people are unable to function without the pain relief they provide.

Although narcotic medications can play an important role in managing chronic pain, many nonopioid pharmacologic options also exist. In addition to NSAIDs, several nonnarcotic classes of medications such as antidepressants, anticonvulsants, and steroids can provide significant relief, either alone or in combination with narcotics, for patients with chronic pain. Neurontin (Gabapentin) is an anticonvulsant medication that has also been approved to manage the neuropathic pain related to post-herpetic neuralgia (Parke-Davis Product Monograph, 2009). In addition, this medication has provided significant relief when used as an off label indication for patients with other neuropathic pain syndromes including diabetic neuropathy and prevention of migraine headaches (Mack, 2003). A pharmacologic approach often works best when combined with physical and/or behavioral interventions to manage pain.

Physical and Behavioral Interventions

Physical and behavioral measures can also be effective for some people with chronic pain. Some patient populations, especially the elderly who worry about falls and medication-related side effects, actually prefer a nonmedical approach to pain management (Lansbury, 2000). Rosenburg et al. (2008) observed that more than half of the 463 people with chronic pain who were sampled in a study reported current use of complementary and alternative modalities (CAM). Some of the modalities reported were vitamins/herbs, massage, chiropractors, meditation, yoga, and accupuncture/acupressure. See Chapter 10, "The Role of Healing and Holistic Nursing in Palliation of Suffering," for additional information about the role of CAM in reducing suffering.

Support to gain control of chronic pain and return to a meaningful lifestyle can best be provided by a multidisciplinary approach (Koestler & Myers, 2002). Pain clinics are especially knowledgeable about the various treatment modalities available to alleviate suffering related to chronic pain. Davies, Crombie, and Macrae (1994) observed that patients who had neurogenic pain for more than 1 year had a significantly better chance of having access to specialized therapies such as adjuvant pharmacotherapy and nerve stimulators when they attended an outpatient pain clinic than before referral to such a facility. The emergence of pain clinics has increased awareness of the scope and need for chronic pain management (Dormandy, 2006).

Case Study 6–4: Chronic Pain in a Hospitalized Woman

I met Ms. B after she had a lysis of adhesions and colectomy for a small bowel obstruction. She was familiar with the hospital routine as she had had a similar surgery just 6 months earlier. Her postoperative recovery was complicated as she developed a prolonged ileus that required Nasogastric (NG) tube drainage and total parenteral nutrition (TPN). She continuously stated that her pain was not well managed despite being connected to a patient controlled analgesia (PCA) pump that delivered a continuous morphine infusion along with the option to self bolus. She had suffered with chronic abdominal pain for several years. After repeated medical evaluation and diagnostic testing, no physical explanation was ever identified for her chronic abdominal pain. Ms. B had been taking MS Contin (controlled release morphine sulfate) at home for over a year. She was a smoker and had a remote history of alcohol abuse.

Ms. B consistently presented a challenge to the hospital staff. Many nurses refused to care for her and referred to her as "the challenging patient" or "the psycho." I will admit that when I heard the report on her, I also cringed a bit. Ms. B repeatedly refused treatments, dressing changes, hygiene, and her clear liquid diet because "it's gross." She often yelled at the staff, and even shouted at her own family. She repeatedly asked for more pain medication, even when dozing off. However, I cringed even more when nurses reported that they were trying to withhold pain medication. One nurse stated, "I didn't tell her that the doc changed her PRN order for oxycodone from every 3 hours to every 2 hours, because I just knew that this would prompt her to ring every 2 hours to bring it in." When Ms. B pulled out her own NG tube, the nursing staff appeared to give up.

The student nurse who was assigned to care for Ms. B was apprehensive yet eager to bring her enthusiasm and fresh perspective to the situation. Immediately the student recognized that the patient was suffering. Ms. B was violently retching, and vomit filled the pink basin she held on her lap. Quite expectedly, the student spent less than 5 minutes in the room and returned to the nurses' station in search of pain medication at the patient's request. The primary nurse, quite unalarmed, repeated what seemed like a well-rehearsed line about being unable to give any further pain medication because Ms. B would vomit the pills, since she was refusing to have her NG tube reinserted. The student looked disappointed and frustrated that she could not offer any intervention to help the patient. The student and I briefly reviewed what options we had at that point.

Clearly, trust was the first issue at hand. Having just met Ms. B we did not want to disappoint her already by appearing not to believe the severity of her pain or fail to bring the pain medication she requested. We had to be intentional about showing her we were on her side without placing blame on her primary RN, who was going to care for her for the next 12 hours (which was 5 hours longer than we would be at her bedside). We decided that fewer nurses at the beside would make the patient feel less intimidated, so the student opted to go in and explain the situation with sincerity. I could hear the student take ownership for the decision not to bring in pain medication. The student consciously showed that she believed the patient was in pain and tried to establish rapport in the new patient-nurse relationship, "It looks like the vomiting is contributing to your discomfort; can you tell me what happened with your NG tube?" The patient relayed a story of accidentally pulling out the tube when she was "half asleep," and her intense fear of the pain of putting it back in; "my nose and throat are so irritated, I couldn't bear it going back in." The student proposed what seemed like a simple solution, "What if we could get some numbing spray for your throat? Would you agree to let us reinsert the tube then?" Quite amazingly, Ms. B agreed.

At the nurse's station the primary RN was startled to learn that this ordinarily hostile patient was willing to let a student nurse reinsert the tube she had refused for several days. The RN and student spoke to the MD about a lidocaine spray order and the possibility of increasing the dose of her morphine PCA. The MD was so pleased that the patient was willing to replace the tube that he willingly ordered the new medications. After the NG tube was inserted, over 1200 mL of gastric drainage was removed.

Questions on the Case Study

1. What was the priority nursing assessment for Ms. B during the first meeting?
2. How else could the nurse establish a therapeutic relationship with Ms. B?
3. List the factors that are contributing to Ms. B's pain.
4. What additional nursing interventions would be appropriate for this woman?

Summary

The emphasis in this chapter has been on the nurse's role in helping to manage the suffering of people with chronic pain. As nurses, we can attend to the pain, but protecting our patients from all suffering is not only unrealistic but it may not necessarily be the goal. Feeling and finding meaning in the suffering, and staying connected to others, is what is important (Gunderman, 2002). One patient with arthritis pain, when asked what was important in living with chronic pain, said, "Having a sense of humor to enable you to laugh at frustrations and keep pressing on with life" (Taylor, 2001, p. 121). Nurses can press for every person to receive a comprehensive and individualized plan to cope with the pain but also to manage the many debilitating symptoms that often accompany chronic pain.

Key Points

1. The experience of pain, especially chronic pain is subjective.
2. Mistrust is not uncommon in the nurse-patient relationship when chronic pain is unrelieved. Listen to the patient. Believe the patient.
3. Patients with chronic pain are likely to have a list of additional distressing symptoms that need to be properly assessed and addressed.
4. Chose an individualized treatment plan that you are prepared to reevaluate and readjust often.

Exercise: One Day Spent Suffering with Chronic Pain

- Reflect on your activities throughout the day today.
- Take a piece of paper and write the hours you were awake in a list format on the left side of the paper, with each hour starting on a new line. These hours will make your first column; draw lines to make a total of three columns across the page.
- Next to each time, write in the second column a short description of what you were doing during that hour, that is, "taking a shower, driving to work."
- Now imagine that you are suffering with intractable chronic back pain that sends sharp "electrical" pain through your arms whenever you raise your arms more than 45 degrees from your body and sends sharp "electrical"

pain through your legs if you sit longer than 10 minutes or stand/walk longer than 10 minutes at a time. Once the pain starts, you need to lie flat for at least 15 minutes to get relief.

- Reflect on the activities you listed in the second column. Put a line through any activity that will subject you to pain.
- In the last column list 15 minutes for each crossed out activity.
- Add up all of the minutes in the third column. This is the time you would need to schedule into your day (in addition to your usual daily activities) if you had chronic pain.
- Reflect on the following questions as you look at your daily schedule:
  1. If you had to add more hours to your day to manage your pain, what would you give up? (e.g., sleep, work, social activity)
  2. What adaptations would help you maintain your normal activities of daily living? (e.g., a shower chair would enable you to alternate between sitting and standing in the shower to prevent pain)
  3. Approximately how much would these adaptations cost?
  4. Explain why daily activity is an outcome indicator when managing chronic pain.

References

ABC News/USA Today/Stanford Medical Center Poll: Pain. (2005). *Broad experience with pain sparks a search for relief.* Retrieved from http://abcnews.go.com/images/Politics/979a1TheFightAgainstPain.pdf

Adams, Plane, Fleming, Mundt, Saunders, & Stauffacher. (2001). Opioids and the treatment of chronic pain in a primary care sample. *Journal of Pain and Symptom Management, 22*(3), 791–796.

Arnstein, P. (2003). Comprehensive analysis and management of chronic pain. *Nursing Clinics of North America, 38*(3): 403–417.

Arnstein, P., Caudill, M. A., & Wells-Federmann, C. L. (2000). Self-efficacy as a mediator of depression and pain related disability in different samples of chronic pain patients. *Progress in Pain Research and Management, 4,* 1105–1111.

Baliki, M. N., Geha, P. Y., Apkarian, A. V., & Chialvo, D. R. (2008). Beyond feeling: Chronic pain hurts the brain, disrupting the default-mode network dynamics. *Journal of Neuroscience, 28*(6), 1398–1403.

Davies, H., Crombie, I., & Macrae, W. (1994). Why use a pain clinic? Management of neurogenic pain before and after referral. *Journal of the Royal Society of Medicine, 87*(7), 382–385.

Davis, G. C., Hiemenz, T. L., & White, T. L. (2002). Barriers to managing chronic pain of older adults with arthritis. *Journal of Nursing Scholarship* (second quarter), 121–126.

Dormandy, T. (2006). *The worst of evils. The fight against pain.* New Haven, CT: Yale University Press.

Gerstle, D., All, A., & Wallace, D. C. (2001). Quality of life and chronic nonmalignant pain. *Pain Management Nursing, 2*(3), 98–109.

Green, C., Wheeler, J., LaPorte, F., Marchant, B., & Guerrero, E. (2002). How well is chronic pain managed? Who does it well? *Pain Medicine, 3*(1), 56–65.

Gunderman, R. B. (2002). Is suffering the enemy? *Hastings Center Report, 32*(2), 40–44.

The Joint Commission. (2001). *Health care issues news room.* Retrieved from http://www.jointcommission.org/News Room/health_ care_issues.htm#9

Kerns, R. D., Turk, D. C., & Rudy, T. E. (1985). The West Haven-Yale Multidimensional Pain Inventory (WHYMPI). *Pain, 23*, 345–356.

Koestler, A. J., & Myers, A. (2002). *Understanding chronic pain.* Jackson: University Press of Mississippi.

Kugalmann, R. (2003). Pain as a symptom, pain as a sign. *Health: An Interdisciplinary Journal for the Social Study of Health, Illness and Medicine, 7*(1), 29–50.

Laccetti, M. S., & Kazanowski, M. K. (2009). *Pain management* (2nd ed.). Sudbury, MA: Jones and Bartlett.

Lansbury, G. (2000). Chronic pain management: A qualitative study of elderly people's preferred coping strategies and barriers to management. *Disability and Rehabilitation, 22*(1/2), 2–14.

Lazarus, H., & C. J. Neumann. (2001) Assessing undertreatment of pain: The patient's perspectives. *Journal of Pharmaceutical Care in Pain and Symptom Control, 9* (4), 5–34.

Lin, E. H. B., Katon, W., Von Korff, M., Tang, L., Williams, J. W., Kroenke, K. . . . Unutzer, J. (2003). Effect of improving depression care on pain and functional outcomes among older adults with arthritis: A randomized controlled trial. *Journal of the American Medical Association, 290*(18), 2428–2434.

Mack, A. (2003). Examination of the evidence for off-label use of gabapentin. *Journal of Managed Care Pharmacy, 9*(6), 559–568.

Matteliano, D. (2003). Holistic nursing management of pain and suffering: A historical view with contemporary applications. *Journal of the New York State Nurses Association, 34*(1), 4–8.

McCracken, L. M., & Iverson, G. L. (2001). Predicting complaints of cognitive functioning in patients with chronic pain. *Journal of Pain and Symptom Management, 21*(5), 392–396.

Meeks, T. W., Dunn, L. B., Kim, D. S., Golshan, S., Sewell, D. D., Atkinson, J. H., & Lebowitz, B. D. (2008). Chronic pain and depression among geriatric psychiatry inpatients. *International Journal of Geriatric Psychiatry, 23*, 637–642.

Meinhart, N. T., & McCaffery, M. (1983). *Pain. A nursing approach to assessment and analysis.* Norwalk, CT: Prentice Hall.

Merriam-Webster Online Dictionary. (2010). Addiction. Retrieved from http://www.merriam-webster.com/dictionary/addiction

National Center for Health Statistics. (2006.) *Health, United States, 2006: With chartbook on trends in the health of Americans.* Hyattsville, MD: Author.

National Center for Health Statistics. (2009). *Health, United States, 2009: With special feature on medical technology.* Hyattsville, MD: Author.

Peolsson, M., Hyden, L. C., & Larsson, U.S. (2000.) Living with chronic pain: A dynamic learning process. *Scandinavian Journal of Occupational Therapy, 7,* 114–125.

Pfizer: Parke-Davis Product Monograph. (2009, April). Neurontin. Retrieved from http://www.pfizer.com/files/products/uspi_neurontin.pdf

Rosenberg, E., Genao, I., Chen, I., Mechaber, A., Wood, J., Faselis, C., Kurz, J., Menon, M., O'Rorke, J. Panda, M., Pasanen, M., Staton, L., Calleson, D. & Cykert, S., 2008). Complementary and alternative medicine use by primary care patients with chronic pain. *Pain Medicine, 9*(8), 1065–1072.

Schechter, N. L., Berde, C. B., & Yaster, M. (2002). *Pain in infants, children and adolescents* (2nd ed.). Philadelphia, PA: Lippincott Williams and Wilkins.

Selye, H. (1976). *The stress of life.* New York, NY: McGraw-Hill.

Song, J., Change, R. W., Manheim, L. M., & Dunlop, D. D. (2006). Gender differences across race/ethnicity in use of healthcare among Medicare-aged Americans. *Journal of Women's Health, 15*(10), 1205–1213.

Taylor, B. (2001). Promoting self-help strategies by sharing the lived experience of arthritis. *Contemporary Nurse: A Journal for the Australian Nursing Profession, 10*(1–2), 117–125.

Thomas, S. (2000.) A phenomenologic study of chronic pain. *Western Journal of Nursing Research, 22*(6), 683–705.

World Health Organization (WHO). (1990). *Cancer pain relief and palliative care: report of a WHO expert committee.* World Health Organization Technical Report Series 804. Geneva, Switzerland: Author.

Wise, E. A., Price, D. D., Myers, C. D., Heft, M. W., & Robinson, M. E. (2002). Gender role expectations of pain: Relationship to experimental pain perception. *Pain, 96*(3), 335–342.

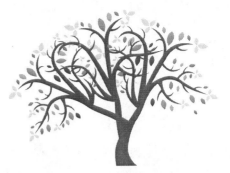

SEVEN

Spirituality and Suffering

■ Mertie L. Potter, Sylvia M. Durette,
and Mary K. Kazanowski

> Suffering is inevitable; misery is optional.
> —Anonymous

Objectives

1. Analyze questions related to challenges of spirituality and suffering.
2. Develop responses to proposed questions.
3. Compare and contrast different religious perspectives on suffering.
4. Differentiate religion, faith, and spirituality.
5. Relate the nurse's role in assessing and addressing spirituality, faith, and religion in clinical practice.
6. Evaluate evidence-based practice in relation to spirituality and suffering.

Student Project

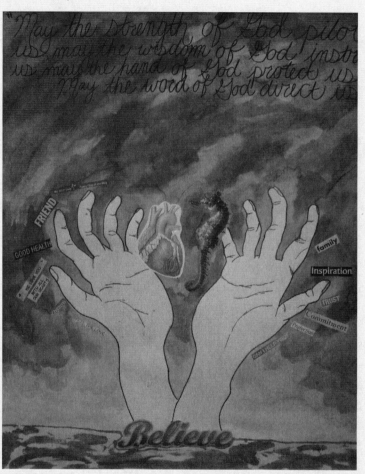

Emily Traicoff's project shows that people can find meaning in suffering through the belief that God values all life and holds all life in his hands as depicted by the hands of God holding a child's heart and a tiny seahorse.

Source: Courtesy of Emily Traicoff, student nurse, 2010.

Case Study 7–1: Robert's* Story

Robert was born in the 1970s. As a young child growing up in a Rwandan middle-class home, Robert always sensed God was with him. He cannot recall a time when he was not aware of God's presence in his life. His parents, especially his mother, practiced a strong Christian faith. At age 15, Robert reports he recognized that "what my mother had been teaching me was true" and "accepted the Lord."

Due to severe and harsh tribal conflicts between Hutus and Tutsis in Rwanda, Robert, at age 17, began a long journey to stay alive. He fled from Rwanda in 1994 and traveled to refugee camps in several countries. During that time, he studied at two different universities for brief periods. He then fled on foot for approximately 7 months and walked "about 1,457 miles in the bush." He and about 347 other people were then deported back to Rwanda.

Robert endured many years of violence and suffering. His father and siblings were burned alive in their home in 1998. He has not been able to determine what happened to his mother. Upon his arrival back in Rwanda, he was held prisoner in a torturing hall for 3 years. Beatings, torture, being forced to eat and drink human feces, and unspeakable treatment of his genitals resulted in recurring bladder infections and other conditions. He witnessed many murders while imprisoned. He saw women raped and have "red pepper put in their private parts and in the eyes of their children."

At the end of 2 years, a grenade was thrown to kill the remaining 67 prisoners where Robert was held. Sixteen died immediately, dozens sustained injuries, and Robert went into a coma due to severe hemorrhaging. The military, thinking Robert was dead, placed his body with the other corpses in a mortuary hall. As was the custom, the Red Cross came 2 days later to collect the bodies for burial. At the morgue, someone realized Robert was alive. They pulled his body out from the others and took him to the Red Cross clinic. Nurses began reviving this presumed-to-be-dead young man who had severe grenade wounds to his right leg as well as additional injuries. The wounds by this time, as he describes them, were "stinking" badly.

*Name changed and information disguised to protect Robert's identity

Robert then began a long road to recovery. He fled from and to different hospitals trying to escape tribal conflicts. He eventually made his way to an African country where he heard through his church of a university he might attend. During that time, he met his "American family" and was able to graduate with a bachelor's degree in communication.

This author came to know Robert in an African country where they served together on a medical mission team. Later that same year, doors opened for Robert to come to the United States and study for his master's degree. His journey to the United States was one of strong faith and perseverance. Robert feels very "blessed" to be in the in this country with a family who grew to know him in Africa and "adopted" him (Anonymous, personal communication 11–21–09).

Questions on the Case Study
1. Why do you think God would allow such suffering in the world?
2. How does suffering challenge *your* religion, faith, or spirituality?

Introduction

In recent years, it has become more widely believed and accepted by nurses and other health professionals that individuals are an integration of body, mind, and spirit (Carpenter, Girvin, Kitner, & Ruth-Sahd, 2008; Chochinov & Cann, 2005). Therefore, the relationship between religion and health is receiving increased attention in research. Religion can be measured fairly readily. However, it is more challenging to measure faith and spirituality.

Spirituality also has become more accepted as an important factor by researchers, educators, and clinicians who provide care for the dying (Chochinov & Cann, 2005). Whenever patients are suffering, but especially near the end of life, their spirituality may give meaning to their suffering. Yet not all patients are able to find such meaning easily and some experience spiritual distress. Thus, nurses may be confronted with how to help patients find meaning in their suffering. Assisting patients in spiritual distress may be challenging for nurses if the nurses are uncertain about their own spirituality (Baldacchino, 2006). Providing spiritual nursing care is both important and complex. The patient's spirituality not only assists in the discovery of meaning but also in attainment of hope—even when the outcomes from the patient's condition may be negative (Greenstreet, 2006).

Definitions

There are discrete definitions for religion, spirituality, and faith. Understanding the distinctions among them assists the nurse in recognizing what the patient is experiencing and expressing.

Religion

Religion can be defined a number of ways:

1. a. Belief in and reverence for a supernatural power or powers regarded as a creator and governor of the universe.
   b. A personal or institutionalized system grounded in such belief and worship.
2. The life or condition of a person in a religious order.
3. A set of beliefs, values, and practices based on the teachings of a spiritual leader.
4. A cause, principle, or activity pursued with zeal or conscientious devotion (*American Heritage Dictionary*, 2006, p. 1474).

Religion generally involves a system of organized beliefs and forms of worship and practices (Emblen, 1992). Most of the major religions share some of the same basic tenets:

- Individuals have a spiritual dimension.
- Individuals have a soul or spirit.
- Life is sacred.
- Life has a higher purpose (Ledger, 2005, p. 221).

Religion can provide answers and help provide meaning to circumstances related to suffering (Greenstreet, 2006). When individuals meet with others of similar beliefs and values or participate in similar faith-based communities, they usually are provided with supportive social networks (Weaver & Flannelly, 2004). Religious traditions generally provide people with community, companionship, and support. Companionship and support help people transcend the suffering experience, often by helping them achieve peace (Smith, 1996, p. 163).

Conflicts may arise between care providers and patients who have different worldviews. As an example, patients may recognize a treatment or intervention as helpful and have no direct objection to the intervention but choose to rely upon their faith or prayer instead of allowing the intervention. Interestingly, not as many conflicts tend to arise if patients decline interventions based upon religious beliefs (Curlin, Roach, Gorawara-Bhat, Lantos, & Chin 2005). Such situations can cause great distress for a care provider. The frustration most likely will not be expressed by the care provider, and understandably so, in order to respect the patient's autonomy and belief system. It is important, however, to be aware that such situations may arise. A delicate balance exists between what can be done and what should be done in certain medical circumstances, and that balance often is impacted by a patient's religious beliefs (Curlin et al., 2005).

Faith

The American Heritage Dictionary (2006) defines faith the in following way:

1. Confident belief in the truth, value, or trustworthiness of a person, idea, or thing
2. Belief that does not rest on logical proof or material evidence
3. Loyalty to a person or thing; allegiance
4. Often Faith *Christianity*—The theological virtue defined as a secure belief in God and a trusting acceptance of God's will.
5. The body of dogma of a religion: *the Muslim faith.*
6. A set of principles or beliefs (p. 636).

Weaver and Flannery (2004) provide a slightly different perspective stating that faith is "a framework for finding meaning and perspective" (p. 1210).

Spirituality

Spirituality is defined as

1. the state, quality, manner, or fact of being spiritual;
2. the clergy;
3. something such as property or revenue, that belongs to the church or to a cleric (*American Heritage Dictionary*, 2006, p. 1676).

Table 7–1   Five Spiritual Needs

Love	Faith	Hope	Virtue	Beauty
Love, affection, commitment, compassion, relationships, community, connection, fellowship, companionship, esteem from others	Faith, worldview, personal philosophy, worship, awe, wonder, reverence, humility, reaching for the transcendent, prayer, contact	Hope, meaning and purpose, courage, perseverance, perspective, vision	Virtue, integrity, morality, ethics, consistency, character, loyalty, goodness, kindness, patience, honesty, humility, wisdom, justice, gratitude	Beauty, art, music, aesthetics, balance, elegance, nature, creativity, expression, imagination, curiosity, exploration, renewal, rest, quiet, meditation, humor, diversion, fun, play, laughter, joy

Source: Adapted from Bartel, 2006, pp. 188–189.

According to Bartel (2004), five major spiritual needs include

- love (community, connection);
- faith (worldview);
- hope (vision);
- virtue (ethics); and
- beauty (renewal) (pp. 188–189).

Within each of these general categories, are broad and fuller elements which are shown in Table 7–1.

Spirit–Mind–Body Connection

In addition to examining various definitions of religion, faith, and spirituality, it is important to have an understanding of what is meant by spirit within the body–mind–spirit connection. Again, exploring definitions provides a helpful starting point. Spirit is considered to be

1. a. The vital principle or animating force within living beings.
   b. The part of human associated with the mind, will, and feelings.
2. The soul, considered as departing from the body of a person at death (*American Heritage Dictionary*, 2006, p. 1676).

One's spirit helps define the uniqueness of an individual. One's spirit also can help an individual transcend beyond his or her suffering at times.

Connectedness Between Religion, Faith, and Spirituality

Examining these definitions, a connectedness between one's religion, faith, and spirituality emerges. Religion tends to be more an organized system of beliefs often connected by an individual's faith or held beliefs to his or her spirituality. Spirituality is more unique to the individual and is the individual's personal journey to find meaning and purpose and a sense of connectedness to a transcendent dimension (Hermann, 2006).

What people believe directs where and with whom they will be most comfortable sharing their beliefs and values. Being with a group of individuals who hold similar beliefs and values can provide companionship and support, as mentioned earlier. Such support also can provide meaning, purpose, and connectedness that may result in comfort to a suffering patient (McEwen, 2005).

What is the relevance of religion, spirituality, and faith when providing nursing care? The interconnectedness of the three impact the individual's spirit or vital force. Nurses can assist patients in drawing upon such strong resources if they themselves are comfortable with their own spirituality. If nurses are comfortable with the topic of spirituality, and especially with their own spirituality, they can promote hope within patients by assisting patients to draw upon their own religion, spirituality, and faith beliefs.

The Relationship Between Spirituality and Suffering

Studies have demonstrated that spirituality can alleviate suffering. Hermann (2006) demonstrates that spirituality fosters coping, hope, and a sense of hardiness. McManus (2006) states that spirituality and religious beliefs promote recovery from illness. Longer survival rates in individuals diagnosed with HIV/AIDS were found to be related to four factors (Chochinov & Cann, 2005):

- sense of peace;
- faith in God;
- religious behavior; and
- compassionate view of others.

Individuals generally handle stress more constructively when they are able to find meaning in their situations (Desbiens & Fillion, 2007). In fact, a greater appreciation of life is associated with a spiritual quality of life, even if one is experiencing pain and fatigue (Brady, Peterman, Fitchett, Mo, & Cella, 1999). Viewing illness solely in light of somatic pathology or psychopathology reveals the limitations of medicine; a person's uniqueness and ability to heal physically and mentally often reside in that person's spirituality (Pavlović et al., 2008)

Conversely, patients' suffering can be exacerbated when they are struggling with spiritual as well as physical causes. In a study of 57 hospitalized patients with end-stage cancer, Mako, Galek, and Poppito (2006) found that patients described their spiritual pain as being in predominantly one of three different realms:

1. intra-psychic (suffering that involves despair, loss, regret, or anxiety; 48%);
2. related to the divine (feeling abandoned by God, being without faith and/or a religious or spiritual community; 38%);
3. interpersonal (feeling unwanted by family members, feeling disconnected from others; 13%).

Intensity of spiritual pain correlated significantly ($r = 0.43$, $p < 0.001$) with depression, but there was no significant correlation between intensity of spiritual pain and either physical pain or severity of illness (Mako et al., 2006).

Spiritual pain or spiritual suffering often is indicative of spiritual needs being threatened or unmet. Bartel (2008, p. 194) describes the experience one has of sensing a discord between an individual's faith and critical events occurring in one's life as "spiritual dissonance." Millspaugh (2005a, p. 920) asserts that spiritual pain or suffering is related to a number of factors. He depicts these factors in the following equation:

$$\text{Spiritual pain or suffering} = \frac{(\text{Awareness of Death} + \text{Loss of Relationships} + \text{Loss of Self})(\text{Loss of Purpose} + \text{Loss of Control})}{\text{Life Affirming and Transcending Purpose} + \text{Internal Sense of Control}}$$

Millspaugh further contends that a larger numerator results in greater spiritual pain, and a larger denominator results in lesser spiritual pain. He equates spirituality overall with "being."

Student Questions

The authors of this book collected questions posed by students who had taken a course about suffering. Students asked questions from their own perspectives and from that of the patients for whom they provided care. Some of these questions were addressed to clergy; some were addressed to the authors. Below is a representation of those questions with answers in italics from the authors. There are no absolute answers to the questions. These are guidelines to help readers begin their own journey toward finding their own answers.

Coping

1. If you cannot relate to a person's suffering, how do you help the individual cope?

    Attentive listening and compassionate care can convey encouragement to patients. Also, by reviewing the literature on suffering and spending time reflecting on the suffering witnessed, the nurse may develop insight to assist with better understanding of the patient's suffering experience.

    Religious literature can provide an appreciation of the human dimensions of suffering. Nurses can obtain resources for themselves and help patients reflect upon and discuss their feelings of suffering, especially with a chaplain or one knowledgeable about the experience; this can also assist in the patient's understanding of the experience (Smith, 1996, p. 163).

2. Do people who are actively involved with religion generally cope better with suffering?

    What some call prayer and others call meditation are practices that can slow a person's heart rate, blood pressure and respiratory rate. These physiologic changes can help the person to cope better with suffering. In addition, the person's ability to cope may be enhanced by the peace they experience through prayer or meditation.

Faith

3. How does a person's faith change as he or she endures suffering?

   There are many ways individuals' faith can be impacted as they endure suffering. For some, their faith will increase because they will sense that God or a Higher Power got them "through it." For others, their faith may decrease or be dismissed if they feel God or a Higher Power did not respond in the way they had hoped.

4. When I think of my faith, I think of my faith in God. Do people express faith in other things?

   Absolutely. Some have faith in their own health, in medical providers, in family members, in money, in power, in themselves, in their pets, and so on. Individuals express their faith in ways that are unique to them. Some may express their faith more closely to traditional religions, and some may express their faith nontraditionally.

5. Does faith play a role with family members involved with a patient who is suffering?

   It is important to assess whether family members practice a faith and if their belief system is the same or different from the patient's. If it is different, there may be conflict. If they share a similar faith, it may help the entire family.

6. How does suffering affect a young child's faith?

   Young children usually take cues from their caregivers, especially parents and guardians. Older children, although still watching for cues from their parents and guardians, take many of their cues from their peers. Therefore, children, no matter what age, will watch how those around them are responding to suffering, focus upon that response, and often try to follow it.

7. Do children have their own faith or is it the faith of their parents?

   As mentioned, children usually watch their parents or guardians for cues. This includes how children develop their belief systems while young. Children may be angry at God or a Higher Power for allowing them to suffer; they may acquire this view if it has been role modeled to them. It would be unusual for children to have completely different views and beliefs from their parents or guardians although it is possible if they admire someone else as much as the parents or guardians.

8.   Why does it seem as though bad things happen to good faithful people?

Bad things do happen to good people. This is a mystery. Often you will hear people say, "Life is not fair." Some would think, regardless of whether they are suffering, that they have been treated very fairly. Others, who may or may not be suffering, might think they have been treated very unfairly. It depends greatly upon one's perspective, that is, a person's view on this topic is well depicted by the saying "Do you view your cup as half full or half empty?"

9.   What is the best way for a nurse to ask about a patient's faith?

Do you practice a faith that is meaningful to you? Do you have specific religious beliefs? Are spiritual matters important to you? Generally, patients will respond in one of three ways: (1) "No, and I'm not interested"; (2) "I used to, but I don't feel worthy any more or I feel guilty about . . ."; and (3) "I couldn't cope if it weren't for my faith." Nurses can take cues from the patients' responses on whether to pursue that topic.

God

10.   Why does God permit human suffering?

There is no simple answer for the existence of suffering in any religious tradition. Some religions believe it is a mystery that will never be completely grasped or comprehended. Different religions have different views. (See discussion on specific religions.)

11.   When people ask why God has allowed them to suffer, what should the nurse say?

Assess whether they have a specific faith tradition and offer to have a chaplain or someone with knowledge of this faith tradition speak with them.

12.   If the nurse does not believe in God, how would he or she respond when a patient asks them for spiritual support? What should the nurse do if a patient asks the nurse to pray with them?

Nurses need to respect the beliefs of patients. If the nurse is not able to provide the spiritual support that the patient is requesting, the nurse needs to arrange for another staff member or clergy to provide spiritual support. It is the nurse's responsibility to facilitate coping and a good outcome. Research demonstrates that for people with faith, praying and having spiritual sup-

port promotes positive outcomes. Nurses need to refer to the Nurse Practice Act of the state in which they are working and the terms of the contract of their employing agency to identify how those documents identify nursing responsibilities.

If there is no opportunity to arrange for another staff member to pray with the patient, at the very least, the nurse should remain with the patient, showing respect for the person's beliefs, while the patient or family prays, unless doing this presents the nurse with an ethical conflict and/or causes moral distress. Nurses generally are held to a standard requiring them to practice essential moral duties, such as doing good, avoiding harm, respecting freedom of choice, speaking truthfully, being loyal, and promoting justice. If the "prayer" of the patient is in conflict with any of these generally accepted values, it may be appropriate that the nurse not participate.

Nurses Sharing Feelings and/or Crying

13. It is not right to be emotionally cold and it is not right to be emotionally attached. Where is the happy medium?

    There is a balance between being emotionally cold and emotionally attached. The areas of self-disclosure and boundaries are related to this topic. In regard to self-disclosure, the nurse needs to determine if it can be limited, helpful to the patient, important to the nurse–patient relationship, and keeps the focus on the patient rather than the nurse. Some nurses are more comfortable than others sharing appropriate feelings with patients. Others are not able to go there, and that is okay.

14. What if I cry in front of a patient?

    It is okay to cry, and in fact some families actually get upset if the nurse shows no emotion. The nurse, however, needs to be able to function. Potter (2006, p. 283) coined the term "therapeutic tear" to describe when a nurse becomes empathically tearful with a patient while maintaining the ability to direct the situation in a meaningful and positive manner.

    The registered nurse (RN) often is the healthcare provider (HCP) who spends more time than any other HCP with the patient. Because RNs witness so much suffering, they must learn how to effectively care for patients' suffering. Regardless of emotions, the nurse must find the strength to meet the patient's needs. The nurse with a strong faith may draw upon that faith to cope with a difficult experience. Often, the nurse is better able to function in such situations than expected.

Nursing Interventions

15. A patient is suffering, and the nurse asks if there is anything she can do to help. If the patient says, "There is nothing you can do," how should the nurse respond?

    The nurse can make a comment on what she is observing, such as, "I sense you are in a lot of pain because I see you wincing. I can try to help by changing your position. I also would like to sit here and be with you if that is okay."

16. How should the nurse respond to those who blame themselves for the suffering they are enduring? Is it normal to feel that one is being punished for wrong done previously?

    It is not uncommon for people to feel that their suffering is punishment and to feel guilty. The nurse can ask what makes them feel they deserve punishment. It is important to validate the person's feelings. The nurse might ask how the patient would treat someone in the same situation. People often are harder on themselves than they would be on others in the same situation.

17. Do you think it is ever permissible to put someone out of pain if it means ending that person's life?

    The American Nurses Association (ANA) and many religions do not support assisted suicide. However, the ANA and many religions support symptom management for pain and support acceptable medical interventions for relief of pain, often when these are aggressive. As long as accepted standards of appropriate doses of medication are followed (even aggressive doses, as long as they are ordered by an experienced HCP, e.g., one with hospice/palliative care training), aggressive management is acceptable. As long as the patient is in agreement with the treatment plan and recognizes that the expected outcome is not death, although death may occur as an adverse effect.

    For example, if a patient has cancer pain, states he wants to die, and is narcotic naive, the HCP should not order 30 mg IVP morphine. That dose could be lethal. The HCP would order an acceptable dose of morphine (or other drug, e.g., 2 mg IV), with orders to repeat it as needed, if the patient's respiratory status and level of consciousness were acceptable (e.g., RR > 10; sleepy but able to be roused).

The higher the dose of narcotic a patient is tolerating (e.g., 200 mg IV morphine an hour), the higher bolus dose the patient can safely tolerate. For example, a patient receiving 200 mg IV morphine each hour could probably safely tolerate one quarter of that dose, or 50 mg IV. There is a manner in which an opioid is safely increased related to dose and frequency; it has to do with half life and drug accumulation.

18. How can you assist patients to get in touch with their spirituality without seeming to denigrate the extent of their suffering?

    Engaging or connecting with patients in such a way that they perceive you truly care for their welfare is key. Reading Spirituality, Suffering, and Illness *(Wright, 2005) will offer specific ideas on how to engage individuals and families in conversations about suffering and spirituality that have the potential to invite healing and diminish or alleviate emotional, physical, and spiritual suffering. Learning how to initiate these conversations is a skill that is learned over time.*

19. Can patients request a particular clergy member to come visit them in a hospital at any time?

    Most hospitals have chaplains to meet with patients who request visits. Patients always can request to see a clergy member, their own clergy, or someone representative of their belief system.

20. What do we tell patients who are worried about not going to heaven after death?

    Ask them what their concerns are. Assist them to determine whether they need/want to do something to be more at peace about that topic or if they would like to speak with someone of their belief system.

21. What are comforting words you can say to a person near the end?

    "You are loved very much by your family here" (if that is accurate and appropriate).

    "You have many things to show for your hard work here (on earth)."

    "Your children are very kind—that says a lot about you and how they feel about you" (if that is accurate and appropriate).

    "I am pleased I was allowed to care for you. I appreciate _____ (your courage, your gentle spirit, your love for your family, etc.)."

    Ira Byock (2004), asserts that people headed into serious medical procedures and facing the possibility of death always are thinking about those they care about. He suggests that care providers encourage such individuals to say what is needed, such as "I love you," "Please forgive me," "I forgive you," "Thank you."

22. How should the nurse respond to a person who blames himself for the suffering he is enduring? Is it normal to feel that one is being punished for wrongdoing done previously?

People frequently express the idea that suffering is a punishment imposed by God or a Supreme Being for past faults. That question continues to plague mankind. It is important to respond kindly and gently to individuals who believe they are suffering for past wrongdoings. Listening to the patient's concerns about such guilt is important, as is respecting their belief system. Acknowledging people's openness and desire to move on are critical. Helping them do so may require connecting them with others of their belief system.

23. I would like to learn ways to help a person who is suffering. It is hard to find time in our busy assignments. Are there ways that are quick but show the person that you care?

Check in on these people often throughout your shift, and ask them what they need. Clearly communicate to them that their needs are important to you. (Often these people are avoided by other healthcare professionals who simply do not have the patience or compassion to listen.)

Validate their feelings. "You sound upset."

If pain is present, offer and obtain medication, and check back to assess its effectiveness.

24. I would like to be more confident in myself and my skills in talking to people who are suffering. Many times I find myself just sitting there and listening, but many times I do not know how to respond. I wish I had more confidence or knew what to say to make the person feel better.

With time, the nurse feels more comfortable in this role. Initially, the nurse can focus upon giving the patient direct attention. The nurse needs to validate patients' feelings. Reading, practicing assisting patients spiritually, and using clinical supervision can be helpful to the nurse.

Assessment of Patient's Spirituality and Religion

Competent nursing care involves addressing the patient's body, mind, and spirit. Nurses are most often comfortable intervening in patients' bodily needs, somewhat comfortable in intervening in patients' mental and emotional needs, and rarely comfortable responding to spiritual needs. Dealing with tangible needs often is viewed as being safe, because nurses often perceive those needs as more acceptable to identify and discuss in Western culture. Mental/emotional needs are sometimes more difficult and seemingly "sensitive" to identify and address as they involve a person's "thoughts" and "behaviors." Because a person's spirit is at the very core of the individual, nurses may or may not feel comfortable trying to work with a patient to identify and address spiritual needs, especially if they have not recognized or examined their own spirituality (Carpenter et al., 2008; Catanzaro & McMullen, 2001; McEwen, 2005).

At times, nurses "silence" patients' spiritual pain. According to Taylor (2007), ways in which nurses may do this include

- redirecting the conversation away from the topic of spiritual pain;
- diminishing the patient's spiritual pain;
- using humor inappropriately;
- answering in a superficial manner;
- imposing the nurse's view or ideas;
- focusing upon tangential information; and
- being overly positive and disregarding the patient's spiritual pain.

Rather than silencing the patient's pain, nurses can and should promote a healing environment so that they can assess the patient's pain. Taylor (2007) states that nurses can do this by

- keeping the response patient-centered;
- remaining neutral and encouraging the patient to share more;.
- exploring contributors to the patient's spiritual pain; and
- assisting the patient to accurately name feelings and examine emotions related to the spiritual pain.

Nurses have a responsibility to meet patients' spiritual and/or religious needs (Chochinov & Cann, 2005; Ledger, 2005; & Pesut, 2008). Where can the nurse begin? Nurses must assess their own spirituality by thinking through what their views are related to religion and spirituality and then realizing how those views may impact their interactions with patients (Carpenter et al., 2008; Pesut, 2008). However, nurses and other care providers need to guard against ever imposing their beliefs on patients (Smith, 1996).

Millspaugh (2005b) examined spiritual pain and suggested pastoral interventions; his work is helpful for the nurse to consider when helping patients who are suffering:

- Self-appraisal: Has the nurse been close to death? What suffering has the nurse experienced? What are the nurse's views on suffering?
- Presence: Is the nurse aware of the power of presence? Is the nurse prepared to journey with the patient through the patient's suffering?
- Key issues in suffering: How well is the patient dealing with purpose and meaning, death, issues of self (loss of known self, awareness of a diminished self) in relation to the suffering?
- Degree of locus of control (external versus internal): How much control does the patient feel she or he has (internal) versus no control (external control)?
- Is the nurse aware of the extent of the patient's suffering? What other areas are being impacted and causing suffering for the patient besides those that are obvious?
- Has the nurse formulated a spiritual plan of care? What is the extent of the patient's suffering? What are the patient's coping skills? Has the nurse looked at the patient's losses and sense of being alone?

Nurses can recognize spiritual distress when patients are

- questioning personal existence;
- being angry toward God;
- being depressed;
- being discontent;
- feeling separated emotionally from others;
- avoiding usual religious rituals and observations; and
- requesting spiritual assistance (McEwen, 2005).

Alleviating Spiritual Suffering Within the Nurse

Another question asked by a student nurse was, "How can we as nurses alleviate suffering in ourselves? We see a lot of things that we do not agree with and sometimes those things are hard to come to terms with. Are there ways that we can help ourselves in our own suffering? I have faith but sometimes faith is not enough."

Specific strategies to intervene with patients and to assist nurses themselves are to have spiritual goals and measure outcomes. Carpenter et al. (2008, p. 18) encourage nurses to contemplate their own spirituality, develop ways to foster their spirituality, acknowledge purpose and meaning in their work, and approach the patient relationship with intention. Spiritual care involves connecting to the patient in relationship. Focusing upon the patient, putting aside distractions, and touching the patient's hand, arm, or shoulder, if appropriate, can help the nurse connect more with the patient (Carpenter et al., 2008).

Pesut (2008) suggests that spiritual interventions take place on two levels:

- supporting religious and spiritual practices—providing privacy for religious rituals, praying, referring to spiritual counselors, enhancing access to sacred materials, and facilitating religious practices; and
- therapeutic use of self—being present, touching, being respectful, giving time, and directing conversation to topics of "meaning, purpose, hope, values, connection, and forgiveness."

One's spiritual dimension often is at the core of providing meaning in suffering and being a springboard for hope (Greenstreet, 2006). Morse and Doberneck (1995) recognized seven aspects of hope that can be used as a springboard to promote hope in patients with chronic illness:

- assessing a predicament or threat realistically;
- imagining alternatives and setting goals;
- preparing for negative outcomes;
- assessing resources realistically;
- seeking mutually supportive relationships;
- evaluating continually signs to strengthen selected goals; and
- resolving to persevere.

Instillation of hope is critical for the suffering patient and for the nurse witnessing the suffering. Nurses must care for themselves proactively, especially because they are witnesses to so much suffering. Selecting self-care strategies that best protect oneself against the dangers of "suffering overload" will help determine how long the nurse can sustain the pressures of bearing witness to suffering in the profession.

Considering the need for forgiveness as part of a nurse's self-care and care for patients is important. The need for forgiveness may arise in situations such as when a nurse has a patient who refuses treatments that could help or family members who displace their anger for their loved one's terminal illness on the nurse (O'Brien, 2011). Healthy relationships with others help promote inner peace and self-acceptance (Mahlungulu & Uys, 2004).

Major World Religions

In order for the nurse to assist patients with their journey through suffering, it is helpful to have some understanding of the different religions patients may practice. It is important to look to the different religions and practices of faith to see how patients and families explain their suffering. Smith (1996, p. 163) states, "At the heart of the religious response to suffering is the search for meaning." The main religions chosen to be discussed include those with the largest number of followers. The U.S. population is representative of many nations, cultures, religions, and spiritual beliefs. However, individuals in the United States identify themselves predominantly with Christianity as shown in Table 7–2.

Within all of the faiths discussed there is an opportunity for growth and hope for patients, their families, and the nurses who take care of them. Murray (2010, p. 57) asserts, "As nursing professionals explore their own sense of purpose and spirituality and discover what gives life meaning, they will become better able to understand and relate to their patients."

Spiritual Assessment

Assessments are utilized to assist nurses in understanding patient beliefs—religious and spiritual. An example of such an assessment is a part of the Functional Assessment of Cancer Therapy-General, the Spiritual Well-being Scale. This

Table 7–2 Religious Affiliations of the United States, 2009

Religious Affiliation	Percentage
Christian	81.0
No Affiliation	11.8
Buddhism, Hinduism, Islam, Judaism, and Others	6.9

Source: Pew Forum on Religion and Public Life, 2009.

Table 7–3   Major World Religions and Summary of Beliefs on Suffering

Religion	Meaning of Suffering
Christianity	Mystery, develop closer relationship with God
Islam	Normal part of imperfect life, self-knowledge acquisition
Hinduism	Natural part of life, opportunity for Nirvana
Buddhism	Due to life's impermanence, result of Karma
Judaism	Natural part of living

Spiritual Well-being Scale gives the nurse information about the patient's religious practices and beliefs and monitors any changes that illness may have caused. The measure assesses behaviors associated with religion, faith, and spirituality, or meaning and purpose (Kruse, Ruder, & Martin, 2007, p. 299). Although an individual assessment is essential as people may not share the commonly expressed views of their religion, each of the major religions has a view on suffering. These views are summarized in Table 7–3.

Christianity

Christianity is the largest of the faith groups to be discussed and comprises five major identified religions: Catholics, Protestants, Jehovah's Witnesses, Orthodox Christians, and Anglicans. By far the largest of all the religious groups, these comprise about 2.1 billion members worldwide (Major Religions of the World, 2007) and account for 33% of the world's population (Islam: The second largest world religion and growing, 2010). All of the religions within Christianity follow specific beliefs, rituals, and traditions that have the potential to bring meaning and comfort to the person who is suffering, the significant others who are witnessing the suffering, and the nurse. Many Christians seek to understand the meaning of their suffering and that of those around them.

Different beliefs surround the concept of suffering. Some followers see suffering as a mystery to believe in but not to solve. Christianity embraces suffering as a mystery that can never be fully grasped or comprehended (Ferrell, 1996). Some within Christianity view suffering as remembrance of the suffering Christ. They turn to the suffering Christ as an example of the innocents who have suffered.

Suffering in this manner becomes a means to live in closer relationship with God through one's own suffering. Patients may express the belief that they deserve to suffer, that somehow they deserve to live with pain or to have a shortened life span.

Identifying with Christ's suffering may bring a patient solace. A family member may find peace in connecting with the patient's religion. A nurse may assist a patient in a Christian ritual as a means to comfort. Still others may not question the reason for their own suffering. One may hear them say, "It is God's will," or "God's will be done." They seemingly accept their diagnoses and the ensuing symptoms without question. In fact, to question the reason for their suffering may bring on undue stress and spiritual discomfort.

Whatever the patient's point of reference, it becomes important for the nurse's relationship with the patient to follow the patient's lead in the discussion. For a patient to feel validated by the nurse, it is important to take one's cues from the patient and significant others as to how they see their suffering.

Providing the patient with support and refuting the beliefs they have held does not help them to overcome their negativity toward their past practices. Consulting with a member of the clergy or a church elder may assist this patient if controversial issues arise.

Christians may have different religious objects near them. Nurses should be aware that all of these objects should be handled with reverence. Some patients will have rosary beads nearby; others may have relics or pictures of Christ and various saints. If patients ask to bring some of these objects with them for tests, it becomes important for the nurse to actively research the feasibility of having some of these objects present. It may not always be possible to have the patient near these possessions, but it is part of the holistic care of our patients to make every attempt to have them nearby. Consulting with clergy, either within the institution or within the community, is done whenever needed and possible.

An important point of clarification is that people may be of different cultures and still share the same faith. Cultural differences in the expression of pain and suffering will be noted even while people may share similar religious beliefs. For example, a Hispanic female suffering with chronic pain may be able to explain her suffering in terms of her faith but her expression of her suffering may be quite different from that of the Asian female suffering with her chronic pain.

Islam

The second great religion to be discussed in terms of suffering is Islam. Approximately one fifth of the worldwide population is Muslim (Haq, 2002). Islam accounts for about 1.5 billion followers (Major Religions of the World, 2007) or 21% of the world's population (Islam: The second largest world religion and growing, 2010). The Koran (Quran, Qu'ran) contains the teachings of this religion, much as the Bible holds the teachings for Christians.

Differences can quickly be noted between the two largest religious groups in relation to their views on suffering. Christians generally seek to understand the mystery of suffering; those practicing Islam do not even ask questions about it. According to the Quran, "Verily, we have created man into a life of pain, toil and trial" (Quran 90:4). Suffering is a part of life and to be expected. Questioning the merits or meaning is seen as beyond the scope of the mere mortal's perspective.

Islam is based on the basic tenets of submission and peace. Because of this, suffering is to be met with patience or "sabr." Suffering is to be expected as a part of life and the response to suffering is noteworthy in that the patient is responding to the expected. It would be very unusual to hear a person who follows this religion (a Muslim) say, "Why me?" Instead, the Muslim patient explains suffering as what is expected in this imperfect life. Muslims believe that a quiet acceptance of their suffering is best and they must do what they must to get well or to accept the end of their life in a peaceful manner.

Another basic tenet is that suffering is not the mere ending of a healthy life. In fact, death is not viewed as an ending but as another dimension of life. What is important to note is that the second dimension of life is lived in direct proportion to how well the first life was lived. Therefore, if patients practicing Islam become terminally ill, the nurse may note a higher level of negative emotions and stress as they reminiscence over their past lived behaviors, especially if those behaviors have not been seen as positive by others. Also, if patients have lived with suffering throughout this dimension of life, they may accept the end of their days with peace and joy as they await a better life in the coming dimension.

Islamic belief involves the idea that suffering is a test for individuals, sent to them from God or Allah. Trials have the potential of allowing the followers to have a better awareness of their own temperament as they witness their response to the suffering at hand. It is important to note here that the Muslims' response to good fortune is as important as their response to suffering.

Muslims pray five times a day. Honor and not incurring any pain to one's fellowman is very important to them. Because of this view, medical information that may be construed as stressful—such as unfavorable test results—should be delivered to an identified person. Giving this news to the suffering patient would be looked at as adding to the person's suffering. Muslims respect the healthcare system in this country; their expectations are high. They expect to be given medications and treatments to take care of a healthcare issue and that follow-up is not necessary because the treatment prescribed will provide a cure or a cure was not meant to be.

A story that is shared by both Christians and Muslims is the story of Job (Ayoub) found in the Old Testament of the Bible and the Quran. Both note Job's response to his suffering and both note him to be an example of suffering as a follower of God and Allah.

Hinduism

Hinduism is the third largest religion, accounting for over 900 million followers (Major Religions of the World, 2007). A belief common to this religion is that suffering is God's will. Hindus do not question the existence of God. They have many arguments proving the existence of God. They go so far as to say that humans are a manifestation of God. The possibility of Nirvana, or a bliss state with God, is possible. Hindus also are known for their belief that suffering exists because of karma. Humankind perpetuates the existence of suffering because of actions and inactions. Tragedies in our world may be due to the imbalance of the systems. They believe the desires of humans that enable them to take more from the world than they return is an issue that brings much suffering to all humans.

For these reasons, these patients may not demonstrate outward signs of discomfort. It may be difficult for the nurse to assess the level of a patient's pain. Patients may refuse to disclose their level of pain and may even deny the existence of pain even though their nonverbal behavior may indicate otherwise. So what is the nurse to do? It becomes important to assess the patient utilizing nonverbal cues. It may also be good practice to consult folk practitioners at the patient's request or to seek advice for a case consultation. Many Hindus maintain close ties with their folk healers and although they may practice Western medicine, they may benefit from these healers.

It also is important to note that this population may accept care for some forms of physical suffering more readily than for psychological suffering. Psychological suffering, conditions Western cultures would list as mental disorders, are not labeled as such in the Hindu religion. People who are showing signs of depression may not be encouraged to seek psychiatric help and their family may become their primary caregivers. Their symptoms may be seen as "God's will" and they accept the symptoms as such and do not seek relief for their symptoms.

Hindus may assume a sick role by changing their social roles, letting others take care of them, and making no attempt to reduce their symptoms. This is acceptable practice in the Hindu religion. Suffering is not seen as an opportunity to demonstrate gratitude or to learn, but more as a consequence of human desires, whether of this particular individual or of the person's ancestors.

Besides being a religion, Hinduism is also a way of life. Some believe because of this, Hinduism becomes very difficult to practice in its truest sense in the United States and Europe.

Buddhism

Buddhism is the fourth category of religions and includes almost 376 million followers (Major Religions of the World, 2007). Buddha has provided this religion with the original teachings called Theravada. This religion does not question the existence of God, and Buddhists are seen as more practical in their approach to life than their Hindu counterparts. They view suffering as inevitable. Buddhists see the potential for suffering in all living activities. There is suffering in birth, in any illness, and of course, in death.

Buddhists also further the concepts of compassion and doing good deeds by following the ethical principle of Ren. It is believed that doing good works and caring for one's fellowman will enable a person to be reincarnated into a better life. Life events are also seen as the result of karma. Those actions taken in an earlier or past life have now come back to influence the quality of the person's present life. It is believed that questioning the reason for the suffering state or to question the past actions of a population are futile. One is to live with the suffering until death.

Buddhists accept different procedures and treatments as possibilities to reduce suffering. They encourage their followers to pursue these activities but not if reducing the suffering changes the person's karma.

Buddhists hold to different concepts that enable them to reach different levels of solace or enlightenment. It is told that Buddha had the ability to live in indulgence and also had the opportunity to live in impoverished environments. Buddha recounted to his followers that when he kept himself with moderation, neither impoverished nor indulgent, there was a better opportunity for enlightenment.

The attitude of moderation lends itself to a better fit with enlightenment. Enlightenment also is possible through meditation. Through meditation, Buddhists will look at the impermanence of life and remind themselves of the inevitability of death. The saying "this too shall pass" encompasses the idea of impermanence. They have the ability to look at life events with a detachment that prevents their getting caught up in the emotion of a situation.

They are reminded in their teachings that the desire and acquisition of possessions may lead them to a state of suffering because they may indeed lose those possessions. They emphasize that the mere desire for some possessions leads them to a state of suffering because at any given time, these possessions may be lost. Possessions for them include relationships with others.

Judaism

Judaism has as its roots the history of Israel and its people. Approximately 14 million people practice this religion and it is the smallest of all of the groups discussed thus far (Major Religions of the World, 2007). As is the case for most religions, Judaism is also a culture. Within Judaism there are different groups: the first group is the Orthodox who follow the traditional rituals and teachings of the Torah; the second group is the Ultra Orthodox or Hasidic; and the third group is the Reform Group which is the most liberal of the three. All three share core beliefs but some such as the Reform Group may practice fewer rituals than the Hasidic Jews.

Overall, this religion ascribes in general to health promotion activities. Followers of Judaism are encouraged to pay attention to their health and place emphasis on healthy practices that will prevent illnesses. "According to Jewish law, individuals may not intentionally damage their bodies or place themselves in danger" (Purnell & Paulanka, 2008, p. 283). The body belongs to God and it must be returned to God intact in death.

Suffering is seen as a natural part of living. Treatment is sought to alleviate suffering. Instructions are followed; continuing treatment is respected. When it becomes obvious that a medical treatment will not meet with success, the Jewish person is allowed to end treatment. Other definitions of the meaning of suffering include (1) the ability to use the experience to build character, and (2) carrying the suffering for other populations. The building of character is seen in other religions in the process of enlightenment and getting to know oneself better. It is thought that the experiences have the ability to help the suffering individuals know more about themselves as they question the process. The act of suffering for others is thought to stem from the history of the persecuted Jews. The long history of ostracism and persecution emphasizes the role the Jews play in providing the world with a role model of living well with suffering.

Respecting the Sabbath is the Jewish custom of honoring a break from work. The Sabbath begins at a set time on Friday evenings and ends at a specific time on Saturday evening. Depending on the group, different healthcare activities are tolerated at this time. For example, those practicing Orthodox Judaism may need to be educated about taking their statin medications as they may construe this activity as work. Work is not to be done on the Sabbath. The nurse should explain to them the necessity of taking this medication as ordered. Jewish patients who are suffering with physical and emotional disorders are exempt from following the fasts and the rituals of Jewish practices.

If suffering becomes overwhelming, committing suicide and remaining in good standing with Judaism do not go hand in hand. The only exceptions to this would be children and those patients deemed to be incompetent. The expression of pain is not denied. Patients who practice Judaism identify pain and expect their symptoms to be alleviated. They expect that their suffering will be recognized by the healthcare providers and that treatment will be available.

Nursing Interventions that Promote Spiritual Care and Alleviate Suffering

It is important to patients that their healthcare providers demonstrate respect for their religious and spiritual beliefs (Chochinov & Cann, 2005; Cohen, Wheeler, & Scott, 2001). Additionally, Pesut (2008, p. 167) asserts that there are three major assumptions related to spirituality and spiritual care in nursing:

- Everyone has a spiritual dimension whether or not it is acknowledged.
- Providing spiritual care is an ethical component of holistic care.
- Many nurses are not prepared to provide spiritual care.

As with other aspects of nursing care, competence in providing spiritual care is necessary. Nursing competencies for providing spiritual care include the following:

- Awareness and use of self dimension
  - Handles own beliefs and feelings professionally with patients of different values and religions
  - Addresses the topic of spirituality with patients from different cultures in a caring manner
- Spiritual dimensions of nursing
  - Collects information related to the patient's spirituality and identifies the need
  - Discusses with patients and team members how spiritual care will be provided, planned and reported
  - Encourages a multidisciplinary effort to meet spiritual needs
- Dimension of assurance of quality and expertise
  - Contributes to quality assurance and improvements in spiritual care within the organization (van Leeuwen & Cusveller, 2004, 241–244).

Case Study 7–1 (continued)

Robert recalls being treated very "empathically" by all his nurses. He remembers they "listened to me," "smiled at me," and "cared for my stinking wounds" without judgment. He was touched when he realized that the nurses of the opposing tribe were "overlooking tribal affiliations" and providing such kind care to him.

Besides nurses from the Red Cross clinic, nurses in other facilities stand out as well. Robert was transferred from the Red Cross clinic to a national hospital run by the opposing tribe. He escaped from that hospital, as he feared for his life. Upon reaching the hospital of another African country to receive further treatment for his wounds, he was moved by nurses who prayed with and for him. When asked how it came about that they prayed with and for him, he does not recall exactly. He speculates they may have noticed he was reading a Bible, a gift he received while in one of the refugee camps. He received a Bible from an organization that distributes Bibles worldwide; he continues "to carry this Bible in all troubles to wherever I went, and until now I still have it."

What Robert does know is that he was comforted by these nurses' compassion and caring in action. They supported his faith and fostered his hope. He notes that "the only way to live life is with faith, because without faith, you can't have hope" and says that Psalms 91 is "the promise God gave me when I was in that torture hall" (Anonymous, personal communication 11–21–09). A portion of that passage reads: "For the Lord says, 'Because he loves me, I will rescue him; I will make him great because he trusts in my name. When he calls on me I will answer; I will be with him in trouble, and rescue him with a full life and give him my salvation.'" (Psalms 91: 14 & 15).

Questions on the Case Study

1. In what ways did the nurses support Robert's spirituality?
2. Try to imagine caring for someone whose wounds are "stinking?" What do these thoughts evoke in you?
3. How would you feel caring for someone whom you always had been told held beliefs and exhibited behaviors totally opposed to yours?
4. What biases do you need to examine to provide care to those whom you might consider to be "enemies?"

Summary

One's spirituality is at the core of one's being. Factors that increase spiritual pain and suffering include awareness of death, loss of relationships, loss of self, loss of purpose, and loss of control. Factors that help decrease spiritual pain and suffering include an affirmed life, a transcending purpose, and an internal sense of control (Millspaugh, 2005a, p. 920).

Many questions arise in relation to spirituality and suffering. The nurse is in a unique position to help patients address their spiritual distress and questions related to suffering and spirituality. Being sensitive to a patient's religion, faith, and spirituality is critical to promoting holistic nursing care, especially in relation to the patient's suffering experience.

Key Points

1. Most of the major religions share some of the same basic tenets.
2. Numerous studies demonstrate a positive relationship between health promotion and spirituality and religious beliefs.
3. One's spirit helps define one's uniqueness.
4. One's spirit can help one transcend suffering at times.
5. Crying with a patient may be therapeutic if done empathically and with the nurse still able to direct the situation in a meaningful and positive manner.
6. Spiritual self-awareness is important for the nurse in relation to helping patients who are in spiritual distress.
7. One's spiritual dimension often provides meaning in suffering and a springboard for hope.

Exercise

Select one of the following questions. Write your response to the question in one or two pages using APA format. Include references to support your response.

1. What is the connection between spirituality and suffering?
2. Discuss your perception of the meaning of the following quotation from the beginning of the chapter: "Suffering is inevitable but misery is optional." What you think that means?
3. How would you respond to a family member of a patient who is suffering and asks, "Why do bad things happen to good people?"
4. How can one's spirituality alleviate suffering?

   Now faith is being sure of what we hope for and certain of what we do not see.
   —Hebrews 11:1

References

American Heritage Dictionary of the English Language (4th ed.). (2006). Boston, MA: Houghton Mifflin.

Baldacchino, D. R. (2006). Nursing competencies for spiritual care. *Journal of Clinical Nursing, 15*(7), 885–896.

Bartel, M. (2004). What is spiritual? What is spiritual suffering? *Journal of Pastoral Care and Counseling, 58*(3),187–201.

Brady, M. J., Peterman, A. H., Fitchett, G., Mo, M., & Cella, D. (1999). A case for including spirituality in quality of life measurement in oncology. *Psychooncology, 8,* 417–428.

Byock, I. (2004). *The four things that matter most: A book about living.* New York: Free Press

Carpenter, K., Girvin, L., Kitner, W., & Ruth-Sahd, L. A. (2008). Spirituality: A dimension of holistic critical care nursing. *Dimensions of Critical Care Nursing, 23*(1), 16–20.

Catanzaro, A. M., & McMullen, K. A. (2001). Increasing nursing students' spiritual sensitivity. *Nursing Educator, 26,* 221–226.

Chochinov, H. M., & Cann, B. J. (2005). Interventions to enhance the spiritual aspects of dying. *Journal of Palliative Medicine, 8, Supplement 1,* S-103–S-115.

Cohen, C. B., Wheeler, S. E., & Scott, D. A. (2001). Anglican working group in bioethics: Walking a fine line: Physician inquiries into patients' religious and spiritual beliefs. *Hastings Center Report, 31,* 29–39.

Curlin, F. A., Roach, C. J., Gorawara-Bhat, R., Lantos, J. D., & Chin, M. H. (2005). When patients choose faith over medicine. *Archives of Internal Medicine, 165,* 88–91.

Desbiens, J., & Fillion, L. (2007). Coping strategies: Emotional outcomes and spiritual quality of life in palliative care nurses. *International Journal of Palliative Nursing, 13*(6), 291–300.

Emblen, J. D., (1992). Religion and spirituality defined according to current use in nursing literature. *Journal of Professional Nursing, 8*(1), 41–47.

Ferrell, B. (1996). *Suffering.* Sudbury, MA: Jones and Bartlett.

Greenstreet, W. (2006). From spirituality to coping strategy: Making sense of chronic illness. *British Journal of Nursing, 15*(17), 938–942.

Haq, I. (2002). Faith and suffering in Islam. Retrieved from http://www.stauros.org/notebooks/articledetail.php?id=284

Hermann, C. (2006). Development and testing of the Spiritual Needs Inventory for patients near end of life. *Oncology Nursing Forum, 33*(4), 737–744.

Islam: The second largest world religion and growing. (2010). Retrieved from http://www.religioustolerance.org/islam.htm

Kruse, B. G., Ruder, S., & Martin, L. (2007). Spirituality and coping at the end of life. *Journal of Hospice and Palliative Nursing, 9*(11), 296–304.

Ledger, S. (2005). The duty of nurses to meet patients spiritual and/or religious needs. *British Journal of Nursing, 14*(4), 220–225.

Mahlungulu, S. N., & Uys, L. R. (2004). Spirituality in nursing: An analysis of the concept. *South African Nursing Association, 27*(2), 15–26.

Major Religions of the World. (2007). Retrieved from http://www.adherents.com/Religions_By_Adherents.html

Mako, C., Galek, K., & Poppito, S. (2006). Spiritual pain among patients with advanced cancer. *Journal of Palliative Medicine, 9*(5), 1106–1113.

McEwen, M. (2005). Spiritual nursing care. *Holistic Nursing Practice, 19,* 161–168.

McManus, J. (2006). Spirituality and health. *Nursing Management, 13*(6), 24–27.

Millspaugh, C. D. (2005a). Assessment and response to spiritual pain: Part I. *Journal of Palliative Medicine, 8*(5), 919–923.

Millspaugh, C. D. (2005b). Assessment and response to spiritual pain: Part II. *Journal of Palliative Medicine, 8*(6), 1110–1117.

Morse, J., & Doberneck, B. (1995). Delineating the concept of hope. *Image: Journal of Nursing Scholarship, 27*(4), 227–285.

Murray, R. P. (2010). Spiritual care beliefs and practices of special care and oncology RNs at patients' end of life. *Journal of Hospice and Palliative Care Nursing, 112*(1), 51–58.

O'Brien, M. E. (2011). *Servant leadership in nursing: Spirituality and practice in contemporary health care.* Sudbury, MA: Jones and Bartlett.

Pavlović, E., Ljubičić, D., Peitl, V., Peitl, M. V., Ljubičić, I. B., & Ljubičić, R. (2008). Dimensions of human spirituality, layman understandings of health and limits of medicine. *Psychiatria Danubina, 20*(4), 508–511.

Pesut, B. (2008). Spirituality and spiritual care in nursing fundamentals textbooks. *Journal of Nursing Education, 47*(40), 167–173.

Pew Forum on Religion and Public Life. *Religious demographic profile: United States.* (2009). Retrieved from http://pewforum.org/world-affairs/countries/?CountryID=222

Potter, M. L. (2006). Loss, suffering, bereavement, and grief. In M. L. Matzo & D. W. Sherman (Eds.), *Palliative care nursing* (2nd ed., pp. 273–315). New York, NY: Springer.

Purnell, L., & Paulanka, B. (2008). *Transcultural health care* (3rd ed.).Philadelphia: F. A. Davis.

Smith, R. (1996). Theological perspectives. In B. Ferrell (Ed.), *Suffering* (pp. 159–171). Sudbury, MA: Jones and Bartlett.

Taylor, E. J. (2007). Spiritual pain. *Advance for Nurses, 7*(22), 21–23.

van Leeuwen, R., & Cusveller, B. (2004). Nursing competencies for spiritual care. *Journal of Advanced Nursing, 48*(3), 234–246.

Weaver, A. J., & Flannelly, K. J. (2004). The role of religion/spirituality for cancer patients and their caregivers. *Southern Medical Journal, 97*(12), 1210–1214.

Wright, L. (2005). *Spirituality, suffering, and illness: Ideas for healing.* Philadelphia, PA: F.A. Davis.

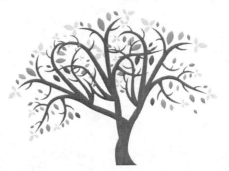

EIGHT

The Search for Meaning in Suffering

■ Kathleen Ouimet Perrin

Objectives

1. Discuss ways in which Holocaust survivors and patients have found meaning in their suffering.
2. Compare and contrast various views on the meaning of suffering.
3. Describe ways to assist a person to find meaning in suffering.
4. Explore the feminist interpretations of the concepts of relationship, compassion, and respect in relation to suffering.
5. Discuss the opinions of prominent people concerning the meaning of suffering.

Student Project

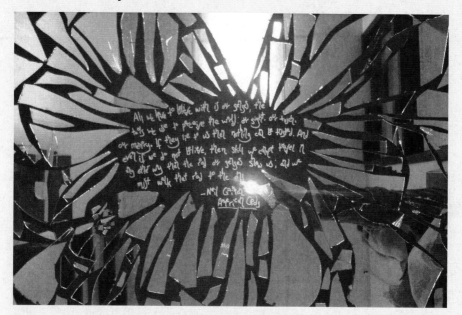

Case Study 8–1

Alan, an 8-year-old boy, was diagnosed with leukemia. After a course of chemotherapy he was in remission for a short period of time; then his leukemia returned. Alan had only one brother who was not an acceptable bone marrow match so the search for an appropriate donor began through the national donor bank and a local telethon. After almost a month the family was thrilled to learn that an appropriate donor had been found. Just as the donor began the necessary workup, Alan developed pneumonia, which led to septic shock. He died a week after the donor had been found. His family and all those who knew him were devastated; they kept asking themselves how and why this could have happened. Why had this young boy gone through so much, come so close, and then died such a difficult death? They cried to anyone who would listen that it was not fair to have their hopes lifted up so high then shattered so abruptly.

Source: Courtesy of Jillian Buratto, student nurse, 2010.

Questions on the Case Study
1. How would you respond to the person or family asking the questions the family did in this case study?
2. How could you help the family members during their distress?
3. Have you ever had a patient or family who felt as if all meaning was gone from their lives and their worlds were shattered?

Introduction

One only needs to be alive to be thrust into situations that may cause suffering. The situations range from individuals' tribulations such as divorce, separation, loss of job, and illness to large-scale catastrophes such as the earthquake in Haiti or the Holocaust. Whether the event is small or large, if it threatens an individual's purpose/goals, values, or beliefs about life (also known as global meaning), it may trigger a new search for meaning (Skaggs & Barron, 2006). This chapter explores what is known about the search for meaning in suffering on two different scales. First it reviews what is known of Holocaust survivors' search for meaning. Then it explores patients' and their families' search for meaning in illness. Ways to assist people in their search for meaning are described. Finally, the feminist perspective—that one should not try to find meaning in negative events; rather, one should try to alleviate them—is explored.

The Holocaust was chosen for consideration in this chapter because it occurred over 50 years ago and survivors have been able to examine their experiences, find their voices, and develop their narratives. Some, like Elie Wiesel and Victor Frankl, have thought and written extensively about the meaning of their experiences as well as the importance of searching for meaning in suffering and in life.

Shattering of Global Meaning

Some events, like being brought to a concentration camp during the Holocaust, are so devastating that they may "shatter" the global meaning the people involved previously held. This may happen whenever a future that had been taken for granted is threatened, when it becomes apparent that life will be cut short or that life will never be the same (Skaggs & Barron, 2006, p. 564). Those involved may begin searching for the purpose of life and wondering what makes life worth living. One of the most poignant examples of such a shattering of a previously held understanding about life is this excerpt from *Night* by Elie Wiesel (2006, p. 34):

Never shall I forget that night, the first night in camp, that turned my life into one long night, seven times sealed.

Never shall I forget that smoke.

Never shall I forget the small faces of the children, whose bodies I saw transformed into smoke under a silent sky.

Never shall I forget those flames that consumed my faith forever.

Never shall I forget that nocturnal silence that deprived me, for all eternity, of the desire to live.

Never shall I forget those moments that murdered my God and my soul and turned my dreams to ashes.

Never shall I forget those things, even were I condemned to live as long as God Himself.

Never.

(Excerpt from *Night* by Elie Wiesel, translated by Marion Wiesel. Translation copyright © 2006 by Marion Wiesel. Reprinted by permission of Hill and Wang, a division of Farrar, Straus and Giroux.)

In *Against Silence*, a compendium of Wiesel's papers, speeches, and interviews (Abrahamson, 1985, p. 52), Wiesel questions the presence of God, asking "Where was God? . . . How could he be silent?" Wiesel admits that he has still not found any way to answer this question. In fact, the more he thinks about it, the more he lives, and the more he remembers, the deeper the question and the mystery becomes for him of where was God.

Despite all this, Wiesel chooses to survive, to tell the world about his suffering and his refusal to give in to it. He asks rhetorically, "When you experience all this suffering, all these questions, and all the despair, what is one to do today? Give up? Go under?" And he answers those questions with a resounding "No" because to give in would be to accept defeat and he is "with all my heart against transmitting defeat to our younger generation, to our children" (Abrahamson, 1985, pp. 52–53).

The Search for Meaning

Viktor Frankl, another survivor of the Holocaust, developed a form of psycho-analysis called logotherapy based on the premise that finding meaning is one of the essential tasks in a person's life. During his experience in concentration camps, Frankl discovered that it was possible to remain humane and act morally in even those most horrendous of circumstances. Frankl (1992) wrote, "There were always choices to make. Every day, every hour, offered the opportunity to make a decision, a decision which determined whether you would or would not submit to the powers which threatened to rob you of your very self, your inner freedom: which determined whether or not you would become—molded into the form a typical inmate" (p.75).

In addition to surviving as a moral human being, Frankl (1992) believed that it was possible to find meaning in these terrifying experiences and a reason to continue living. He believed that if it was a person's destiny to suffer, the person must accept that the suffering was unique to him alone and realize that no one could bear the burden of his suffering for him (Frankl, 1992, p. 86). This did not mean that one had to bear suffering that could be alleviated; Frankl believed that if suffering could be alleviated, it should. In fact, he said it was masochistic to undergo unnecessary suffering. However, he had been in circumstances in which there was no possibility of alleviating suffering and believed that when it was impossible to change a situation that caused suffering, the sufferer could still change his attitude (p. 148). At dawn one morning, after a forced all-night march against an icy wind, Frankl realized, "In a position of utter desolation when man cannot express himself in positive action when his only achievement may consist of enduring his sufferings in the right way—an honorable way—in such a position . . . man can achieve fulfillment" (pp. 48–49).

Ways to Find Meaning

Frankl (1992) believed that there are three ways by which man could achieve fulfillment and arrive at meaning in life. The first was by creating a work or doing a deed and the second by being in love and experiencing or encountering someone intimately. However, he believed the most important avenue to finding meaning in life was for a person to rise above a hopeless situation that he could not change and grow beyond himself. In that way he could turn a personal tragedy into a triumph (pp. 146–147). From his own experience, Frankl believed that those concentration camp victims who found a purpose and set a goal were more likely to survive the experience.

Attributes of Holocaust Survivors

White, Newbauer, Sutherland, and Cox (2005) studied Holocaust survivors. They concluded that these individuals possessed attributes that made them able to consciously assign meaning and purpose to their lives. The researchers believed their findings supported Frankl's observation that the search for meaning enhanced fulfillment and survival. Moreover, they noted that even though the popular image of the Holocaust survivor was as a victim, that was not what they found. Instead, they noted that these people, far from being psychologically broken by all that they had experienced, had often been successful. They stated, "These survivors' stories are often success stories" (p. 37).

White and others (2005) utilized a lifestyle narrative to attempt to understand how 30 Holocaust survivors conceptualized their world and the world at large. The researchers also examined how the survivors chose to belong to the world and what impact they chose to have on it. From the interviews the researchers found the following themes descriptive of the survivors:

- First born or only child
- Responsible psychological position
- Higher socioeconomic status
- Focus outside family of origin
- Devaluing of religion
- Belief in importance of education
- Strong goal and future orientation
- Demonstrating flexibility/resiliency
- Belief in the importance of the arts and creativity

After extensive review of the narratives and themes, the researchers concluded that these successful survivors were self-directed and consciously future oriented. They adapted quickly to their environments. They were reflective and thought extensively about the meaning of their experiences. Finally, the researchers concluded that the survivors had a "strong inclination to ascribe meaning and purpose to their lives."

Many philosophers, nurses, and researchers believe that such catastrophic suffering can never be meaningful in itself: it is inherently negative. However, they believe that one may learn from suffering, one may grow from it, and one may choose to find a new meaning or direction for one's life after experiencing suffering. That is what Wiesel, Frankl, and the 30 Holocaust survivors from the previous study appear to have done.

Illness as a Source of Suffering

Illness is a catastrophe too, but on a much smaller scale (Klienman & Benson, 2006). Just as a person's identity, role, and purpose in life were threatened in the Holocaust, they are also threatened by illness. Klienman and Benson observe that illness is a profoundly moral experience since sufferers have so much to lose.

Learning the Meaning of the Illness to the Patient

Klienman and Benson (2006) believe that what the patient may be the most afraid of losing from illness varies across ethnic, racial, and cultural subgroups. For that reason, Klienman developed a series of questions for healthcare providers to ask patients so that the healthcare provider could begin to understand what the illness meant to the patient and how the patient might be suffering. The questions were these:

- What do you call this problem?
- What do you believe is its cause?
- What course do you expect it to take?
- How serious is it?
- What do you think this problem does inside your body?
- What do you most fear about this condition?
- What do you most fear about the treatment?

The questions were intended to open lines of communication and allow healthcare providers to learn what the illness episode meant to the patients. Other authors might call this helping the patient to tell his story. However, Klienman and Benson (2006) were disappointed with the results because when healthcare providers utilized these questions, they tended to see the responses as static so the questions served as conversation stoppers. Rogers and Cowles (1997) note that "the silence and secrecy that hinder providers' attention to suffering and that removes suffering from polite and even professional discussion may interfere with the suffering person's acknowledgement and expression of the experience as suffering as well" (p. 1052). In fact, they went so far as to call the inability of health-care providers and patients to discuss suffering "a conspiracy of silence" (p. 1048).

Silent Sufferers

Bjorn, Fredniksson, and Eriksson (2001) agree that people often suffer in silence. They believe that suffering can mute the voice of the sufferer especially when the suffering is new; the very newness of the experience may prevent the sufferer from finding a voice. Later, sufferers may fail to speak because they fear that no one will listen and hear what they are trying to say. Sufferers may also remain mute because they believe the nature of their suffering is one that should never be spoken aloud (such as in the sexual and genital abuse in the narrative in Chapter 7). In the instance of such unspeakable suffering, the sufferer may also be hesitant to speak since he may fear that hearing the story will cause others to suffer needlessly.

Jones (1999) argues that healthcare providers, nurses included, may actually deny suffering people the opportunity to voice their suffering. She notes that mute sufferers may actually speak of other issues, banter, or even laugh; they are simply unable to give voice to their suffering. Nurses may fail to recognize the suffering underlying the banter and therefore never encourage the sufferers to tell their stories. Or the healthcare provider may subtly discourage the "strange voice" (p. 827) of pain and distress. The patients then turn to defense mechanisms such as repression and denial, becoming mute instead of voicing their authentic suffering and telling their stories.

Despite the reluctance of people to speak about their suffering, researchers have concluded that finding a voice, specifically telling the story of their suffering, developing an illness narrative, and integrating the experience into a life narrative can help sufferers to find meaning in the experience and in their lives. Similarly, Eifried (1998), in an interpretive phenomenological study, found that nurses used the strategies of being present, calling forth a voice, listening, and being a guide to help patients speak about their experience of suffering and find meaning in it.

Wounded Storytellers

Frank (1995) explains this concept slightly differently; he calls a patient a wounded storyteller and believes that when a person becomes ill, the person's body sets in motion the need for new stories. He believes that patients need to tell their stories to construct new maps and develop new perceptions (similar to what others call a search for meaning). Frank believes that as patients tell their illness stories they are listening to both the story itself and to the responses of the listeners. The telling of the story and the responses of the listeners help patients to make sense of what is occurring to them and to begin healing.

In order to heal, Frank (1995) believes patients should shape their own narratives. This is difficult in the current healthcare system since patients often surrender their narratives to the authority of healthcare providers. This happens when patients permit the medicalization of their illnesses by allowing physicians to take sole responsibility for their care and letting their medical charts become their stories. When patients are able to shape their own narratives, Frank states that the narratives usually fall into one of three different types: restitution, chaos, and quest. Restitution narratives anticipate getting well again and emphasize the technology of cure. In contrast, in chaos narratives, the illness stretches on interminably with no obvious end or redeeming insights. Quest narratives are about finding meaning in the illness as the person is able to reshape his or her journey and become someone new.

In a similar vein, Råholm (2008) states, "As people tell their stories, they start to hear their life anew through the hearer; they fabricate, explain, elaborate, exaggerate, minimize, silence themselves, and give themselves away. It transforms a destructive experience into a process for health, well-being, and wholeness" (p. 66).

Value of Stories/Narratives

Bjorn et al. (2001) distinguish between stories, narratives, and life histories (sometimes called life narratives) and believe that in reflecting on the stories and developing a narrative, the suffering patient may be on the path to health. They provide the following definitions:

- A story is an informal, provisional accounting of events that includes the meanings that the person gives to the events.

- A narrative is a consciously formulated, coherent account of the experience. To become a narrative the experience must be conceptualized, restressed, and completed. It usually has a point or lesson learned from it.
- A life history (or life narrative) is a chronological person-centered case study using a narrative that offers sociocultural dynamics and offers a long and comprehensive view of the person.

Patients' Stories

In order for this potentially healing process to occur, patients must find their voice and begin to tell their story. An essential part of the patient's finding a voice and beginning to tell the story is the presence of a sensitive listener, someone who will respond to the tentative voice of the patient, a voice that is not calling out and demanding attention. When a healthcare provider responds to the patient's call to listen to the story, the provider should be cautious not to take over the role of "hero" or rescuer in the patient's story. If the patient is to develop some understanding or find some personal meaning from the story, then as Frank has stated, it must be the patient's own story and not a medicalization of the story. Bjorn et al. (2001) concur, saying that patients must be preserved or restored as the authority on their experience of illness and suffering.

A patient's story is like any story: it has a central theme that includes a problem to be solved with actions and events aimed at resolving the problem. According to Bjorn et al. (2001), the first step for the patient in the potentially healing process is telling the story. Younger (1995) notes that in this early phase, some patients may lament, voicing their own innocence while exploring how this could have happened to them: However, other patients may hold themselves to blame for their afflictions or lash out in anger at others during this phase (Gunderman, 2002). Giving vent to these feelings of guilt, anger, and possibly horror prevents patients from simmering away destructively inside (Bjorn et al., 2001). Although the responses of lamenting and lashing out are very different, the patients are trying to do the same thing—establish why this catastrophe was visited upon them. The crucial questions for patients during the phase of story development are Why me? and Why now?

A nurse may help suffering patients to develop their stories simply by asking open-ended question such as, How did it all start? This is similar to the open-ended question proposed by Klienman and Benson (2006): "What do you believe is the cause of your problem?" Researchers have found that before most people can move ahead, they need to establish how the problem came about (Bjorn et al., 2001). During the storytelling phase, the patient is attempting to clarify what happened, how things are now, what he or she needs, and what the current struggle involves. Arriving at this understanding will likely take more than just one telling of the story as the patient considers and reworks the experience. Developing the story is essential preparation for reflection and narration, the next phase (Bjorn et al., 2001).

Patients' Narratives

During the second part of the process, development of the narrative, the patient is able to order the events in the illness in sequence and is beginning to reflect on them. Organizing the story and making some sense of how the events are interconnected allows the patient to experience a feeling of some control. Bjorn et al. (2001) agree with Klienman and Benson (2006) that this is extremely important, especially if the healthcare system has begun to erode the patient's sense of responsibility for his or her own illness story. Hawkins (1993) likens the narrative to the function of a myth—it allows the patient to begin to create order out of chaos. She argues that patients often talk in mythological terms about going on journeys, engaging in battles, awaiting death, or being reborn to a new experience. This is in contrast to the three types of narratives that Frank (1995) describes: the restitution narrative, the chaos narrative, and the quest narrative. Bjorn et al. (2001) recommend that since there is no consensus in the research literature about how to use these general patterns to help a patient, each patient should first be treated as an individual.

During the narrative phase, patients may use metaphors to describe their experience. Metaphor has the potential to open up new views and meanings for patients. Thus when they use metaphors to describe their illness, the nurse should explore the meaning of the metaphor. Patients might delve into various art forms finding they aid in developing metaphors for their illness and help them arrive at new understandings. During this stage in the process the nurse might ask, What have you been experiencing? What were the major events during the course of your illness? How would you characterize what has been happening? What has this illness meant to you? Asking these questions allows the nurse to begin to understand the patient's situation, perspective, and vulnerability—understandings that Råholm (2008) argues are essential to ethical action. Although asking these questions is important, even necessary, it is not clear how much detail a healthcare provider should go into with any individual patient, how long the process should take, or how in depth the process with each person should be. However, it is apparent to Bjorn et al. (2001) that for the potential for healing to occur, the person will need to enter the third step in the process.

Patients' Life Histories/Narratives

The third stage in the process is the connection of the illness or suffering experience with the person's life history or narrative. When this occurs, the person may begin to ask, "What is to be learned from this period of suffering? How can I use it to create a new period of wholeness—a new meaning for my life?" Although Bjorn et al. (2001) acknowledge that reflecting on the period of suffering may be threatening to some people, they believe that it is important for individuals to incorporate the experiences into their life histories and proceed to either a new level of health or a peaceful death. Morse and Carter (1995) believe that survivors find meaning and integrate suffering experiences into their lives by telling, interpreting, and incorporating the event into their lives intermittently over a period of time. It may even be a lifelong endeavor.

Pathway to Healing

Bjorn et al. (2001) also caution that the process of incorporating the suffering event into the life narrative is not necessarily a straight path. Most patients follow a convoluted route to make sense of their suffering. Frank (1995) agrees that the process is not linear, noting that patients use the three types of narratives he has identified at varying times throughout an illness, retracing experiences and reworking the narratives depending on their needs. However, as noted earlier, the researchers who interviewed the Holocaust survivors were able to demonstrate that these survivors were reflective, had thought extensively about the meaning of their experiences, and had a "strong inclination to ascribe meaning and purpose to their lives" (White et al., 2005, p. 37). The findings from these successful Holocaust survivors' lifestyle narratives clearly parallel what Bjorn and colleagues believed should occur for the suffering person to return to health.

Aesthetic Experiences

Råholm (2008) notes that narratives have aesthetic elements as well as an ethical component. She believes that to tell a story well is an art form. Steeves and Kahn (1987), nursing researchers with a long history of exploring the effects and meaning of suffering on patients and their families, have noted that during their illnesses some people have aesthetic experiences that change their thoughts about suffering. They summarized, "Patients were having critical experiences that they felt were bringing them into contact with forces greater than themselves and fundamentally changing the way they viewed suffering." During and following these experiences, the patients had a sense of well-being and order that resulted in a sense of peacefulness and contentment (Steeves & Kahn, 1987, p. 114).

The incidents the patients described were

- self-contained;
- involved a change in the way the person experienced reality;
- always positive;
- centered around an activity or object outside the patient that was time limited;
- closely tied to suffering;
- experiences of meaning; and
- had a strong link between suffering and an aesthetic experience.

Ordinary Nature of Experiences

The critical experiences that Steeves and Kahn identified in 1987 were not unusual and spectacular events in themselves. Usually, they were ordinary events in the individuals' lives that had an extraordinary effect on their experience of suffering. These experiences were only identified in people who seemed to be coping well with their suffering. The patients and their family members who were not coping did not appear to be experiencing similar events. Steeves and Kahn provide the following experience of one woman whose husband was dying of lung cancer:

> As she dug in the soil, time passed and she did not think about her problems. . . . She became peaceful and content. . . . Through her involvement with the soil and living plants she felt in contact with forces great than herself and her fundamental relationship with reality changed. She was aware that the world had not changed; all the reasons to suffer remained, but she was content somehow with her condition because she was experiencing it differently. (Steeves & Kahn, 1987, p. 114)

Steeves and Kahn (1987) suggest that these experiences might be viewed as aesthetic experiences that allow the person to see reality as a whole rather than just seeing its parts. Therefore, the aesthetic event is experienced with the mind, body, emotions, and spirit and not understood by the mind alone. Or in the example of their research participants, the experiences brought them in touch with something that they considered to be greater than or outside themselves that altered the way they experienced themselves.

What Steeves and Kahn are describing is similar to an event that Frankl (1992) describes just before he concludes that man may endure his suffering in an honorable way and find meaning in suffering. As noted earlier, Frankl had been on a forced nighttime march from one concentration camp to another. A horrible situation had been made even worse by the icy wind and the guards driving the detainees by striking them with gun butts. However, he clearly had an aesthetic experience that dramatically changed his perception of himself and the world. He wrote that as the stars began to fade and the light of morning began to dawn, he could imagine his wife with extreme clarity, even hear her answering him. He concluded:

> Real or not she was more luminous than the sun that was beginning to rise. A thought transfixed me. . . . In a position of utter desolation when man cannot express himself in positive action, when his only achievement may consist of enduring his suffering in the right way—an honorable way—in such a position—through contemplation of his beloved—man can achieve fulfillment. (Frankl, 1992, pp. 48–49)

There are questions that remain about such aesthetic experiences. Do the experiences have a long-term effect on the patient and family as Frankl's appeared to? Does the suffering allow the experience to happen or is the experience an act against the suffering and a means of rising against it? (Steeves & Kahn, 1987).

Assumptions About Aesthetic Experiences

Steeves and Kahn (1987) proposed five assumptions about experiences of meaning. The first is that meaning is experienced by individuals. The person does not think about the experience as it is happening and may not ever have a rational explanation about it. The experiences themselves are all absorbing and complete. The second assumption is that experiencing meaning is a positive thing. Hospice patients and their family members cope better with suffering when they have had such an experience. The third assumption is that experiences of meaning are often tied to suffering. The experiences usually change how the individuals view the suffering as well as how they cope with it. The fourth assumption is that certain conditions are necessary but not sufficient for the experience of meaning. These conditions include

- access to and capability of perceiving objects in the environment;
- free time and solitude; and
- freedom from pain that totally consumes one's attention.

These conditions are important to the fifth assumption, the goal of nursing. Steeves and Kahn (1987) state that the "goal of nursing is to establish and maintain those conditions that are necessary for and helpful to experiencing meaning. . . . Nurses cannot create the experience of meaning or participate in someone else's, but through awareness they may help to create an atmosphere calm enough in the midst of suffering to allow the phenomenon to occur" (p. 116).

Is Suffering All Bad?

Gunderman (2002) poses the essential question about suffering. Can we really claim that suffering is all bad? He argues that the tragedies of Sophocles and Shakespeare invite us to share in the suffering of others and to learn from them. He suggests that patients and their caregivers should seek out these examples and gain wisdom "because suffering is pregnant with the insight that there are at work in the world forces even beyond our ken" (p. 43). From the patient's own suffering or the vicarious suffering of others, Gunderman believes we can learn the art of caring. He reaches the conclusion that to inflict suffering would be cruelty, but we must recognize that suffering cannot always be relieved. When it cannot be relieved and must be shared, he believes it calls us to the humane in us, shows us how to love, and allows us to become wiser than we are.

Feminist Response

Nel Noddings (1989) completely disagrees with Gunderman's (2002) answer to the question. She adamantly affirms that suffering is all bad. She argues that suffering has no inherent meaning and suffering does not gain meaning merely because some people might learn, grow, or find meaning through it. She acknowledges that the humanities are steeped in a tradition that searches for meaning in suffering. However, she prefers the existentialist countertradition that suggests that meaning is created by human beings "in their struggle in a universe otherwise devoid of meaning. Suffering in itself has no meaning and is not redeemed simply because it triggers a search for meaning in those who encounter it" (p. 75).

Noddings's (1989) objection to the common view of suffering is that it encourages people to seek justification not only for their own suffering but also for the suffering they might inflict upon someone else in order to make the other person grow. For example, years ago, teachers were allowed to hit the hands of students with a wooden ruler when they gave a wrong answer to a question so that the student would learn the material and would not answer incorrectly in the future. She notes that when "we believe that God teaches us something or cures us of something through pain, then we feel justified in inflicting pain on others in teaching or curing them" (p. 75).

Noddings is not alone in stating that suffering has no meaning and there can never be any justification for it. Levinas (1988), a Jewish philosopher, rejects the possibility that suffering has any meaning. He specifically speaks about the Holocaust and says that suffering of such magnitude and such uselessness can never be absorbed into a justifying narrative. Noddings (1989) concurs with Levinas when she says: "Why should any man, woman, or child have to seek meaning for his or her own life in the horror of the Holocaust. Who would dare to speak to Elie Wiesel of justice? We all know that such things should never have happened and should never happen again. Talk of justice and meaning is out of place in the context of such horror" (pp. 76–77).

Georges (2004), examining suffering from a critical feminist self-reflective approach, agrees with Noddings. However, she speaks more specifically about nurses and says that as nurses we are deeply entrenched in a European metanarrative that encourages us to search for meaning in suffering. This metanarrative has limited what we study and understand about suffering. She believes that the predominant metanarrative teaches us that suffering happens to someone else in a distant place and is perpetuated by distant people (and never by us as nurses). But, she cautions, we are part of the community that may cause suffering and in the very least we have ignored known sources of suffering. She recommends continued and expanded work on the political context of suffering.

Do We Contribute to Suffering?

Both Noddings and Georges agree that we need to critically examine the metanarrative to understand how we as nurses have contributed to suffering in the name of health or cure. Noddings (1989) says we need to pursue a response to suffering suggested by the ethics of caring. We should actively resist allowing the inevitability of suffering to lead us into a search for meaning or justification of the suffering. Rather, we should work to alleviate the suffering that we are witnessing, eliminate its causes, and educate people so that they will not willfully or negligently cause suffering in people or other sentient beings in the future (p. 76).

Responses to Suffering

Noddings (1989) speaks of how both men and women ought to respond to suffering in a chapter called "Woman's Answer to Job." Although she speaks of women specifically, she hopes that men will learn to respond compassionately in the same way. Noddings's (1989) words are an inspiration; she says that women's answer to suffering is given in their personal, caring presence. Noddings believes that the first part of a caring response is to say, "I am here. Let me help you." What follows is just as important; women responding to suffering should not judge or condemn or dominate with commands. They should not turn their attention away from the human beings who are the most likely present source of help and solace, toward some eternal search for meaning. Instead, women should offer concrete help by feeding the suffering and helping them reconcile among themselves.

Even though Noddings (1989) expects women to concentrate on these essential details, she still advocates their visualization of the larger picture. She says, "We need a framework, a theoretical or spiritual perspective that will keep our hearts and minds directed toward eliminating moral evil, toward the responsibility of caring for each other. We need a perspective that will help us to find meanings in our relations with fellow human beings not one that separates us in a search for "meanings" (pp. 76–77).

Georges (2004) agrees that suffering should be eliminated but advocates examining and eradicating the root causes. She looks at how political, economic, and institutional power promote suffering. She recommends beginning with the feminist assertion that the personal is political and suggests that we start with ourselves and learn what we have done to promote suffering and what we can do to remove the root causes of it.

She notes that nurses in Nazi Germany were able to use traits of "distancing" and "free-floating responsibility" to dissociate themselves from what they were doing. The nurses distanced themselves emotionally from the women in the concentration camps by seeing them as "others," people who were very different from them and barely human. The nurses used free-floating responsibility when they reassured themselves as they worked with condemned women that "At least, I'm not actively doing the killing." They also reassured themselves that there must be a law that allows this and therefore, they felt they were not responsible for their actions. Georges argues that these traits allowed the nurses to participate in and perpetuate the suffering without feeling responsible for it. Georges asks each of us as nurses to examine what we are doing to perpetuate suffering by continuing these behaviors of distancing and free-floating responsibility. She believes that when we fail to investigate the political and power dimensions of suffering, we risk perpetuating that suffering.

Research on Gender and Cultural Issues

On a larger scale, Georges (2004) believes that we cannot begin to develop interventions for suffering until we can represent that suffering. She believes that most of the research that has been done about suffering to this point has failed to examine the political and power factors that underlie the suffering, and the interventions that have been developed have failed to take into account the root causes (Georges, 2002). She recommends that nurse scholars design studies that examine the role of gender and cultural issues in suffering as well as how the use/misuse of power contributes to suffering. Despite disagreeing with much of what has been written about meaning and suffering, she does appear to believe that narrative and storytelling are part of the process of healing the sufferer, stating that "from a womanist perspective, remembering and retelling, resisting, and redeeming characterize suffering" (Georges, 2002, p. 84). She believes that we need to reenvision suffering in a much larger context, one that goes beyond the individual person disconnected from the rest of the world. Finally, she recommends that this new search for understanding of suffering be done via an interdisciplinary, critical humanities approach.

Identification of Power Imbalances

What would Georges's approach mean for nursing practice? She believes that the nursing approach to suffering should be to identity and alleviate the conditions that put oppressed people at risk and give rise to suffering. The nurse caring for a suffering patient would need to take into account the power differential between her position as a healthcare provider and the sufferer as a patient. Each interaction between sufferer and nurse would be highly individualized, with the human cost of the suffering at the heart of the interaction. Emphasis in the relationship would be on creating an authentic feeling of presence and being with the sufferer. In such a relationship, the nurse would be highly involved and would not be able to distance herself from the patient's suffering, would be shaped by the suffering, and would likely be unable to perpetuate the metanarrative that one can "learn" from suffering (Georges, 2002).

Presence and Awareness of Power Imbalances

Ferrell (2005) also talks about the necessity of the nurse being present in the relationship with each patient. However, her focus is on the dynamics of the relationship when a patient is experiencing pain and notes that there is an element of uncertainty in the relationship. The patient is certain of the pain; it is present and it is palpable. However, the nurse may be doubtful because she is only hearing about the pain and possibly witnessing some of its manifestations. This doubt on the part of the nurse can result in power imbalances between patient and nurse. According to Ferrell, feminist ethicists have noted the overwhelming power imbalance between the patient in pain and the nurse who has been asked to provide relief. This imbalance can become even more profound when the person suffering is a child, a woman, or someone who does not speak English. Ferrell cautions nurses providing care to suffering patients to be conscious of these power imbalances and aware of how vulnerable the patients are.

Compassion

Ferrell (2005) argues, as Noddings does, that the appropriate response, and she calls it a feminist response, to pain and suffering is compassion. However, her conviction is even stronger than Noddings's as she states that there is a moral imperative to respond to the patient in pain with compassion. Ferrell continues that nurses, because of their intimate place in caring for suffering patients, have the opportunity to give voice to patients' suffering. She, like most of the other nurse authors discussed in this chapter, encourages nurses to listen to their patients, learn their stories, and work with them to alleviate their suffering.

Ferrell (2005) references *The Female Face of God in Auschwitz* by Raphael (2003) describing the compassion, respect, and caring for each other that developed among female inmates in untenable circumstances. Raphael describes how women cared for each other and helped each other to survive in Auschwitz noting that even small gestures were against the rules and were punishable. These simple caring activities were acts of resistance in that foreboding place. Following this line of thought, Ferrell wondered: Are nurses the face of God in pain management and is advocating pain relief for those who cannot voice their own needs a "courageous act of resistance"?

Summary

Although there is agreement among authors that suffering is intrinsically evil, there are differences of opinion on whether and how suffering individuals and others should respond to suffering. There are philosophers, psychologists, and health-care providers who believe that helping individuals who are suffering to find meaning in their suffering will help them to integrate it into their lives. Another view, often espoused by feminists is that suffering is often a result of the misuse of power. Therefore, an appropriate response to suffering is to look for the root causes and try to obliterate them. However, both groups appear to agree that reflection and narrative can help the suffering individual. The first group suggests that telling their stories and having an empathetic listener may help the sufferers to find meaning in the experience. The other group believes that narrative may help the sufferers to remember, retell, resist, and redeem.

Key Points

1. Sufferers benefit from telling their illness story and beginning to integrate the story into their life narrative.
2. Nurses can help patients to find their voice by being present, acknowledging the patient is suffering, asking a few simple open-ended questions, and actively listening.
3. People will often begin to heal themselves as they tell, retell, and integrate the story of their suffering. Through this process, some people will find meaning in their suffering.

Exercises

1. Consider what you believe about suffering by doing the following:
    Find a quotation concerning suffering from one of the following two websites:
    http://wisdomquotes.com/cat_suffering.html
    http://www.brainyquote.com/quotes/Keywords/suffering.html
    or from an author of your own choosing.
    A. Write a brief statement about the background of the person being quoted and consider whether the author's background influenced his or her view of suffering.

    B. Write an additional paragraph or two stating whether you agree with the quotation and explaining why you agree or disagree.

    C. Be prepared to discuss your exercise.

2. Read the following:

Hatthakit, U., & Thaniwathansnon, P. (2007). The suffering experiences of Buddhist tsunami survivors. *International Journal for Human Caring, 11*(2), 59–66.

    A. How is suffering seen in Buddhism?

    B. How do the findings concerning religion in this article compare with those in the article by White and others on Holocaust survivors?

    C. What are the two Buddhist tenets that affected survivors' views on the tsunami?

    D. How long did it take survivors to begin to heal compared to what is a generally accepted time frame?

Questions for Reflection and Journaling

1. When you cared for a person who was suffering, did the person or a family member ever wonder about the meaning or reason for the person's suffering?

2. If so, how did they express their concerns to you?

3. Did you respond to their concerns? If so, how?

4. Have you ever wondered why a patient, family member, or someone in your personal life was suffering? What were your thoughts and feelings during the experience? What are your thoughts and feelings about the experience now?

Case Study 8–2: The Sufferer's Story—the Lament

The way people respond to learning that someone has a serious diagnosis, such as cancer, can either be hurtful or helpful. I had experiences with people responding both ways. An example of a hurtful response was when someone immediately turned to me and asked "When was your last PAP smear?" When I said I had missed one, she said "Aha!" When I said it appeared I had found the cancer early and would be having surgery in 2 weeks, she said, "Well, are you sure you don't need an MRI? You could have metastases and need chemotherapy first." In contrast, a helpful response was from the person who put his arm around me and said, "What can I do to help you? We will take care of everything so that you just focus on getting well."

I imagine both are extreme responses—yet I felt no compassion at all in one. There was no attempt to convey concern; instead, there was an attempt to blame me, the patient, who had developed the cancer. Yes, I had missed a PAP smear, but that is not how my type of cancer is usually found. Yes, I ultimately did need chemotherapy, but not because the cancer was in a late stage; rather, it was because it was a rare form of cancer found in an early stage.

Healthcare providers and institutions can also choose to create either a compassionate and caring environment or one where people are treated like objects. At one oncology center where I went for evaluation, the patients enter and stand in long lines to obtain a restaurant-style beeper. When it buzzes, they can enter the next door to have their vital signs taken by an LNA. While taking the vital signs, the LNA must ask "Do you feel safe at home?" and "Are you having any pain?"—which each LNA did with her back to me, mumbling each word. I wondered what she would have done if I had said yes to either question. I was then hustled into another exam room to wait for a physician.

The physician arrived, introduced herself, stood with arms crossed, and stared at me. When I asked whether the treatment would be of benefit to me or not, she replied, "Well, it's what the tumor board recommended; I don't discuss chances with any patient, it's too hard—it's either 0 or 100% survivability for each person. Here is the chemotherapy we will give you; this paper lists the side effects for all the chemotherapy agents we use, not specifically the ones we will be giving you. I'll be back with the consent form, and the nurse practitioner will bring some prescriptions. Do you have any questions? You need a CT of the thorax and blood work before your first treatment. We'll be in touch with you with the date and the times of your appointments for your first therapy."

I decided not to receive chemotherapy at that illustrious institution. At the facility where I eventually received my chemotherapy, as my husband and I entered the waiting area, the receptionist said, "Hello, my name is Stephanie, how may I help you?" After taking my name, she said, "Tracey, the nurse, will be with you in just a few moments; would you like to take a seat?" The nurse found us in the waiting area, introduced herself, and brought us into an exam room where she took my vital signs then sat down face to face with me and asked me some health history questions. When the physician arrived, she also sat down to ask me questions. Without being asked, she said, "It's unusual for us to see people with your stage of cancer; most of the surgeons keep these patients to themselves or just offer radiation. It was the tumor board's unanimous recommendation that you receive chemotherapy and I think it is a forward-looking recommendation." We reviewed what would be happening and my specific chemotherapy and prescriptions. Then Tracey returned to review the medications again, show me the infusion room, and talk with me about how I might want to prepare and what I might want to bring with me for my scheduled treatment.

Certainly in health care, time is money. Yet, the second visit took no longer than the first one. In less time, when the healthcare providers took the few moments to sit and talk with me, I provided more usable information to them and I learned much more about my own care. More important to me, I felt as though the providers at the second institution saw me as an individual with distinct needs and concerns. I would argue that all patients should be treated as humans with distinct needs because they deserve that respect. However, even if one does not believe that, then one could argue that one should treat patients as individuals so that their health care can be appropriately planned and managed. Treating a vulnerable patient as a human being rather than a number is not just a respectful, caring approach; it's also a way to assure that the patient receives appropriate health care.

Illness Narrative: Meaning

In the realm of suffering, mine is a very small, personal piece. I'm only one person feeling some discomfort, frustration, anxiety, sadness, and uncertainty. It's not the Holocaust, or Hurricane Katrina, the tsunami in Thailand, or the earthquake in Haiti. There are not thousands of people lost, hurt, in pain, and without apparent recourse. In fact, I've been cared for and loved during this process. Believe me, as a nurse, I have seen individuals who have suffered far, far more than I have, and I know how fortunate I have been. So, is there any reason to look for meaning in personal suffering?

I suppose everyone wonders at some point when they receive a difficult diagnosis, Did I do something wrong? Is this a punishment from God? I certainly have made my share of mistakes in my life, and a God who believed in punishment could, I suppose, choose to punish me. Fortunately, my religion does not espouse a God who dispenses earthly punishment for past sins. That might not stop me from wondering about the possibility of punishment at 2 AM when I am sleepless and anxious, but in general, I have not allowed this potential source of anxiety to overwhelm me.

However, there are other questions: Should I be learning something from my small share of suffering? Has this experience been visited upon me so that I can learn something about myself and alter my relationship with the people in my world? Or, beyond that, should I be looking at my world and envisioning ways to expand it? Have I been too selfish in the way that I view and respond to the world? Nell Noddings would say "No." I should not be the primary person learning from my suffering. Rather, I should be receiving care, support, and sustenance from those around me, just as I have been. I do agree that the support of those around is essential, but I don't know that I agree that nothing is required of me.

I have this time—a very self-centered bit of time—when I might look at how I interact with my world. There is a pattern in my behavior in response to certain types of people, people who recur in my life, that is not constructive. The way I respond is not beneficial either to the other people or myself. Since this is a recurrent problem and I am encountering these people during my illness, is this a time when I should learn how to change my response? Does my illness give me an opportunity to change long-established and possibly unhealthy ways of relating to others? If I were able to do that, would there be meaning in my illness?

Beginning Integration of Illness into the Life Narrative

It's a year after my initial diagnosis, and I'm not quite sure what I am. Am I healthy? Am I ill? Am I recovering? While I was receiving treatment and for the first few months after treatment, I was clearly still recovering. Now, I am physically healthy, but right at the moment, at this year anniversary of my diagnosis, I am unsettled emotionally. I've moved on with life, returned to work, and assumed the role of supporting another woman recently diagnosed with a similar cancer who is receiving chemotherapy. But I haven't yet integrated this illness episode into my life. I think partially that is because I'm still not sure how the episode will end. I'm still living with uncertainty.

Most days I can sort of brush everything to the back burner; I can even not think about my prognosis while I'm following the treatment regimen required several times a week after my radiation therapy. I think that's part of what you have to do to make things manageable. That's not to say I don't think about what's happened. I had not thought ahead when I bought my wig, and I bought one that did not work well in the hospital setting. So, I stopped wearing the wig and went about my life with very, very short hair. The result was that many of my patients and their families knew I had been treated for cancer. Although I have always tried to be present for my patients and families, I think I have been much more aware of how I interact with them. Focusing very carefully not just on what I say when I am with them, but how quickly I move. I'm more aware now that when I am busy and hurrying on to the next patient and the next task, I may be conveying something very different from what I intended to those around me.

I had hoped to improve my relationships and my way of interacting with some of the people in my life. I'm still working on that. I can't say that I have resolved any of the relationship issues, but my illness really accentuated the problems in these relationships. I wish I could say I have been following a consistent and therapeutic communication pattern with these people, but some days it's just more than I can manage. Changing my pattern of interaction is one of my goals for the next year.

At this year anniversary, there are two things that keep presenting themselves to me: Can I make this illness experience an opportunity for growth? Can I cope well with the ongoing uncertainty. As an ICU nurse, I know how unexpected and uncertain life can be. However, with this illness I have experienced that uncertainty firsthand. Mark Nepo (2007), a cancer survivor, says it best in *Facing the Lion, Being the Lion, Finding Inner Courage Where It Lives*: "I feel compelled to inquire into the art of facing things—facing ourselves, each other and the unknown. It is something we cannot do without for facing things is what the courage at its most fundamental level is all about. Without this, we replay and pass our sufferings on to others repeatedly. It is time for me to face the uncertainty and go forward" (p. 17).

Questions on the Case Study

1. What was the patient lamenting about in her story? Did she have a reason to be upset or was she displacing some of her anger about being ill?
2. What questions could you ask her to help her consider how her story was developing?
3. What questions could you ask her to help her anchor her story in reality?
4. Do you think the author is really searching for meaning in the experience in her narrative? Why or why not?
5. What types of questions might help her to organize the experience and begin to find meaning?
6. When might sufferers begin to integrate the experience into their life narrative? Is a year too soon?
7. What suggestions would you have to help a person live with the uncertainty of an illness like cancer?

References

Abrahamson, I. (1985). *Against silence: The voice and vision of Elie Wiesel.* New York, NY: Holocaust Library.

Bjorn, A., Fredriksson, L., & Eriksson, K. (2001). The patient's narrative of suffering: A path to health? *Scandinavian Journal of Caring Sciences, 15*(1), 3–11.

Eifried, S. (1998). Helping patients find meaning: A caring response to suffering. *International Journal for Human Caring, 2*(1), 33–39.

Ferrell, B. (2005). Ethical perspectives on pain and suffering. *Pain Management Nursing, 6*(3), 83–90.

Frank, A. (1995). *The wounded storyteller.* Chicago, IL: University of Chicago Press.

Frankl, V. E. (1992). *Man's search for meaning.* Boston, MA: Beacon Press.

Georges, J. (2002). Suffering: Toward a contextual praxis. *Advances in Nursing Science, 25*(1), 79–86.

Georges, J. (2004). The politics of suffering: Implications for nursing science. *Advances in Nursing Science, 27*(4), 250–256.

Gunderman, R. B. (2002). Is suffering the enemy? *Hastings Center Report, 2*(2), 40–44.

Hawkins, A. H. (1993). *Reconstructing illness: Studies in pathography.* West Lafayette, IN: Purdue Research Foundation.

Jones, A. (1999). Listen, listen trust your own strange voice. *Journal of Advanced Nursing, 29*(4), 826–831.

Klienman, A., & Benson, R. (2006). Alexander Richman commemorative lecture: Culture, experience, and medicine. *Mount Sinai Journal of Medicine, 73*(6), 834–839.

Levinas, E. (1988). Useless suffering. In R. Bernasconi & D. Wood (Eds.), *The provocation of Levinas: Rethinking the other.* London, UK: Routledge.

Morse, J., & Carter, B. (1995). Strategies of enduring and the suffering of loss: Modes of comfort used by a resilient survivor. *Holistic Nursing Practice, 9*(3), 38–52.

Nepo, M. (2007) *Facing the lion, being the lion, finding inner courage where it lives.* San Francisco, CA: Conari Press.

Noddings, N. (1989). Woman's answer to Job. In R. Taylor & J. Watson (Eds.), *They shall not hurt: Human suffering and human caring.* Boulder: Colorado Associated University Press.

Råholm M. (2008). Uncovering the ethics of suffering using a narrative approach. *Nursing Ethics, 15*(1), 62–72.

Raphael, M. (2003). The female face of God in Auschwitz. New York, NY: Routledge.

Rogers, B., & Cowles, K. (1997). A conceptual foundation for human suffering in nursing care and research. *Journal of Advanced Nursing, 25,* 1048–1053.

Skaggs, B. & Barron, C. (2006). Searching for meaning in negative events: concept analysis. *Journal of Advanced Nursing, 53* (5), 559–570.

Steeves, R. H.,& Kahn, D. L. (1987). Experience of meaning in suffering. *Image: Journal of Nursing Scholarship, 19*(3), 114–117.

White, W., Newbauer, J., Sutherland, J., & Cox, C. (2005). Lifestyle strengths of Holocaust survivors. *Journal of Individual Psychology, 61*(1), 37–46.

Wiesel, E. (2006). *Night.* New York, NY: Hill and Wang.

Younger, J. (1995). The alienation of the sufferer. *Advances in Nursing Science, 17*(4), 53–72.

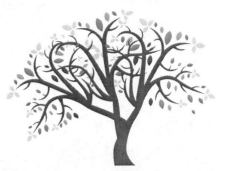

NINE

The Nurse as Witness to Suffering

■ Kathleen Ouimet Perrin

Objectives

1. Describe the responses of nurses and students to patients' and families' suffering.
2. Compare and contrast enduring and suffering.
3. Identify ways to assist healers to cope with their patients' suffering.
4. Analyze ways that you have responded to a patient's suffering.

Student Project

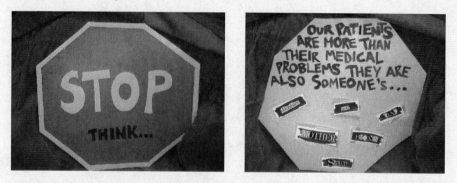

The stop sign reminds us to stop and see each patient as someone's father, mother, brother, sister, or child.

Source: Courtesy of Kaitlin Farley, student nurse.

Case Study 9–1

Mrs. G was very pale and always seemed to look as though she was in pain. She had a naso-gastric tube, Foley catheter, and IV which probably caused her discomfort. To make her situation worse, she could not talk and she could not move on her own, not even to use her call bell. Because of this she, could not let anyone know if she wanted or needed anything. She was a diabetic and her blood sugars were taken every 6 hours, with insulin shots following. She also had to go to dialysis at least three times a week and one week, she went every day. However, worst of all, she had recently had an above the knee amputation that had dehisced and the entire leg was completely open. She had to endure painful dressing changes when gauze would be packed into the wound and wrapped around her leg. She was NPO and being fed by tube feeds through her NG; however, she continued to have frequent and sometimes constant diarrhea. Because her amputation was so high, the diarrhea would get into her dressing. No matter how many pads the nurses used to protect the dressing, it always got dirty. Her incontinence also caused many open sores on her bottom, which made changing her extremely painful. Her world was filled with all types of physical pain. When the nurses were changing her she could not express any of the physical pain that she was experiencing because she could not talk. She could not yell or scream or tell us to stop, like any of the other patients.

Source: Courtesy of Shaylin Kirby, student nurse.

Questions on the Case Study

1. What types of suffering is the patient experiencing and how do you know that?
2. What can the caregivers do to acknowledge to the patient that they recognize her suffering?
3. Does her caregiver appear to be suffering? If so how?

Introduction

Mark Nepo (2000) describes how African Bushmen greet each other when one becomes aware of the other coming out of the bush. The one who first notices calls out to the other, " I see you," and the other responds, " I am here." Nepo believes that the way these Bushmen are bearing witness to each other is simple yet profound because it speaks directly to the desire that all people have to be seen as they are and for those who see them to acknowledge the journey that has brought the traveler to where he is.

Bearing Witness/Not Bearing Witness

The idea of seeing and acknowledging an individual as he or she journeys through suffering is a similar concept, often called bearing witness. Most authors indicate that the act of bearing witness to suffering includes not just the component of seeing the person but also, like the Bushmen, letting the person know that he was seen. For patients, being seen by a nurse means that the patients recognize that the nurse sees beyond their disease and vulnerability to the human individuals that they are at that moment. Arman (2007) describes these two parts of bearing witness as witnessing as seeing and witnessing as telling or acting. These two parts are further developed into four aspects that indicate what the caregiver should do after witnessing the sufferer. The four aspects include the caregiver

- witnessing the entire situation including the patient's suffering;
- telling the patient that the situation has been seen and understood;

- acting to improve the situation and alleviate the suffering; and
- shining the light of hope on the situation by being open and caring.

Ethical Aspects of Bearing Witness

Cody (2007) states that nurse researchers worldwide are exploring what is involved in bearing witness to suffering, which he believes is a fundamental part of being human. His focus is on the ethical aspects of bearing witness or not bearing witness. According to Cody, bearing witness means being present with the suffering person and in so doing accepting the risk of suffering alongside the person. In contrast, turning away from suffering and refusing to bear witness devalues human connectedness. He explores the issues that arise when caregivers try to maintain a balance between the two. He summarized one of his studies by saying that although bearing witness to suffering was challenging, painful, and at times an emotionally costly decision, all of the caregivers eventually reached a place of comfort and peace. His definition of bearing witness, like Arman's (2007), went beyond merely seeing the suffering and included attesting to the reality of the patient's experience by being present. Unlike Arman who specified that the caregiver should shine the light of hope on the situation by being open and caring, Cody specified personal presence as the appropriate response.

Cody (2007) believes that bearing witness is a moral act. He suggests that when a nurse chooses to bear witness to a person's suffering experience, the nurse is committing to the values of respect for human dignity, veracity, nonmaleficence, and fidelity. He states that the nurse bearing witness is committing to listening to the patient's description of the experience and accepting the meaning the patient ascribes to it. Bearing witness also means acting to minimize patients' fears while facilitating their wishes and preferences.

Naef (2006) also believes that bearing witness is the moral way of relating to a patient. She describes bearing witness as listening to, being present for, and staying with the patient. Naef lists the specific behaviors required to bear witness as being attentive to the person's lived experiences and truths, honoring the person's uniqueness by respecting the person's choices about how to live, believing that people know themselves best and will make the most appropriate choices, and recognizing the interconnection between people. She equates bearing witness to giving testimony to suffering that has taken place or is taking place and believes that it is a "gesture of ethical resistance" (p. 149) and a well-articulated and particular way to provide care through living true presence.

Not Bearing Witness

Unfortunately, Cody (2007) believes that not bearing witness is common in patient care. He notes that healthcare professionals can be prevented from bearing witness by the dominant paradigm in the current healthcare system. Not bearing witness is turning away from the patient, dismissing what the patient experiences as not real or not important. He believes that in addition to failing to respect the human dignity of the patient, it creates the potential for errors because of the failure to pay attention to the patient.

Naef (2006) raises a question suggested by Cody: If bearing witness is such an ethical responsibility, why do some nurses turn away, leaving their patients to travel their journey through suffering alone? Answering her own question, Naef responds that nurses are turning away from intense moments of struggling, questioning, and the changing of life patterns. She calls not bearing witness a mistake or a missed opportunity and believes that the experience may return to haunt the nurse who chose to turn away because the face of the patient in her vulnerability will not go away. By not bearing witness to a patient, the nurse may experience moral distress.

Why therefore, would a nurse choose not to bear witness? Arman (2007) explains that bearing witness is in itself an act of courage because it makes the caregiver open and vulnerable to experiencing suffering with the patient. Bearing witness means being present for the patient despite being too busy because of working conditions or an atmosphere that favors completion of tasks rather than attention to patients. Cody (2001) notes that nurses may be too busy bearing witness to technical tasks to be present with their patients. As noted in Chapter 8, Georges (2004) states that some nurses may utilize distancing to remove themselves from the uncomfortable elements of patient care so that they do not have to question the suffering that they may be causing as they provide care.

Distancing Techniques

Whatever the reason, there are numerous techniques that nurses may use to distance themselves or disembody themselves so that they are not present, not bearing witness to their suffering patients. Maeve (1998) described a variety of behaviors that nurses use to temper their involvement with patients, such as setting limits/boundaries, coming to love/not love a patient, embodiment/disembodiment, and using humor. Setting limits in Maeve's definition was what Georges (2004) would call distancing; it meant clearly recognizing that what was happening was occurring in the patient's life and not the nurse's. Coming to love/not love meant coming to terms with how much the nurse cared about each individual patient and recognizing that she could not care equally about each of them. Maeve defined disembodiment as dissociating oneself from one's body so that one is not truly present in the situation and not fully bearing witness to the patient's suffering during the experience. Finally, humor was sometimes used to temper involvement when the nurse needed to bolster courage to face something truly awful.

Communication Strategies Nurses Use with Suffering Patients

In a classic article from 1992, reprinted in 2006, Morse, Bottorff, Anderson, O'Brien, and Solberg identified and described communication strategies that nurses employ with patients who are suffering. They were able to identify two broad characteristics: whether the nurse became engaged with the patient, or whether the nurse's communication style was disengaged from the patient.

Patient-Focused

Morse and colleagues note that when the nurse is engaged with the patient's suffering experience, the patient's suffering is embodied by the nurse and the suffering experience is shared. In addition to whether the caregiver was engaged in the situation, the responses were also categorized by whether they were focused on the patient or the caregiver. Here are few examples of patient–focused, engaged responses by nurses that Morse and others (2006) believe may result in comfort for the patients:

- *Consolation:* "I am working with you" or other easing, soothing expressions of encouragement. This response is initiated by the patient but led by the nurse; the patient is passive. It usually results in a temporary reduction in the patient's suffering.
- *Compassion:* Sensitivity to the other's plight shown by listening and echoing the patient's sentiment. The response is initiated by the patient and both the patient and the nurse participate.
- *Commiseration:* Sharing of mutual predicaments. This is more often found in support groups and involves listening to tribulations, expressions of agreement, and a shared response.

However, nurses are not always able to be engaged and patient-focused. For example, a nurse may need to limit her sharing of the experience so that she can move on and care for other patients or to avoid becoming emotionally drained and exhausted. In such circumstances, a nurse who is patient-focused may use second-level responses that are professional learned responses that do not require engagement. According to Morse and others (2006), these second-level responses keep the nurse somewhat detached, objective, and at a distance (although just a short one) from the patient. These responses, although occasionally off target, are usually therapeutic. Listed here are a few examples of such patient–focused, learned, professional responses:

- Therapeutic empathy, which is a learned empathetic response that maintains the nurse at a distance from the patient.
- Informative reassurance, which is a purposeful attempt on the part of the nurse to reduce the patient's feeling of uncertainty and produce a state of calmness. Usually the nurse attempts to accomplish this by providing information and explanations.
- Humor.

Self-focused
Morse and others (2006) have determined that caregivers who need to protect themselves from engagement may utilize self-focused responses to suffering patients. These responses help to create or maintain the distance that the caregiver needs to remain unengaged and therefore are also known as distancing behaviors. Nurses may use such responses when they are exhausted, burned out, or overcome by the stress of dealing with a specific situation. First-level, reflexive responses that are caregiver-focused include presenting a front to the patient that all is well and as it should be. This response may be therapeutic as it may protect the patient if a situation is particularly unpleasant and the patient is watching the nurse for any indication of just how terrible the situation really is. However, if the patient eventually realizes that the nurse is hiding the truth of the situation, it may erode the trust between nurse and patient.

When nurses or other caregivers need to continue working but are unable to bear their patients' suffering, they may employ responses that are self-focused and not engaged (Morse, 2006). In such situations, the patient may be treated as a case or a stranger rather than a person. The provider may appear mechanical, absent-minded, or even callous in responses. Typical responses used by caregivers that are self-focused and not engaged include failure to listen to the patient, false reassurance, rote learned responses that fit the patient into a known pattern, and false pity. In these circumstances, Morse and others believe the patient may be in jeopardy because the patient's needs are ignored, the caregiver is unable to provide the necessary care, and there is no one who can or will serve as an advocate for the patient.

Morse (2006) cautions that although engaged patient-focused responses to the suffering patient are beneficial to the patient, it is not possible for a nurse to connect in such a way with all patients at all times. To do so would be problematic for the nurse. In some situations, other types of relationships may protect the caregiver or be needed by the patient and appropriate for the situation. Morse (2001) believes that the caregivers' responses should be matched to the behaviors displayed by the patient to achieve the desired outcome.

Morse's Model of Patient Suffering

When we speak about witnessing suffering, we talk about understanding the suffering but, like the Bushmen, what we see is the actual person as she emerges from the suffering experience. As we are looking at the person, it is crucial that we recognize and acknowledge the behaviors that indicate suffering. Morse (2001) was concerned that although nurses were giving voice to patients' stories of suffering and responding to suffering, there was no accurate research-based description of the behaviors that patients displayed while suffering. More important, she believed that there were no research-based studies describing how nurses should respond to the specific behaviors patients were displaying. Therefore, she undertook a series of discrete research projects funded by the National Institutes of Health and the Medical Research Council of Canada to explore various aspects of suffering and how best to comfort suffering people. The model of suffering that she developed from these projects is based on interviews and videotapes of trauma and burn victims, patients with chronic conditions, oncology patients, and patients in palliative care. It allows nurses and other caring professionals to identify and respond to the cues of suffering.

Morse's revised model (2001) is composed of two behavioral states: enduring and emotional suffering. In the first phase, enduring, patients suppress all emotions so they can get through whatever extraordinary psychological or physiological shock has caused their suffering. They are not capable of consciously or deliberately selecting responses; their energy is focused solely on getting through the situation. This means that they cannot weigh alternative responses, hope is paralyzed, and they just exist. In the second phase, emotional suffering, the suffering patients begin to grasp the situation and are able to acknowledge that what has happened is real. Only when they begin to have a realistic appraisal of the event can emotional suffering begin; then they may seek emotional support or consolation and may begin to move ahead.

Enduring

Morse (2001) describes enduring as a natural and necessary part of the response to suffering that helps people survive the initial impact of the threat to themselves. It is a blocking of emotional response so they can focus on what must be done in the present moment and allows them to accomplish what they believe must be done. Morse states that "individuals intuitively sense that they must be strong or they will not be able to support others and do what needs to be done" (p. 57). For example, a mother might have to inform a child that the father had been injured in an auto accident and then drive to the hospital to be with her spouse. The capacity to endure allows her to inform others of the injury and, more importantly, to safely drive to the hospital if no one is available to drive her. The mother's emotions are suppressed as she goes through the motions of informing people, finding someone to provide child care, and driving to the hospital.

According to Morse (2001), enduring can occur at differing levels of intensity depending on the level of the threat. In the most extreme example, the person will appear emotionless and have a masklike expression. Other visible signs and behaviors that a person enduring may display include

- erect, upright posture with shoulders back and head up;
- mechanical movements and a robotlike gait;
- lack of eye contact and an unfocused gaze;
- little movement of mouth and face while speaking and a monotone voice; and
- short sentences with many sighs.

The person usually remains alone and aloof, nonverbally sending the messages "Leave me alone, stand back, I'm okay" (Morse, 2001, p. 54). In a family group, if the family is enduring, there are spaces between the family members;

they do not touch each other, maintain eye contact, or talk with the person who is enduring the most. To support the person who is enduring the most, they may talk for him and will stand on either side of him, but will not touch him.

It is important for nurses to remember that this blocking of private grief allows for performance of public behavior during events such as funerals, but it does not bring relief to the patient or family. Additionally, those enduring, although they rate themselves at the time as functioning well, are not functioning well, cannot make well thought-out decisions, and do not realize how poorly they are functioning and thus how poor their decisions are likely to be. In addition, enduring may result in such emotional suppression that the person does not recall the event or any information that was provided.

The person who is enduring is living only in the present; she is not aware of the past or the future. This allows the person to keep going minute by minute or second by second. To get through the threat, the person may utilize strategies that help her to hold on, such as marking the time by counting things such as seconds or breaths.

Releases from Enduring

The energy and emotion suppressed while a person is enduring must eventually be released. The pent-up emotion is the reason patients and families may have emotional outbursts, expressing anger at some trivial or tangential issue and blowing it completely out of proportion. For example, a patient who had had serious medical problems following a mitral valve replacement needed a bedpan at change of shift. The patient's daughter found several nursing assistants who had their coats on and were leaving the unit. She yelled at them for several minutes for leaving when her father needed the bedpan even though an incoming staff member was already attending to her father. As Morse believes is typical, after the few minutes the tirade lasted, the daughter returned to enduring.

Escapes from Enduring

Morse (2001) believes that people who are enduring occasionally need an escape from enduring. These escapes are mind-absenting behaviors since they allow the person to think about something other than what is occurring. They may include strategies that direct the mind, like crossword puzzles, engaging in strenuous physical exercise, or laughing hysterically. Morse believes that these escapes, like enduring itself, are instinctive behaviors that are helpful since they help the person to protect herself from the threatening event.

Another example of escape from enduring occurred with the daughter described previously. Immediately after her father's admission to the hospital, the family was informed that a balloon pump had been inserted and their father would need an aortic valve replacement. More problematically, the surgeon had informed the family that he was gravely concerned about the sudden onset of valvular dysfunction, suspected endocarditis, and anticipated a poor prognosis. The family had been asked to leave the patient while he was situated in the intensive care unit. Because it was evening and no one had eaten all day, they asked for directions to the cafeteria from a woman working in the gift shop. The woman was foreign, and she suggested that they follow the signs with the "fork" on them. Her mispronunciation of the word "fork" had the daughter laughing hysterically—all the way down the hall into a packed elevator. When the people in the elevator stared at her, she merely repeated the mispronunciation and laughed even harder. After the hysterical laughter, she returned to enduring.

Types of Enduring
Morse et al. (2006) has identified three types of enduring. These are enduring to survive, enduring to live, and enduring to die. Enduring to survive occurs in situations like burns and trauma and enables patients to focus on getting themselves through the trauma. Morse and Carter (1995) call this endurance because these people have such a tenuous hold on life. During this type of endurance all of a patient's concentration and energy are needed just to live through the moment. Reality may seem too incredible to understand. Enduring to live occurs in untenable life situations such as those described by Frankl and Wiesel in Chapter 8. These situations are still deplorable, but the person is usually not physiologically threatened. In this type of enduring, all of the person's energy is focused on maintaining psychological integrity and protecting the self. Enduring to die occurs as the patient is dying. Enduring requires less energy than emotional releasing so dying individuals may endure to conserve energy and remain focused on what is most important to them at the end of life. Morse et al. (2006) believe that as their condition deteriorates, fatigue will overwhelm them and they will slip from enduring and surrender to death.

Morse (2001) states emphatically that those who are enduring should have their enduring supported. They should not be touched, as that will give them something else that they must "resist if they are to maintain control—another thing to resist and to be endured" (p. 57). When a nurse realizes that a patient or family member is enduring, the nurse can be supportive by such verbal statements as "You're holding up well." Even if the person seems unaware of the nurse's presence, being with the patient in silence may be supportive to the enduring person. Any support provided should be focused and, according to Morse, empathy should not be used. Enduring people are emotionally unavailable and an empathetic statement or statement may break through the enduring. Morse calls this "side swiping" (p. 57), as enduring people are trying to maintain control, and empathy makes it more difficult for them to do so.

Failure to Endure

Through research with patients and families who have had endured a traumatic injury, Morse (2001) has uncovered six patterns of behavior that indicate that either the patient or significant others are failing to endure. The first four states are unconscious, relaxed/normal, scared, and afraid. According to Morse, these states signify that there has been some degree of relinquishment for the care from the person or family to the healthcare providers. Nurses will find information about strategies for comforting patients exhibiting these four behaviors in Chapter 11, Conveying Comfort. Some of these comfort strategies may also be helpful for the patient or family member in the fifth state, terrified. Unfortunately, neither Morse nor other healthcare providers have identified nonpharmacological comfort strategies for patients who are failing to endure and are in the sixth state, loss of control. Morse describes these patients as screaming and unable to hold still, and usually needing pharmacological management or restraints for delivery of needed care to proceed.

Morse (2001) states, "Those who are enduring do not move from enduring to emotional suffering until they are tentatively ready to accept their loss" (p. 52). However, people may move slightly beyond enduring and "taste emotional suffering, then sense the possibility of emotionally disintegrating and instantly move back to enduring" (p. 52) or they may move back and forth between enduring and emotional suffering depending on the context of the situation, their energy level, or the amount of support available to them. Nurses and other healthcare providers need to recognize that moving from enduring to emotional suffering is not a linear process, so they must be careful to assess each person to determine what phase the person is in at each moment and what response is appropriate.

Emotional Suffering

Emotional suffering is described by Morse (2001) as a very distressed state in which emotions are released. The person is filled with sadness and displays the sadness by crying, sobbing, or moaning constantly. The emotionally suffering person may

- assume a stooped posture;
- have a face that is lined and a drooping facial expression;
- look as if he or she will fall apart;
- talk with whoever will listen, repeating his or her illness story over and over.

Telling the illness story repeatedly helps sufferers to make the story their own, affirm the story, and understand what has really happened. Morse notes that patients may say something like, "When I tell you, it makes it seem real."

During the emotionally suffering phase, the person recognizes the significance or meaning of whatever is changed or lost and there is recognition that the future is irrevocably altered. Still, this phase marks the beginning of healing. Gradually, hope begins to seep in, possible alternative futures are imagined, realistic goals are established, and strategies are developed. Note, this is the same function that telling the story served for the sufferer and was described in Chapter 8, The Search for Meaning in Suffering. Telling the story helps sufferers to move from the state of despair to being able to reformulate themselves.

Escapes from Emotional Suffering

Just as there must be escapes from enduring, there must also be escapes from emotional suffering (Morse, 2001). After experiencing a taste of the release of emotional suffering, people may fear that they will lose control to the emotions that overwhelm them and they may move back to enduring temporarily. The expression of emotion, the crying, moaning, and sobbing require an incredible expenditure of energy. After a period of such energy expenditure, they may be depleted of energy and may move temporarily back to enduring. Otherwise, they may employ some strategies that help them temporarily escape from the work of emotional suffering. These strategies are usually mind-numbing strategies and include such things as

- mindless watching of television;
- excessive sleeping, drinking, or eating; and
- conservation of physical energy.

In short, emotional suffering is an exhausting stage and people usually cannot continue in it for a protracted period of time before needing a break from it with a return to enduring. Morse (2001) has identified two major factors that influence people's movement between enduring and suffering. These are cultural and behavioral norms for enduring and suffering and the environmental context of the suffering. Davitz and Davitz in 1980 clearly found differences among patients', families', and nurses' beliefs about what was an appropriate display of emotion during suffering, depending on the patients' ethnic group. Nurses need to be aware that there are varying cultural norms about how to display suffering when caring for a patient and find a way to observe or tactfully ask what the families' expectation of suffering involves. There are also differences in environmental context for where a family member may emotionally suffer and where one may endure. Morse gives an example of the difference between the family in the patient's room and the family in the waiting room. Families may endure while in the patient's room because they fear that displaying the full extent of their suffering will have a negative impact on the patient. For example, the daughter of the patient with valvular disease described previously escaped from enduring or displayed emotional suffering only when she was out of her father's sight.

Responses to Emotional Suffering

Emotionally suffering individuals are easy to identify because their distress is so visible. This highly visible suffering usually calls forth an appropriate response from those who witness it. Unlike the response to the person who is enduring, the response to the person who is emotionally suffering usually involves touch. The touch may involve surrounding the person in an embrace, providing a support for the person to lean on, or offering consolation by stroking or holding the person's hand or arm. In any case, Morse (2001) recommends that the touch should be firm.

Morse (2001) suggests that the voices and words of the caregiver should be consoling. People who are emotionally suffering need to talk and tell their story, so caregivers should make every effort to listen attentively to what they have to say. At this stage, Morse recognizes that empathy is an appropriate response to the sufferer's behaviors. If the person is seeking reassurance, she states that it is appropriate for the caregiver to provide it as long as it is realistic. For example, "I'll be there for you" (Morse, 2001, p. 57). Mobilizing assistance with daily tasks, providing comfort, food, and emotional support are also important at this time. Morse believes that the stage of emotional suffering is a prerequisite for healing. She also believes that suffering can result in growth for the people involved, saying, "People who have suffered reconstitute their lives, and they describe themselves as richer for the experience of suffering. They have an urge to 'give back' to help those who are suffering to help them get through the experience" (p. 53).

What Do Nurses Do with the Suffering They Have Witnessed?

Years ago at a National Endowment for the Humanities Summer Institute in Nursing Ethics, Andrew Jameton, a philosopher who was writing a nursing ethics text, remarked that he thought of hospitals as places where there was endless human suffering and he envisioned nurses as the people who swept up all that suffering. Then he would wonder, what do the nurses do with the suffering after they have gathered it all up? Years later, his question still remains: How do nurses personally respond to the suffering that they have witnessed? Does it change them? If so, how and why? Nursing researchers have looked at which stressors impact nurses the most and identified some ways for nurses to respond to the suffering that they have witnessed.

Findings from Nurses Working with AIDS Patients

Sherman (2000) examined the ways that nurses were affected by the stress of providing care to patients who were very ill and dying from acquired immune deficiency syndrome (AIDS). She found that one of the major sources of stress for nurses occurred early in the AIDS epidemic when they would repeatedly see young people suffering and dying and the families dealing with loss and depression. She noted that the nurses had more difficulty providing care to these dying patients if they had unresolved personal losses. Nurses also experienced stress because they felt as if their senses were being bombarded by the sights and smells of the dying patient with AIDS. The patient might have copious diarrhea or severe and draining wounds. The nurses noted that dealing with the offensive sights and odors was more difficult because they had to guard their responses. They did not want the patients to believe the nurse found them repulsive. The nurses also noted that connecting with these patients was often a source of emotional stress. If they developed a close attachment, they felt the pain when they performed a painful procedure and they experienced pain when the patient died. Conversely, the patients they found it most difficult to care for were the ones they felt they could not connect with, no matter what they tried.

However, Sherman (2000) did not just look at sources of stress (or suffering) of nurses involved in AIDS care; she also described some ways that the nurses had learned to alleviate the emotional stress they were experiencing. She recommended that nurses establish a balance between their personal and professional lives. This included first and foremost finding time for laughter and taking care of themselves. It also included acknowledging unresolved losses; sharing with colleagues, family, or a counselor; and obtaining assistance and emotional support when necessary. She recommended releasing the pain by speaking about it, crying about it, or portraying it in some format so that it did not become trapped inside. Finally, she noted that it was important to acknowledge when help was needed and to ask for it.

Threats to Healers

Rowe (2003) also examined the distress that nurses might experience when caring for suffering patients and made recommendations on how to prepare nurses to cope with both their patients' and their own suffering. He was especially concerned that nursing students were not prepared to cope with the suffering they saw and sometimes caused. He believes that part of the difficulty is that nurses went into the profession to be healers, not to cause suffering, and thus causing suffering while providing care can be a real threat to the intactness of the nurse. He identified a variety of threats that can lead to the suffering of the healer:

- *Reverberations from the past.* These are events in the nurse's own past that have caused suffering and are similar to what the patient is experiencing. Sherman (2000) identified a similar concern but called it unresolved personal issues. For example, a nurse might find it very difficult to care for a patient with Alzheimer's disease while she was providing care to her mother with the same disorder. A nurse who might otherwise be able to care for a dying patient might just have learned of the suicide of a friend and might not be able to provide appropriate care around that time.

- *Expectations.* The nurse might have high or unrealistic expectations for herself. For example, a new ICU nurse caring for her first patient who had suffered cardiac arrest found herself running into the bathroom when the patient started to hemorrhage from all his IV sites and every orifice during CPR. She was distraught later that she had not remained with the patient throughout the code.

- *Guilt.* The threat to the intactness of the nurse when she makes a mistake may cause guilt. For example, a nurse who had been working for 6 years without a single error was giving insulin in the era before writing a U for Units was banned. She interpreted a 10 unit dose as 100 units and administered 100 units of insulin. Fortunately, the patient was not harmed because she realized her mistake and the patient received IV glucose. But the nurse felt so guilty that a month later, she had still not returned to work.

- *Vulnerability.* The realization that as a healthcare provider the nurse can be harmed while providing care can feel threatening. This might happen from a needle stick, a splash injury, or violence in the hospital. Another most common reason for nurses to experience the threat of vulnerability is providing care to another healthcare provider who is suddenly ill with a life-threatening illness.

- *High cost of empathy.* As noted in Sherman's (2000) study, caring too much causes pain while caring too little can result in discomfort and even distress. How much can a nurse care for each person? Are some situations just too difficult to bear?

- *Inflicting pain.* For nurses in some settings, such as intensive care units, much of what they do is painful. For example, suctioning, turning, or changing the dressings on a patient may cause pain. A nurse's identity as a healer may be threatened when she is frequently causing her patients pain even if the pain is intended to aid in their cure.

- *Silence.* Frequently a new healthcare provider's efforts to speak about the burdens inherent in the experience are met with the comments such as "You just can't let it get to you" or "Don't take it home with you." How one is supposed to do that is never addressed (Rowe, 2003, p. 18)

- *Threats to the healer's spiritual or philosophical beliefs.* Just as the patient is searching for the reason and meaning in the suffering, the nurse may be searching as well. The nurse may wonder why this suffering was allowed to happen. It may cause the nurse to search for meaning and to experience distress if she is unable to resolve the search.

Rowe (2003) wonders how nurses and other healers respond to their own suffering. He believes some healthcare providers choose to ignore their own suffering. Instead, they may focus on the scientific aspect of what is happening to their patients, failing to see the patients as persons at all. Or, as Cody (2007) said, they may focus only on the tasks that have to be accomplished. Rowe, like Morse (2001), believes that something of incredible value is lost when this happens because he believes the "healer ceases to heal in order to avoid suffering" (p. 19). Perhaps even more important, he believes that a nurse who overcomes suffering has the potential for personal and professional growth.

Rowe examines the phases of suffering in healers. He describes phases that are comparable to the phases described in Chapter 8 for people suffering for other reasons. He states that suffering healers in phase one are mute. They are unable to talk about what is causing their pain and may turn the emotion inward resulting in depression. Like any depressed person, they may develop submissive behavior, withdrawal and apathy. They are not capable of engaging with patients and appear to be going through the motions when at work

As they enter phase two, Rowe (2003) states that nurses find their voice and are able to lament and to communicate about their suffering. At first, the lamenting, similar to that described in Chapter 8, may include blaming or anger. Just as it is important to have ill patients tell their illness story in order to integrate it and grow, it is important to have the wounded healers tell their stories as well. Just as suffering patients need someone to listen in order to fully develop their story, the wounded healer needs an understanding and empathetic listener. After the story has been told and as it is being integrated, Rowe recommends that the technique of reframing be suggested. The technique involves changing the healer's perspective on the event so as to reduce the threat. For example, if the threat that caused the suffering was unrealistic expectations of themselves, the nurses might redefine what is reasonable in the situation. Thus, the nurse who left the ongoing code and was ill might talk with another nurse and realize that it was an especially horrible code so that it was not surprising to feel distressed about it. Leaving was not a sign of failure but a sign of legitimate distress at a horrible event.

Rowe (2003) believes there are a number of other ways that healers can come to terms with their own suffering but cautions that healers usually need assistance to be successful. They may need to come to terms with either their own or the institution's limits. All healers need to learn at some point that they cannot save every single patient and all educators need to realize at some point that they cannot reach every single student. If the suffering has involved threats to the healer's personal philosophy or spirituality, then the person may need to engage in a time of wrestling with his or her faith. Most significantly, Rowe (2003) stresses the importance of communication once the healer has arrived at this stage and has found a voice. This might include debriefing after an event or participation in support groups. In fact, Rowe states that such activities should be considered essential for all healthcare providers.

In the third and final phase of suffering as described by Rowe (2003), the recovering healer begins to work to change the existing structures. Healers who originally imagined that they were suffering alone learned in phase two that they were not alone. Now, in phase three, they are able to work with others in similar situations to bring about change. Rowe recommends that healers in this stage utilize two methods to bring about change: research and political action.

Rowe (2003) concludes by reemphasizing the importance of healthcare workers learning to share their suffering with each other. When healers refuse to speak about their suffering or listen to the suffering of their colleagues, they only worsen the suffering. Rowe states, "The single most important element in reducing the suffering of the healer is to reduce isolation. Isolation is an essential element in the first stage of suffering, and overcoming that isolation is an essential element in moving through the second and third stages" (p. 20).

Nurses' Narratives About Patient Suffering

Long before Rowe (2003), Kahn and Steeves (1994) had determined that nurses volunteer and share very little about the suffering they witness. However, if asked, nurses are able to provide detailed, embodied descriptions of the types of suffering their patients experience. Steeves and Kahn published detailed narratives from nurses describing how they had been affected by the suffering of their patients. Nurses' narratives about suffering usually begin with a description of physical pain. Freshman nursing students usually see pain as the most potent contributor to suffering (Davitz & Davitz, 1980). Yet, after their first clinical course, nursing students, like practicing nurses, see other dimensions as equally or more important in suffering and view suffering as having multiple dimensions and problems, perhaps including social embarrassment or unacceptability mixed with discomfort. The more problems the patients had, the more their suffering increased. Davitz and Davitz noted that nurses were more concerned about the suffering associated with a broken arm in a cleaning woman who could not work, had no "sick time," no health insurance, and no other means of support for her three children than an executive with a similar broken arm.

Kahn and Steeves (1994) believe that when nurses personalize the suffering of patients, it has a strong effect on the nurses and may make them despair of their profession. In an unpublished doctoral dissertation, Perrin (2001) found that experienced ICU nurses began to talk about their patients by describing the patient's deteriorating physiologic status. For example, "his BP was 70/30 on maximum drips, his urine output was 20 mLs all day, and he had four plus pedal edema." However, the nurses quickly supplemented this picture with information about the human costs of their patients' illnesses. Although the nurses would try to relieve each patient's physical and mental suffering, sometimes they were unable to and they would have to bear witness to the patient's anguish. Nurses stated, "It became unbearable to watch the suffering any longer, although we were really free with our medication" or "He looked like the painting, 'The Scream.' " (Perrin, 2001).

After listening to the nurses' narratives of suffering, Kahn and Steeves (1994) noted that the nurses had clearly developed an understanding of the suffering they witnessed in their clinical practice. They wondered, like Jameton (1983) had earlier, what do nurses do in response to the suffering they witness. They believe that nurses have a special obligation in their role as witnesses to patient suffering to act as moral agents and to speak out about what they had witnessed. Note how similar this is to the process of witnessing by Arman (2007) that was discussed earlier in the chapter.

However, the four aspects of bearing witness that Kahn and Steeves (1994) describe for nurses are slightly different from those suggested by Arman (2007). The first aspect they describe emphasizes the importance of the nurse as a first-hand observer of the events. Because nurses have directly observed the events, Kahn and Steeves have found that they recall the events in detail, their remembrances are vivid, and they seldom resort to professional jargon when describing the events. This means they are able to clearly inform others of what they observed. Kahn and Steeves note that if asked, nurses will usually speak readily about what they have witnessed. They argue that to remain silent is to deny its seriousness and impact. They fear that by remaining silent the nurse only distances herself from the patient and situation, and that may result in depersonalization and dehumanization for both nurse and patient. This position corroborates what Rowe (2003) said concerning the importance of healthcare providers speaking up about what they have witnessed.

The second aspect of witnessing, the ceremonial role described by Kahn and Steeves (1994), is not as prominent in other authors' discussions. This aspect of witnessing may be less evident because it is not well developed in the Western world. However, Kahn and Steeves argue that it is practiced and visible in hospice. They argue that in their role as hospice nurses, they have served as ceremonial witnesses to patients' and families' gradual realization that the patient is declining and dying.

The final two aspects of Kahn and Steeves' (1994) witnessing are serving as an expert witness and bearing witness. They believe that nurses, because they can speak as firsthand witnesses, should serve as expert witnesses and testify in public healthcare forums about areas in which they have specific expertise so as to improve the healthcare system. For example, a nurse might speak about what can done to improve pain management or to initiate hospice care earlier in a terminally ill patient's care. The final aspect of witnessing that Kahn and Steeves describe is bearing witness. They believe that the nurse who bears witness is a visionary, one who speaks out about the suffering that she has encountered and works with others, both patients and healthcare providers, to help create an environment in which no person's suffering is ignored. Rowe (2003) consolidates these two aspects in his final phase of suffering of the healer when the recovering healer begins to work to change the existing structures.

Student Nurses' Responses to Patient Suffering

Rowe (2003) believes that efforts to help a healer cope with suffering should not wait until the person begins to experience distress. Rather, he hopes that nursing students will learn to discuss the suffering that occurs all around them in health care with their peers and their faculty. Gunby (1996) and Eifried (2003) both explored nursing students' experiences as they cared for patients who were suffering.

Gunby (1996) interviewed undergraduate nursing students about what it was like to care for an individual who was suffering. Students in her qualitative study rarely had to be asked any question after the first because they were so eager to talk.

Although they appeared anxious at the start of the interview, students remarked at the end that they were relieved to have been able to share their experiences and thanked the interviewer for allowing them to talk. The students participating in the study identified many of the themes identified by practicing nurses. They noted that the meaning (or lack of meaning) that the sufferer attributed to the suffering experience profoundly affected the outcomes. They believed that people who are suffering need someone to listen and to be truly present for them. Unfortunately, the students participating in Gunby's study reported that they had learned this on their own and they did not believe sufficient information about how to care for suffering patients or how to care for themselves was available from professional sources.

Student Nurses' Experiences of Bearing Witness

Eifried (2003) examined the lived experience of nursing students as they cared for patients who were suffering. She noted that nursing students, just like the professional healers in Rowe's study (2003), brought with them experiences from their past that reverberated with their patients' suffering. She uncovered six subthemes that captured the essence of how nursing students were able to bear witness to the suffering of their patients:

- *Grappling with suffering*: Many of the students in the study mentioned being nervous about the tasks they were trying to accomplish for the suffering patient. Others noted that they sometimes felt helpless to manage their patients' pain. All of the students described struggling to come to grips with the suffering experience and the many feelings suffering evoked. Similar to what Rowe (2003) determined about practicing nurses, what was worse than the helplessness or the inability to find meaning for the students in this study was their feeling of being alone in the struggle.
- *Struggling with the ineffable (the unspeakable)*: After being shocked by their patients' experiences, students often felt compelled to pose questions such as "why do patients have to go through this?" If they could find no explanations, students began to question their own beliefs about the role of suffering in people's lives and the ability of nurses to alleviate suffering.
- *Getting through*: The suffering of their patients often provoked feelings of hopelessness or loneliness in the students in Eifried's 2003 study. One way they were able to "get through" their experiences was to confide in others.

They described obtaining comfort from confiding in fellow students. A caring circle of fellow students would form and prevent the student from being isolated. However, faculty members were rarely included in this circle of support and students rarely told faculty of their emotions if they were not asked directly. Most students feared that it would be risky to let their faculty member learn they felt inadequate to care for the patients. When feeling overwhelmed and unable to find support during clinical, students reported hiding to collect their thoughts and emotions before returning to the bedside. Any isolated space, such as a bathroom or utility room, might serve as the hiding place.

■ *Being with patients who are suffering*: Despite all they were experiencing, most students in Eifried's study described finding the inner strength to pull them through so that they could focus on what the patient needed. As one student noted, "I wasn't going to let her down, so I stayed and it worked out really well. It's just getting over that hump, that fear, that anxiety that says "RUN" (Eifried, 63).

■ *Embodying the experience of suffering*: Students reported recognizing when their patients were in pain and almost feeling their patients' pain. They noted that even though the experience was painful, they learned through the embodiment of suffering.

■ *Seeing possibilities in suffering*: All of the participants in Eifried's study reported seeing the patient's courage and strength during the suffering. From this they learned to see possibilities in the suffering such as acceptance of limitations, finding meaning in one's own life, and learning about love.

Faculty Responses to Student Suffering

The students usually found a way on their own to see possibilities in the suffering. In fact, some of the students in Eifried's study actually said they felt abandoned by faculty when they encountered suffering in the clinical setting. They believed that it would have made them feel less inadequate and alone if faculty had been present with them to witness their patients' suffering, letting them know that it was okay to cry and helping them to feel supported. They suggested that there should be time at the end of the clinical day to discuss these experiences of suffering and foster closeness among the clinical group so that it could serve as a support group.

Similar to concerns that Rowe (2003) expressed about both nurses and students, Eifreid (2003) is troubled that students often care for patients in an environment that is both lonely and shrouded in silence. She wonders if this is the intent of faculty and asks whether faculty knowingly throw their students into a baptism by fire. She believes that this is not what faculty want to do or see themselves doing. Therefore, she recommends that faculty examine their own behavior to see how they are handling suffering in the clinical setting and suggests four approaches to create a caring community in which students could learn about the suffering experience:

Recommendations for Nursing Faculty
- First, redesign the clinical experience to include time for reflection and dialogue about suffering on the day of the experience. Be explicit about the topic for reflection as students are unlikely to open the topic of suffering on their own.
- Next, find a space in the clinical setting that is a "sacred space" where students can give voice to what they have been experiencing. They might need time there alone or with a caring other to listen to their story.
- Third, introduce students to writing narratives similar to the ones discussed in Chapter 8 to express emotions, reflect on experiences with suffering, and begin to integrate those experiences into their lives.
- Finally, encourage students to share experiences and bonding.

Experiences of Nursing Faculty
Peters (2006) explored the development of compassion during the everyday experiences of nursing faculty. She stated that the first attribute of compassion is "the deep feeling of connectedness or emotional response to the experience of human suffering" (p. 38). To experience compassion, a faculty member needed to understand the perspective and the meaning attached to the experience by the person suffering. Peters found that nursing faculty identified three types of sufferers: patients, students dealing with patients' suffering, and students dealing with their own suffering. Unlike what the students noted in Eifried's (2003) study, the faculty members in this study stated that they entered the suffering experience with the student and assisted the student in dealing with the suffering.

Peters (2006) uncovered six themes that conveyed the experiences of compassion of the faculty members in her study. The first of the themes was forming connections with others including both the student and the suffering patient. The second theme was walking a mile in another's shoes and involved understanding the student or patient experience by recalling a similar situation in which the faculty member had been involved. The third theme was recognizing needs, burdens, and sufferings. Peters believed this theme was distinctive because the faculty member stepped outside herself to examine the person's needs and suffering from a perspective that was not the faculty member's own. Fourth, faculty believed that they embraced the emotional response to suffering, opening themselves up to the sufferers' worlds sometimes by crying with their students. Fifth, faculty experienced an urgent desire to relieve the suffering and believed that they acted to make it better. Finally, faculty identified that they gave the gift of themselves, explained as what was more than was normally expected of them in such circumstances. In return they received notes and letters of appreciation from students.

Peters' (2006) study of how nursing faculty believe they respond to suffering is in dramatic contrast to the way that nursing students viewed faculty in the study by Eifried (2003). Since both were small-scale, qualitative studies, no conclusion can be reached about how nursing faculty as a whole respond to student suffering. However, what is common to both studies is that students and faculty believe faculty should respond to patients and students suffering in similar fashions. Perhaps, as Eifried suggested, faculty should examine their responses to be certain they are conveying what they intend.

Summary

Suffering individuals, whether patients, nurses, or students, need to have their suffering witnessed. Different researchers and authors have described variations on the specific aspects of bearing witness to suffering, but the essence remains the same. People who suffer need to have someone witness their suffering, assist them to tell the story of their suffering, assure them that the suffering has been seen and understood, act to improve the situation by alleviating the suffering, and shine the light of hope on the situation by being open and caring (Arman, 2007). This chapter has explored ways that nurses, students, and faculty members can bear witness to the suffering that surrounds them.

Key Points

1. Nurses should be aware of whether they are responding to patients with a patient-focused or a nurse-focused response.
2. Nurses may use distancing techniques so that they are not embodying the suffering of each of their patients. They should be aware of when they are using these techniques and if using them is benefiting them or their patients.
3. Morse believes that people who are suffering may be in either the phase of enduring or the phase of emotional suffering.
4. Nurses should be able to identify the behaviors associated with each of these phases of suffering and know how to respond appropriately to the sufferer in both of the phases.
5. Caregivers need to be aware of their own responses to suffering and determine whether they are mute, able to talk about it, or ready to actively begin to alleviate some of the sources of suffering.

Exercise: Witness to Suffering

Warm-up

Using crayon of any color of your choice,

Draw (without taking your crayon off the paper) Joy.
Select another crayon and draw Fear.
Select another crayon and draw Loneliness.
Select another crayon and draw Compassion.

Next: Take a crayon, draw what you imagine in your brain—the source of your intellect.

Take a crayon, draw what you feel in your heart—the source of your emotions.
Take a crayon and draw what you feel in your gut—the source of your instinct.
Take a crayon, draw what you feel in your backbone—the source of your support.

Finally: You may do whichever you prefer first, but should do both:

> Draw how you feel about your experience while caring for patients today.
> In writing, reflect on your experience caring for your patients.

Which format of expression did you prefer? Why?

Questions for Reflection and Journaling
1. How involved do you believe nurses should be with their patients?
2. Have you ever intentionally distanced yourself from a patient? Think about the patient: Why do you believe you needed to distance yourself from that patient? What behaviors did you employ to distance yourself from the patient? What were the consequences of your behavior?
3. Do you believe you have ever gotten too involved with a patient? Why do you think that? What were the consequences of your involvement?

Case Study 9–2: Bearing Witness

Before I could leave the room, Lucille suddenly turned her head back toward me and her eyes caught mine. I saw again the deep suffering she was undergoing within them. She reached out for my hand and held it tightly, and I sensed that she was not just frustrated but scared and lonely. While the nurse made her rounds, I stayed at the bedside, holding her hand and trying desperately to think of what I could do to alleviate her pain. No medicine or nursing intervention I knew could heal such suffering or bridge the gap left by the unspoken words between mother and son. I spoke softly to her and told her that she had a beautiful family, that she must be a wonderful mother to have raised such a kind and devoted son. Then I said that I understood it frustrated her to be unable to speak with him and that she must be feeling lonely too. Her eyes held mine in understanding and she began to cry. As the tears ran down her face, I felt the tears well up in my own eyes. I could not think of any words that would comfort her, and at the same time was surprised at myself. I was supposed to be the strong one, the one keeping it together so she didn't have to. Instead, I did the only natural thing there was to do. I held her hand and cried with her. I felt like the only thing I could do was share her pain, help her cry, and be with her. She kept eye contact with me the entire time, and as she cried, I felt a sense of peace come over her. It was as if being understood was all that mattered and perhaps in that moment, she felt as though I did. Even though no words were spoken, I never felt so connected to a patient as I did that night, and the memory of her eyes and the tight grasp of her hand remain vividly with me today.

Stroke

Silent sufferers

Trying desperately to

Reach

Out

Know they are understood

Eyes cannot hide their pain

Source: Courtesy of Erin Latina, student nurse.
The final definitive version of this material has been published in the *Journal of Holistic Nursing, 25*(3). By Sage Publications Ltd./Sage Publication, Inc. All rights reserved.

Questions on the Case Study

1. Do you believe that this student nurse embodied her patient's suffering? Why or why not?
2. How was the patient able to reach out to the student?
3. Do you believe that the student was able to help this patient? Why or why not?
4. Have you ever connected with a patient in a similar way? How did you feel about it? Would you connect with a patient in such a way again?

References

Arman, M. (2007). Bearing witness: An existential position in caring. *Contemporary Nurse, 27*(1), 84–94.

Cody, W. (2001). The ethics of bearing witness in health care: A beginning exploration. *Nursing Science Quarterly, 14*(4), 288–296.

Cody, W. (2007). Bearing witness to suffering: Participating in cotranscendence. *International Journal for Human Caring, 11*(2), 17–21.

Davitz, L., & Davitz, J. (1980). *Nurses' responses to patients suffering*. New York, NY: Springer.

Eifried, S. (2003). Bearing witness to suffering: The lived experience of nursing students. *Journal of Nursing Education, 42*(2), 59–67.

Georges, J. (2004). The politics of suffering: Implications for nursing science. *Advances in Nursing Science, 27*(4), 250–256.

Gunby, S. (1996). The lived experience of nursing students in caring for suffering individuals. *Holistic Nursing Practice, 10*(3), 63–73.

Jameton, A. (1983, June). Panel discussion at the National Endowment for the Humanities Summer Institute in Nursing Ethics, Medford, MA.

Kahn, D., & Steeves, R. (1994). Witness to suffering: Nursing knowledge, voice, and vision. *Nursing Outlook, 42*(6), 260–264.

Maeve, M. K. (1998). Weaving a fabric of moral meaning: How nurses live with suffering and death. *Journal of Advanced Nursing, 27*, 1136–1142.

Morse, J. (2001). Toward a praxis theory of suffering. *Advances in Nursing Science, 24*(1), 47–59.

Morse, J., Bottorff, J., Anderson, G., O'Brien, B., & Solberg, S. (2006). Beyond empathy: Expanding expressions of caring. *Journal of Advanced Nursing, 53*(1), 75–90.

Morse, J., & Carter, B. (1995). Strategies of enduring and the suffering of loss: Modes of comfort used by a resilient survivor. *Holistic Nursing Practice, 9*(3), 38–52

Naef, R. (2006). Bearing witness: A moral way of engaging in the nurse-patient relationship. *Nursing Philosophy, 7,* 146–156.

Nepo, M. (2000). *The book of awakening*. Berkeley, CA: Conari Press.

Perrin, K. (2001). *How ICU nurses interact with physicians to facilitate discussion of patient preferences about resuscitation* (Unpublished doctoral dissertation). Union Institute and University, Cincinnati, OH.

Peters, M. A. (2006). Compassion: An investigation into the experience of nursing faculty. *International Journal for Human Caring, 10*(3), 38–46.

Rowe, J. (2003). The suffering of the healer. *Nursing Forum, 38*(4), 16–20.

Sherman, D. (2000). Experiences of AIDS dedicated nurses in alleviating the stress of AIDS caregiving. *Journal of Advanced Nursing, 31*(6), 1501–1508.

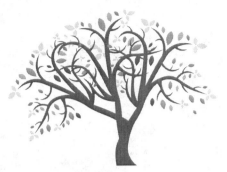

TEN

The Role of Healing and Holistic Nursing in Palliation of Suffering

■ **Maureen M. Gaynor, Mary K. Kazanowski, and Mertie L. Potter**

Objectives

1. Analyze the concepts of healing and holism as they relate to suffering.
2. Compare and contrast allopathic and holistic models of healthcare delivery.
3. Describe the practice of holistic nursing and its role in palliative care.
4. Examine the psychophysiology of body–mind healing.
5. Recognize the implications of body–mind interactions for clinical practice.
6. Explore select integrative modalities and their impact on suffering and healing.
7. Examine legal and ethical issues related to holistic nursing care.

Student Project

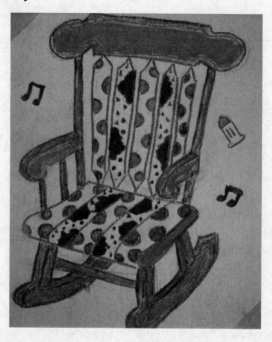

The infant was failing to thrive, so I spent the day rocking her, humming to her, and stroking her.

Case Study 10–1

I was working in the nursery as the nursery nurse for the day. This particular day, we had a boarder baby, a baby whose mother had unfortunately become very ill after giving birth and was now intubated in the ICU. Although attempts had been made to bring the baby to the mother, the mother decompensated each time the baby was brought to her bedside so the ICU nurses had asked that we discontinue visits until the mother stabilized. Although the father had visited at first, as his wife's illness progressed he came less and less often to visit with his newborn. At this point, this little baby had been staying in the nursery for almost 2 weeks with very few visitors, if any at all. Although she was physically healthy, she was definitely showing signs of withdrawing emotionally as she was missing out on the parent–infant bonding experience and even just physical touch and stimulation. To facilitate healing, I attempted to be a healing presence by spending every available moment I had with her during the day. I also tried to create a healing environment. I found a rocking chair in the back room and spent the day holding her in my arms, touching her, stroking her, and rocking her back and forth while talking and humming to her.

Source: Courtesy of Madelyn Cantarow, student nurse, 2010.

Questions on the Case Study

1. How do we know that rhythm, touch, sound, and physical presence are so crucial to infant maturation?
2. Are these modalities also important to the health and well-being of adults? Why or why not?
3. Which of the mentioned types of healing modalities could we also provide for older children and adults?

Introduction

This chapter introduces the concepts of holism and healing while identifying specific holistic nursing theories that support holistic nursing practice. Complementary and alternative medicine (CAM) is now being utilized by an increasing number of American consumers to help manage or prevent the onset of illness. Complementary and alternative medicine focuses on the mind–body–spirit of an individual and on healing the whole person. A variety of holistic modalities are defined and explored and their appropriateness in patient situations is identified. These holistic approaches offer nurses another tool to promote individuals' sense of comfort and well-being. In addition, there are select exercises included for nurses to utilize in their everyday nursing practice.

Concept of Healing

The origin of the word "heal" is the Anglo-Saxon word "Haelan," which means to be or to become whole (Dossey & Keegan, 2009). The basic assumption in healing is that human beings are open systems, with energy flowing in and out of the system, producing balance within the body. Just as suffering is multidimensional, so too is healing. Healing occurs not only in the physical domain but also in emotional, cognitive, and spiritual domains. Healing is defined as a process of being or becoming whole; "the process of bringing together aspects of one's self, body–mind–spirit, at deeper levels of inner knowing, leading toward integration and balance with each aspect having equal importance and value" (Dossey & Keegan, 2009, p. 48).

"If you become whole again," Kubler-Ross observed, "you're healed." Regardless of how serious the illness or suffering experience, the potential to be healed exists for all individuals. Healing occurs when nurses assist patients, families, and communities to move toward harmony and balance. Holistic nursing focuses on the patients' experience through their illness and assists patients in transcending their suffering in order to move toward new patterns of self-actualization (Dossey & Keegan, 2009). The focus of care of holistic nursing is not on recovery from illness but on integration of the illness (suffering) experience. This, too, is the focus of palliative care nursing. Integration and "healing," however, are a challenge because the Western model for health care does not always support this paradigm.

Healing and curing are different processes. Curing is an external approach focused on the elimination of disease. Curing, however, does not necessarily address the emotional, psychosocial, or spiritual suffering that may have accompanied the disease. Unfortunately, Western medicine has primarily focused on cure, and healing and care have not been valued.

Holistic Nursing

Holistic nurses providing palliative care provide person-centered care. In this process the nurse is fully present and gives his or her undivided attention to the patient. The nurse's presence honors and respects the totality of the patient. Paterson and Zderad defined presence as a "relational style within nursing interactions that involve being with, rather than doing to" (Paterson & Zderad, 1976, p. 122). "Being with" is the true essence of the nature of the nursing presence. It integrates intention with the sacredness of the present moment.

Definition of Holistic Nursing

Holistic nursing is defined as "all nursing practice that has healing the whole person as its goal" (Dossey & Keegan, 2009, p. 4). The foundation of holistic nursing practice focuses on the concept of holism, which views the person as an interrelated whole comprising bio-psycho-social-spiritual dimensions. Recognition of the integrated whole of the person encompasses the belief that the whole is more than and different from the sum of its parts (Dossey & Keegan, 2009). The practice of holistic nursing enables nurses to facilitate people's responses to achieve wholeness or heal. Suffering, can hinder a person's ability to achieve and maintain wholeness, or heal.

Holistic Nursing Theories

Several nursing theories support holistic (and palliative care) nursing. The American Holistic Nurses Association (AHNA) states, "Holistic nursing practice draws on knowledge, theories, expertise, intuition, and creativity" (Mariano, 2007, p. 166) Theory provides practitioners with the ability to contemplate current practice and provides guidelines in the development of a specialized body of knowledge. Nursing theory enables nurses to think about and guides decisions concerning their work.

Beginning in the 19th century, Florence Nightingale wrote in her text *Notes on Nursing* "that nursing's role is to put the patient in the best condition for nature to act upon him" (Nightingale, 1860, p. 75). Nightingale's philosophy reflects the concept of holism. She understood that the focus of nursing care encompassed the attributes of body, mind, spirit, and the environment. Her theory emphasized the interrelationship of the environment and the patient. Nightingale believed that healing involved both the internal and external environment of the person and it was the nurse's role to create this healing environment (Macrae, 2001).

Nightingale proposed and implemented a number of measures that included color, light, noise control, privacy, cleanliness, music, relaxation, and nutrition that supported a healing external environment. Her philosophy also focused on the internal or psychological state of the patient and its impact on the person's physical health. She observed that internal processes, such as anxiety and worry, robbed the body of energy necessary for healing (Macrae, 2001). The caring and therapeutic presence of the nurse reflects an important component of the internal healing environment that Nightingale believed was essential for promotion of health of the person. Nightingale also believed that nursing works in collaboration with the natural laws of the universe to promote human wholeness, which is the integration of body, mind, and spirit.

Jean Watson, in her theory of transpersonal caring, established caring as the most valuable attribute that nursing has to offer to patients and described the "caring occasion." These caring occasions provide an opportunity for the patient to experience unconditional positive regard and self-acceptance. These situations occur "when nurse and patient come together in unique ways such that there is a truly transformational encounter" (Watson, 1988). This development of a caring relationship between the nurse and the patient is health promoting, according to Watson. As part of the caring relationship, nurses focus on understanding patients' subjective experiences and acting to assist patients to achieve a higher degree of harmony within themselves (Watson, 1988).

Rosemary Rizzo Parse's theory of human becoming supports the concept of the person being viewed as a unified, whole being. Health is seen as a process of becoming. Parse (1992) believed that patients' reality is the result of the culmination of their own life experiences. Our experiences can take on different possibilities according to what we have learned throughout our life. Nurses assist patients to participate in making different choices in their lives. The nurse's presence is an important concept inherent in Parse's theory.

Martha Rogers's theory, the science of unitary beings, described person "as a unified whole, the person is viewed as an energy field" (Rogers, 1970). Rogers describes the environment as an open system that is ever changing and dynamic. A characteristic of the environment is that it is diverse and complex. Human beings are viewed as open and complex systems that are in constant interaction with the environment. Dora Kunz and Dolores Krieger expanded on Rogers's work to develop the treatment modality of therapeutic touch. The overall health and well-being of the person depends on a continuous flow of energy within the body, interacting with others, and the universe itself. When this flow of energy is disrupted, the belief is that the disruption can lead to disease and illness. The goal of nursing is to seek to promote a cohesive interaction between the person and the environment.

Comparison and Contrast of Allopathic and Holistic Models of Care

A number of contrasts exist between the conventional/allopathic model of care and the holistic model of care. The focus of Western medicine historically has been based on the allopathic model. Allopathic/conventional interventions are those that include medical, surgical, noninvasive, and invasive diagnostic procedures (Dossey & Keegan, 2009). Within this model the body is viewed in a reductionistic manner, as a machine with functioning parts. The holistic model focuses on and takes into account the whole individual. The holistic model supports the view that the individual is made up of bio-psycho-social-spiritual components. In the allopathic model, the body and mind are viewed as separate components, with the mind having a secondary role in organic illness. In the holistic model, the focus is on the interconnectedness between the body–mind–spirit. The mind and body equally play a role in illness. Illness, disease, or symptoms in the allopathic model are seen as disruptions to be treated/eliminated or cured. Illness, disease, or symptoms in the holistic model are viewed as having their origins in the biological, psychological, social, and spiritual realms. In the allopathic model, the patient is viewed as being dependent upon the practitioner, and pain and disease are viewed as negative components that are to be eradicated or cured. In the holistic model, pain and disease are viewed as signals to be aware of, often indicating an underlying stressor between the internal and external environments. The body is viewed as ever changing, fluid, and dynamic. In the holistic model, the focus is on the body–mind perspective and is honored in all interactions. In the allopathic model, the healthcare professional is viewed as the authority in all things. In the holistic model, the patient and healthcare professional are engaged in a partnership; therefore, the patient is viewed as autonomous. The focus of care in the allopathic model is to cure illness, and death is seen as a failure to be avoided at all costs, even to the detriment of the person being cared for. In the holistic model, death is viewed as a natural process of life. Within this holistic/healing model, death has the potential to be viewed as a release of the individual from suffering and pain. Because of the holistic nature of palliative care, it is imperative that nurses providing palliative care adopt the values and characteristics of holistic nurses.

Characteristics of Holistic Nurses

Barbara Dossey has identified the characteristics of nurse healers and has stated that holistic nurses are "instruments of healing" (Dossey & Keegan, 2009, p. 722). Holistic nurses promote compassion and respect for themselves as well as for their patients. Holistic nurses are highly aware of the focus of the interaction between themselves and patients. This focused intent is at the core of holistic nursing and energy theory. It is also a prerequisite for creating a caring and healing field from which the holistic nurse and patient effect change. This creation of a caring and healing field involves intentionality. Intentionality affects the direction of the exchange between the nurse and the patient. When the nurse is intending purposefully to promote and facilitate growth in another, the effect can be powerful. Some research has shown that intentionality, even when the two participants are separated by distance, can have a positive effect on the well-being of the recipient of the intent. Barbara Dossey identified the following key characteristics of holistic nurses:

- Utilizing (or understanding the concept of) nursing presence
- Being intentional
- Being compassionate
- Honoring the self through the continual process of self-care
- Being aware of his or her personal response to the clients' experience
- Listening and being mindful
- Respecting clients
- Role-modeling self-care for clients
- Exhibiting unconditional acceptance
- Acknowledging that the client is the expert within their illness experience
- Being insightful
- Advocating and empowering clients to make the best choices for themselves
- Not being attached to outcomes
- Establishing healthy boundaries with others (Dossey & Keegan, 2009)

Presence

There are many ways that nurses provide presence to their patients. Through the provision of physical care, nurses provide physical presence to their patients. It is challenging for nurses to focus intentionally on providing care for the patient. It is challenging for nurses to let go of their own personal issues and problems in order to be physically present to each patient. As nurses, it is important to assist patients to find meaning in their illness experience. Nursing interventions that provide comfort and support to patients involve the concept of psychological presence. In active listening and therapeutic communication, nurses create a climate in which the patient feels supported. With active listening and therapeutic communication, the nurse conveys respect; genuine, positive regard; and empathy toward the patient. Psychological presence provides the venue for the patient to be able to understand and give meaning to life events.

Therapeutic presence is defined as "the nurse relating to the patient as whole being to whole being, using all the resources of body, mind, emotions, and spirit"

(Dossey & Keegan, 2009, p. 724). To become more mindfully present, nurses can use breath to center themselves. Centering is a conscious state of inner quietude. Through the process of centering one can find an inner reference of stability. With intentionality and mindfulness, nurses can use common activities to become more fully present for the next patient encounter. The use of the breath as an anchor assists the nurse to center. So simply pausing during a busy day to center and focus, and stepping back from a confusing, distressing situation in order to reemerge from a point of calmness are skills that nurses can develop to attend to their own spirit and the needs of their patients. It is through this process that nurses can be more fully present to themselves so as to be instruments of healing for their patients.

The Science of Psychoneuroimmunology

The science of psychoneuroimmunology (PNI) can help nurses to better understand the mind–body interaction. The concept was introduced by Ader and colleagues in their landmark book *Psychoneuroimmunology*. It was through pioneering research done by Ader and his colleagues (2007) that the term "psychoneuroimmunology" was coined.

Psychoneuroimmunology is the scientific study of the linkages between the nervous system, the endocrine system, and the immune system and their impact on an individual's health. Ader (2007) hypothesized and believed that there is a connection between our state of mind and the state of our health. The basic premise is that every thought, emotion, idea, or belief has a neurochemical response. Stress represents a challenge to the individual and requires physiological, behavioral, and psychological changes to be successfully met by the individual (Fricchione, 2004). This stress in individuals' lives, whether good or bad; the individuals' coping patterns; and their beliefs and emotions all impact the neuro-endocrine system as well as their immune systems. The limbic system and the hypothalamus, in particular, are the areas in the brain that primarily deal with emotional issues. This follows the mind–body connection that ultimately affects individuals' quality of life and physical health.

An individual's thoughts/images elicit emotions. These emotions are transduced into chemicals (neurotransmitters, neurohormones, and neuropeptides) that circulate throughout the body and convey messages via cells to various systems within the body (McEwen, 1998). These systems are directly influenced by a person's mental state. The stress response is a good example. This response produces profound physiological alterations in the body—a direct result of the interaction between the hypothalamic-pituitary-adrenal axis and the sympathetic nervous system. The resulting biochemical substances involve a number of neuropeptides that are not only produced in the brain but also by cells throughout the body. These neuropeptides include such substances such as adrenaline, acetylcholine, interleukins or cytokines, insulin, angiotension, dopamine, endorphins, and serotonin. Research by Candace Pert (1997), a neuropharmacologist, demonstrated that these neuropeptides are present not only on the cell walls in the brain but also in the immune system. Pert states that memory is encoded in cells at the receptor sites. The discovery that these chemicals, neuropeptides, are also on the cell walls of the immune system illustrates the connection between emotions and health.

The field of stress medicine has focused on the concept of allostasis, literally meaning maintaining stability through change. This refers to the capacity of the individual to adapt or constantly change in order to adjust to ever shifting environmental conditions. The wear and tear that the body experiences through adaptation and change exposes the individual to repeated cycles of allostasis. This is referred to as allostatic loading. Stress and allostatic loading have been shown to contribute to the onset and exacerbation of many disabling diseases with high mortality and morbidity: hypertension, coronary artery disease, cardiomyopathy, insulin-resistant diabetes mellitus, metabolic syndrome, autoimmune disease, anxiety, and depression.

Can mind–body approaches reduce this allostatic loading? The answer to that question is still forthcoming. However, knowledge of psychoneuroimmunology can provide the basis by which nurses enhance their understanding so they can promote healing/well-being in health care.

Implications of Mind–Body Interactions

Centering is an integral part of any healing intervention. Centering is a conscious state of inner quiet. Becoming centered, both physically and psychologically, is finding within oneself an inner reference of stability. Such experiences can take many forms: counting the breath, focusing on the breathing process, reciting sacred words. The holistic nurse seeks and focuses on the desire to function from the center. Coming from a centered place, practitioners can feel more secure and in control of their own energies and can focus more on the intent of the healing intervention. Remaining on center can also prevent them from over-helping or becoming too involved in the patient's difficulties or problems. Too much involvement can lead to compassion fatigue or burnout. The most effective and widely known effect of centering is the relaxation response.

Relaxation Response

Herbert Benson, at the Harvard Mind/Body Institute, has extensively studied the relaxation response and teaches patients how to elicit the phenomenon. Benson cites four elements that are common to all relaxation responses: quiet environment, mental device, passive attitude, and a comfortable position (Benson, 1975). Consciously taking a breath and slowly repeating one neutral word with each out breath, such as the Sanskrit word "om," or "one," or "calm," "quiet," or "peace," can promote this centered, relaxation response. Direct benefits of promoting the relaxation response are decreased metabolism, heart rate, and rate of breathing. These changes are the opposite of what is observed when an individual is under stress. Promotion of the relaxation response has been shown to be an effective therapy in a number of disease states, including hypertension, chronic pain, anxiety, anger, and hostility. The following exercise is an example of one way in which a nurse can elicit the relaxation response.

Exercise: Eliciting the Relaxation Response

Sit on the floor or on a chair in a comfortable position.

Lay your hands on your lap and gently rock your body from side to side an inch or two to put your body in alignment with your center of gravity.

Find yourself in a stable and comfortable position.

Close your eyes and take several deep breaths, relaxing the muscles in the back of your neck, checking that your extremities are relaxed.

If you feel any sense of tension, release it, just letting it go.

Be aware of your breathing, breathing deeply, slowly and easily.

Be aware of energy flowing between your shoulders, and in the back of your neck.

Try to go more deeply within your consciousness. The human mind has a wonderful capacity to recall an experience, and individuals can simulate this experience of centering and relaxation any time they choose.

Promoting the relaxation response and centering, through breathing exercises, enables the practitioner to let go of outcomes of the healing intervention. An individual may experience feelings of heaviness, warmth, and lightness, which are indications of a deep and profound relaxed state.

Difficulties and Challenges

However, not every person is able to enter such a state. Instead, the person may encounter one of the difficulties and challenges associated with the practice of relaxation. These difficulties and challenges may include

- limited time;
- chattering mind;
- emotions coming to the surface;
- being restless, fidgety;
- falling asleep;
- outside distractions from environment, for example, noises; and
- questioning whether the exercise is being done correctly.

Other techniques used to elicit the relaxation response include sound, prayer, meditation, mindfulness, yoga stretching, contemplation, body scan, diaphragmatic breathing, imagery/visualization, muscle relaxation, repetitive movement, self-hypnosis, and dedicated silence (Webster, 2004).

Applications and Benefits

There are many potential benefits to the practice of promoting the relaxation response in patients. Its usefulness in clinical practice are as follows (Webster, 2004):

- Alter physical symptoms, such as hypertension, irritable bowel syndrome, nausea, or insomnia.
- Decrease pain and the use of pain medications.
- Decrease anxiety.
- Alleviate depression and anger.
- Prepare for and experience medical procedures, treatments, and tests.
- Promote healing and recovery.
- Increase feelings of well-being, comfort, and control.
- Increase self-awareness.
- Change negative thought pattern and
- Promote a peaceful transition at end of life.

Complementary/Alternative/Integrative Therapies

The National Institute of Health and Human Services, the Centers for Disease Control and Prevention, and the National Center for Health Statistics reported that in 2002, more than 50% of all Americans used mind–body approaches for improving their health. Complementary therapies are those used in conjunction with conventional medical practices, while alternative therapies are those that are used instead of conventional medicine. Integrative therapies combine conventional medicine and CAM modalities.

Imagery

Imagery is a good example of the mind–body approach. The mind plays a powerful role in impacting the psychophysiological response. Certain emotions, thoughts, or images stimulate a certain physiological response in the body. Imagery is a therapeutic approach that facilitates working with the power of the imagination to affect mental attitudes positively, elicit positive outcomes, and activate innate healing within the body (Reed, 2007). Imagery is a natural process involving the mind and the right side of the brain. Imagery in this way can be viewed as a form of self-hypnosis. Guided imagery refers to the use of devices to assist in image formation and promotion of relaxation. These devices include verbal suggestions, music, pictures, aromas from oils or candles, or a voice on an audiotape or compact disc that guides the imagery process. The use of imagery in palliative care has the potential to relieve acute or chronic pain, suffering, anxiety, nausea, or depression, and to minimize side effects of medications used for management of symptoms of distress. Visualization or guided imagery can also be utilized to promote relaxation or when seeking guidance or insight. An example of a guided imagery exercise that a nurse might use herself or might use with the patient follows.

Guided Imagery Exercise

Assume a comfortable position.

Start at your own pace, with a general relaxation; focus on your breath.

With each in breath, imagine that you are taking in calmness and relaxation.

With each out breath, imagine that you are releasing tension, discomfort, and worry.

Picture yourself in a beautiful place (real or imaginary).

Allow yourself to experience this place and the relaxation.

Imagine yourself on a sunny beach.

Breath in and smell the fragrances all around you, feel the texture of the surface under your feet, hear all the sounds of nature, see all the different sights.

The sun is warm and welcoming. The sand beneath your feet is soft and soothing. You can hear the sound of the waves breaking on the shore. As you walk along the beach you feel relaxed, refreshed, and carefree. You feel the cool, gentle breeze against your face and the smell of the salt air. Allow all of these sights, sounds, and sensations to relax you more and more.

When you are ready, you can gently bring your attention back to the room, realizing that you may return to this place whenever you wish.

Energetic Healing

Energetic healing is a term used to describe healing that alters the flow of energy within and around a person. This energy flow is called by many names: chi, Qi, mana, and prana. Chi Kung, Qigong, and Reiki are healing traditions from China and Japan.

Therapeutic Touch (TT)

Therapeutic touch is based on the work of Dolores Krieger, a faculty member at New York University's Division of Nursing, and Dora Kunz, a natural healer. This healing practice has evolved from several spiritual and ancient healing practices. The practice of TT is based on the fundamental assumption that there is a universal life energy that sustains all living organisms. This energy, called the human energy field (Krieger, 1979), surrounds and penetrates the body. Therapeutic touch is a compassionate and intentional use of the human energy field to help or heal others who are in need. Therapeutic touch is an interaction between the practitioner and patient for the purpose of finding and correcting imbalances in the patient's energy field. The practitioner focuses on intention to direct the process of energy exchange and uses the hands to mobilize areas in the client's energy field that appear to be congested or sluggish. This modality focuses on re-patterning and balancing the client's energy field (Krieger, 1979).

Acupuncture

Acupuncture is a form of Chinese medicine. It is based on the philosophy that a person has a vital life energy, which is called Qi (pronounced chee). Access to Qi is achieved by inserting sterile, fine needles at acupuncture points for the purpose of adjusting the flow of Qi/energy within the person. Pain and illness are thought to be caused by a blockage or congestion in the flow of Qi. Acupuncture serves to increase or stimulate the flow and relieve obstructions in the flow of energy. A benefit of acupuncture has been demonstrated in the release of endorphins, the body's own pain-killing chemical (NCCAM, 2004).

Aromatherapy

Aromatherapy involves the use of essential oils from plants to heal the body and mind. Essential oils can be inhaled or applied topically to the body. Aromatherapy can be used to manage stress and relieve pain, nausea, or insomnia. There are, however, guidelines that should be followed when using essential oils; these include avoiding their use in those who are allergic to the ingredients in the oils (Wholehealthmd, 2005). The therapeutic value of some common essential oils is applicable for holistic nursing practice. These would include lavender for insomnia, depression, and exhaustion; peppermint for its anti-nausea properties; and frankincense for relaxation (Lee & Lee, 2006).

Music Therapy

Music therapy is defined as "the behavioral science concerned with the systematic application of music to produce relaxation and desired changes in emotions, behavior and physiology" (Guzzetta, 1995, p. 670). Music therapy creates a relaxed state of mind that allows the listener to become open and receptive to healing. A nurse utilizing music therapy alone or with guided imagery can assist a patient into a relaxed state, which is the condition desirable for natural healing. Music therapy promotes the relaxation response in patients. Music therapy can be adapted to fit the patient's needs. For maximum effect it is often used in conjunction with other healing modalities, such as guided imagery, therapeutic touch, meditation, or exercise. Clinical studies demonstrate the outcome of music therapy in decreasing anxiety, blood pressure, and heart rate, and meeting the multidimensional needs of hospice patients and families. When using music therapy in the clinical setting, remember to

- allow the patient to control the session by using the patient's choice of music;
- use earphones when possible; and
- use guided imagery as a catalyst to the music therapy.

Meditation

Meditation provides a means for patients to center and relax. There are many forms of meditation. In some practices, such as the relaxation response discussed earlier, the individual learns the art of quieting the mind by focusing on an object of meditation, such as a word, sound, or image. In the practice of meditation, use of a mantra, a syllable, word, or name that is repeatedly said aloud achieves the effect.

Other practices, such as mindfulness meditation or insight meditation, involve individuals' focused ability to become more aware of their own thoughts, emotions, and physical sensations. Through this growing awareness, an individual can gradually become more attuned to habitual thoughts, worries, and emotional reactions. Jon Kabat-Zinn, director of the Stress Reduction Clinic of the University of Massachusetts Medical Center, believes that mindfulness helps patients live more fully in the present moment (Kabat-Zinn, 1990).

Reiki

Reiki is an ancient Japanese hands-on healing practice. Reiki practitioners focus on the universal life force, which they believe is an energy field that surrounds all beings. Reiki uses a gentle laying on of hands to support and balance the energy pathways of the individual. The practice of Reiki can contribute to bolstering the immune system, a general sense of well-being, and reducing stress.

Massage

Massage by definition is the systematic and scientific manipulation of the soft tissues of the body. Massage can provide relief from symptoms of anxiety, tension, depression, insomnia, and stress, as well as back pain, headache, muscle pain, and some forms of chronic pain. Self-healing can occur through massage through the activation of the immune system. There are many specialized techniques for therapeutic massage such as reflexology, Rolfing, shiatsu, and Amma.

Prayer

Prayer is a spiritual discipline, practiced by various traditions and cultures. Because prayer is a part of holistic care, the nurse should explore patients' need for prayer as well as their beliefs in prayer. Prayer has been a part of human history for many centuries and it has various definitions. Prayer is an expression of the spirit, which is expressed in many different ways such as speaking, silence, singing, chanting, and moaning. Prayer also can be described as communion with

God or the Absolute. Prayer from Florence Nightingale's perspective "is the process of linking the outward personal self with the inward divine spirit" (Macrae, 2001, p. 93).

Humor

Nurses may avoid using humor with patients for fear of offending the patient or not seeming professional, or being unsure when and how to use it effectively. Dean and Major (2008) found commonalities in studies conducted in two unique settings: an intensive critical care (ICU) setting and a palliative care (PC) setting. The themes that arose included

- team work;
- emotion management; and
- human connections.

The researchers found anecdotally that patients reported stress-lowering effects with humor, as well as increased levels of "optimism, hope, and happiness" (p. 350).

Humor has been compared with mild exercise as a means of increasing serotonin release and synthesis and improving mood. Researchers are looking at how humor impacts quality of life by moderating areas such as stress, anxiety, depression, discomfort, and functioning (Christie & Moore, 2005).

Oncology nurses' recognition and response to humor initiated by patients was explored with 47 nurses (Adamle, Lucwick, Zeller, & Winchell, 2008). Findings indicated that there were two predictors of nurse recognition and response to patient-initiated humor: verbalizations of patients and intonations used by patients. As the researchers noted, humor is variable by nature, person, and circumstance. However, if humor is initiated by a patient, recognizing it within the patient and responding to what the patient is trying to communicate are important.

Research has suggested links between humor and health in relation to emotions, pain, cardiovascular effects, and immunity (Christie & Moore, 2005; McCreaddie & Wiggins, 2008; Wilkins & Eisenbraun, 2009). As with other complementary/alternative/integrative therapies, more research will assist nurses in providing holistic and healing care based on evidence.

Evidenced-Based Practice

In a large survey (N = 31,000) conducted in 2002 by the Centers for Disease Control, National Center for Health Statistics, 62% of adults stated that they had used complementary or alternative modalities in the past 12 months. Much of the current research on integrative therapies has applied the theory of psychoneuroim-munology, which hypothesizes that touch therapies promote the parasympathetic response in the direction of relaxation. Evoking the relaxation response can there-fore reduce allostatic load causing a reduction in anxiety, pain, and stress, and pro-moting a sense of well-being. Current National Institutes of Health funding is supporting research that focuses on the physiological and behavioral impact of energetic therapies.

In summary, there are many outcomes for a healing intervention that could relieve patients' suffering. These outcomes occur in different realms: physical, emo-tional, cognitive, and spiritual. Within the physical realm are decreased perception of pain, enhanced sense of well-being, and increased energy. In the emotional realm are reduced feelings of anxiety and increased ability to be open to life. In the cognitive sphere these outcomes are opening the mind to new experiences and expanding hori-zons and visions. In the spiritual realm there is a sense of connectedness with all of life, offering hope, courage, trust, and forgiveness to self and others. All of these out-comes are appropriate for and goals of people engaged in palliative care.

Tending to the Nurses' Spirit

Mother Teresa once said, "To keep the lamp burning, we have to keep putting oil in it." It's that simple. Tending to and nurturing our spirits will assist us in keeping the lamp burning brightly in our lives. The practice environment for nurses is uncertain, complex, and ever changing. Dealing with change continuously, as we do in our profession and in the workplace, can be taxing on the body, mind, and spirit. Nurses, as witness to patients' suffering, loneliness, and pain, are invited into the personal journey of the patients' illness. Nurses cannot avoid becoming "entangled to some degree with our patient's pain." According to Longaker (1997), there are three common sources of burnout or compassion fatigue in healthcare providers: loss of perspective; accumulation of grief; and unfinished business, exhaustion, and stress. These may lead to feelings of irritability, anger that is fre-quent and intense, depression, hostility, helplessness, and fatigue. Several factors contribute to this phenomenon. There have been dramatic changes in the structure of healthcare organizations and in the way that care is delivered. There is an increased use of unlicensed assistive personnel, increased acuity of illness in patients with short hospital stays, increased technology, and a shortage of practic-ing nurses.

Awareness of and care of the self is an integral aspect of holistic nursing care. Through the maintenance and nurturance of our own spirits we can intervene with others in a healing way. It is in the process of self-care that we recognize and honor our humanness and vulnerability. Self-care leads to integration, wholeness, and balance of the individual. Strategies to incorporate self-care would include establishing and maintaining a healthy support system, use of humor, making time for rest and to celebrate life, creating our own rituals, avoiding perfection, having healthy boundaries, learning to say no, and learning some relaxation techniques.

Ethical and Legal Issues

Ethics provides a framework for professional behavior. The Position Statement on Holistic Ethics from the American Holistic Nursing Association states, "All events and ethical decisions become part of the unfolding of a harmonious order and a realization of potentialities" (Dossey & Keegan, 2009, p. 129). The fundamental responsibility of the holistic nurse is to promote health, facilitate healing, and alleviate suffering. This is the same for nurses in palliative care.

There are several ethical considerations to become aware of when implementing holistic interventions:

- Maintain confidentiality of the individual.
- Provide holistic interventions with permission.
- Provide informed consent.
- Respect patients for where they are in the healing process.
- Establish clarity about healing modalities used.
- Obtain consent to use direct physical touch.

Many integrative therapies are within the scope of nursing; these include herbal therapy, aromatherapy, massage, music therapy, guided imagery, meditation, therapeutic touch, and stress management.

To determine whether any given healing modality falls within the parameters of a legally identified profession, a careful reading of a state's licensure status is required. State boards of nursing are a source for interpreting licensure laws and provide direction to nurses who wish to integrate these modalities into their professional practice. The nurse should look to evidence that the modality is within the scope of nursing practice. Evidence would include these: Is the modality included in accredited educational and training programs? Is the modality recognized in professional journals? Is the modality supported by professional organizations? Has research been conducted to support the modality?

The nurse in palliative care should strive to provide all patients with access to integrative modalities that can assist them on their journey. These tools and the therapeutic presence of the nurse, using self as an instrument of healing, is what comprise the true spirit of holistic nursing.

Summary

This chapter is an introduction to holistic nursing and an overview of several holistic nursing modalities. These holistic modalities support the mind–body–spirit connection and the innate ability of the body to heal.

The chapter examined imagery, therapeutic touch, acupuncture, aromatherapy, music therapy, meditation, Reiki, massage, prayer, and humor. In addressing a patient's suffering and pain, nurses must become familiar with these modalities in order to assist a patient toward healing and wholeness.

Key Points

1. The holistic model of care espouses the view that the individual is made up of bio-psycho-social-spiritual components.
2. The National Institute of Health and Human Services, the Center for Disease Control and Prevention, and the National Center for Health Statistics reported that in 2002, more than 50% of all Americans had used mind–body approaches for improving their health.
3. Focused intent is at the core of holistic nursing and energy theory. It is a prerequisite for creating a caring and healing field from which the holistic nurse and patient effect change.
4. When a nurse is present with the patient, the nurse relates to the patient as whole being to whole being, using all resources of body, mind, emotions, and spirit.
5. Centering, creating the conscious state of inner quietude, can assist nurses to be more fully present in each patient encounter.
6. Types of CAM include acupuncture, aromatherapy, humor, imagery, massage, meditation, music therapy, prayer, Reiki, and therapeutic touch.

Case Study 10–2

Cindy is a 36-year-old female with advanced sarcoma that has metastasized to her lungs, brain, and bones. Despite daily episodes of pain rated 6 on a 0–10 scale, Cindy does not like to take medications such as opioids. She states that opioids are "unnatural chemicals," which make her feel out of control.

A comprehensive assessment of Cindy's symptoms by the palliative care team indicates that she is particularly bothered by the fact that she "cannot control her pain" and she feels alone. The nurse caring for Cindy recognizes that Cindy's pain level of 6 may very well cause not only physical suffering but also psychosocial and spiritual suffering, which would impede Cindy's ability to experience a good quality of life. Of particular concern is the negative impact untreated pain could have on Cindy's endurance and ability to address other issues that may need resolution as she nears death.

Several integrative therapies have been shown to decrease and control physical pain as well as the emotional, psychological, and spiritual dimensions of the experience. Given the fact that integrative therapies are characterized as being "natural," Cindy's palliative care nurse provided her with information on various therapies and suggested that she try one. The nurse explained that the effectiveness of many integrative therapies is thought to be related to the active role that the person receiving the therapy plays in the "healing experience." Cindy's desire to control her pain also supported introducing her to integrative therapies, which can empower patients to control their symptoms of distress.

After the discussion of the integrative therapies, Cindy agrees to have the nurse administer therapeutic touch (TT). Cindy states that she is very relaxed after her treatment and that her pain is noticeably less. Visits from the spiritual coordinators of the palliative care team are also arranged to assess Cindy's spiritual needs.

Cindy was discharged to her home with palliative care services, which arranged for a home hospice volunteer to visit twice a week to provide TT. With therapeutic touch, relaxation, prayer, and the ability to remain in her home with her family (and pets), Cindy managed to experience good quality of life without pain and suffering until her death.

Questions on the Case Study
1. Do you believe that the modalities offered to Cindy (TT, relaxation, prayer) could benefit anyone in need of care?
2. How can we advocate that healing modalities be incorporated into a patient's plan of care?
3. What do you think the nurse's role was in helping Cindy to heal?
4. How would you define her healing experience?

Questions for Reflection and Journaling
1. Did you try the two exercises, and did they promote relaxation?
2. In the clinical setting, before a patient interaction, did you ever practice centering/ deep breathing?
3. What holistic modalities would you consider for your own personal and professional development?

References

Adamle, K. N., Ludwick, R., Zeller, R., & Winchell, J. (2008). Oncology nurses' responses to patient-initiated humor. *Cancer Nursing, 31*(6), E1–E9.

Ader, B. (2007). *Psychoneuroimmunology* (4th ed.). New York, NY: Elsevier.

American Holistic Nurses Association (AHNA). (2007). *American Holistic Nurses Association standards of holistic nursing practice.* Flagstaff, AZ: Author.

Benson, H. (1975). *The relaxation response.* New York, NY: Avon Books.

Centers for Disease Control (CDC), U.S. Department of Health and Human Services, National Center for Health Statistics. (2004). Complementary and alternative medicine use among adults: United States 2002. *Advance Data from Vital and Health Statistics, 343,* 1–20.

Christie, W., & Moore, C. (2005). The impact of humor on patients with cancer. *Clinical Journal of Oncology Nursing, 9*(2), 211–218.

Dean, A. K., & Major, J. E. (2008). From critical care to comfort care: The sustaining value of humour. *Journal of Clinical Nursing, 17,* 1088–1095.

Dossey, B. M., & Keegan, L. (2009). *Holistic nursing: A handbook for practice* (5th ed.). Sudbury, MA: Jones and Bartlett.

Fricchione, G. (2004, December). *The potential for illness prevention via spirit–mind–body approaches.* Presented at Spirituality and Healing in Medicine: The enhanced importance of the integration of mind/body practices and prayer. Sponsored by Harvard Medical School and the Mind/Body Medical Institute, Boston.

Guzzetta, C. (1995). Music therapy: Healing the melody of the soul. In B. Dossey, L. Keegan, C. Guzzetta, & L. Kolkmeier (Eds.), *Holistic nursing a handbook for practice* (2nd ed.). Gaithersburg, MD: Aspen.

Kabat-Zinn, J. (1990). *Full catastrophe living: Using the wisdom of your body and mind to face stress, pain, and illness.* New York, NY: Bantam.

Krieger, D. (1979). *The therapeutic touch: How to use your hands to help or to heal.* New York, NY: Prentice Hall.

Lee, I., & Lee, G. (2006). Effects of lavender aromatherapy on insomnia and depression in women college students. *Taehan Kanho, Hakhoe Chi, 36*(1), 136–143.

Longaker, C. (1997). *Facing death and finding hope: A guide to the emotional and spiritual care of the dying.* New York, NY: Broadway Books.

Macrae, J. (2001). *Nursing as a spiritual practice: A contemporary application of Florence Nightingale's views.* New York, NY: Springer.

Mariano, C. (2007). Holistic nursing as a specialty: Holistic nursing—Scope and standards of practice. *Nursing Clinics of North America, 42*(2), 165–188.

McCreaddie, M. & Wiggins, S. (2008). The purpose and function of humor in health, health care, and nursing: A narrative review. *Journal of Advanced Nursing, 61*(6), 584–595.

McEwen, B. S. (1998). Protective and damaging effects of stress mediators. *New England Journal of Medicine, 338,* 171–179.

National Center for Complementary and Alternative Medicine (NCCAM). (2004). *Get the facts: Acupuncture.* Bethesda, MD: National Institutes of Health.

Nightingale, F. (1860). *Notes on Nursing.* London, UK: Harrison.

Parse, R. R. (1992). Human becoming: Parse's theory of nursing. *Nursing Science Quarterly, 5,* 35–42.

Paterson, J. G., & Zderad, L.T. (1976). *Humanistic nursing.* New York, NY: John Wiley.

Pert, C. B. (1997). *The molecules of emotion: Why you feel the way you feel.* New York, NY: Charles Scribner's Sons.

Reed, T. (2007). Imagery in the clinical setting. A tool for healing. *Nursing Clinics of North America, 42*(2), 261–277.

Rogers, M. (1970). *The theoretical basis for nursing.* Philadelphia, PA: F. A. Davis.

Watson, J. (1988). *Human science and human care.* New York: National League of Nursing.

Webster, A. (2004, December). *Teaching techniques for inner stillness.* Presented at Spirituality and Medicine: The enhanced importance of the integration of mind/body practices and prayer. Sponsored by Harvard Medical School and the Mind/Body Medical Institute. Boston.

Wilkins, J., & Eisenbraun, A. J. (2009). Humor theories and the physiological benefits of laughter. *Holistic Nursing Practice, 23*(6), 349–354.

Wholehealthmd.com. (2005, May 20). *Aromatherapy.* Retrieved from http//:www.wholehealthmd.com.

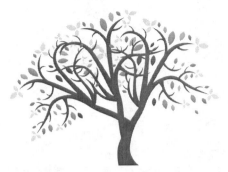

ELEVEN

Conveying Comfort

■ Kathleen Ouimet Perrin

Objectives

1. Explain why some nurse researchers believe that comfort should be the primary focus of nursing.
2. Compare and contrast nursing interventions for patients who are enduring and experiencing emotional suffering.
3. Describe nursing interventions that may promote comfort.

Student Project

Figure 11–1 Mosaic

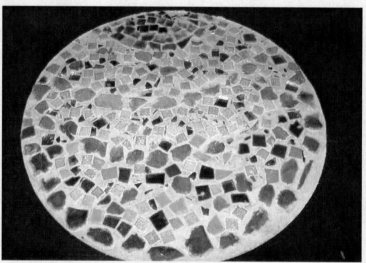

Case Study 11–1

A hospice nurse was returning to the home of a recently deceased 42-year-old husband/father for a bereavement visit. The wife and children were distraught. The experienced nurse listened to their keening but felt powerless to alleviate the pain that encompassed the family. They kept returning to how their husband/father had been the light of their lives, the center of their family life. The hospice nurse recalled a "mosaic stone" that had been created to portray just such a loss, and she happened to have it in her car. She showed the stone to the family, explaining it as the person who had created it had done.

The yellow represents the person you lost, who was at the center of your life. The waves of warm colors flowing out from that point show how he touched people, both those immediately close to him like your family and those much farther away. Just as in this stone, he will always be present because he has touched and warmed each of you. Like the waves of colors that flow from him on the stone, you will always be different from what surrounds you because the light of his being has reflected on you. On warm sunny days, you will be able to feel the radiant beams of happiness shining down and guiding your path.

The wife suddenly relaxed a bit; she brought the nurse to the garden and showed her a series of stones that she had laid in the ground. She begged to keep the stone because it was a concrete reminder of how her husband had touched those around him and it already had a perfect place in her garden.

Source: Courtesy of Megan McMahon, student nurse, 2008.

Questions on the Case Study

1. Should it have been a priority for the hospice nurse to offer some comfort to this grieving family?
2. How did the nurse identify the need of this family for comfort?
3. How did nurse use the mosaic to convey comfort to this family?

Introduction

As far back as 1859, Florence Nightingale identified increasing patient comfort as one of the goals of nursing. Unfortunately, during the subsequent century, comfort was cited frequently but not defined (Kolcaba, 2001). The complexity of the concept of comfort made it difficult for researchers to operationalize and study it until more recently when nursing theorists/researchers responded to the challenge. Janice Morse (1992) defined comfort as the end state of therapeutic actions for a patient. Morse argues that comfort is a state of well-being that may occur during any stage of the health-illness continuum. She believes comfort can serve as a goal of nursing because providing comfort incorporates both the concept of caring and the procedural tasks performed by the caregiver. Katharine Kolcaba (1992) developed a mid-range theory of comfort and describes comfort as a multidimensional, personal experience that has differing levels of intensity. She defines holistic comfort as "the immediate experience of being strengthened through having the needs for relief, ease, and transference met in four contexts of experience (physical, psychospiritual, social, and environmental)" (p. 6). The basic assumption underlying both of these theorists' approaches is that comfort is a desirable state for patients.

Why Should Nurses Focus on Providing Comfort?

In 1992, Morse recommended that the ultimate purpose of nursing was to promote comfort for the patient rather than to care for the patient. She believed that shifting the focus from providing care for the patient to promoting comfort also shifted the emphasis from nurse as provider of care for the patient to the patient and how the patient responded to care. In Morse's view, caring is an essential component of promoting comfort, but comfort should be the primary focus of care. Caring is present as the feeling of moral responsibility for nursing actions and the affect that is present while promoting comfort. Morse believes this shift in focus enhances the potential for nursing research because patient comfort is a variable that is both physically and psychologically measurable—unlike care, which is not directly measurable.

Morse (1992) identified two criticisms of the construct of comfort. First, the term "making the patient comfortable" implies that the nurse is always the actor and the patient is a passive recipient of care. This interpretation fosters patient dependency and discourages self-care. However, Morse states that such a phrase describes only one portion of the range of strategies that promote comfort. In her definition, this range extends from providing comfort measures for the patient to strategies that support a patient's attempts to promote his or her own comfort. The second criticism is that most nursing procedures, like endotracheal suctioning or inserting a nasogastric tube not only due not promote comfort but actually cause discomfort. Morse argues that the discomfort is short-lived and the transient discomfort is acceptable given the long-term likelihood of enhanced comfort from the procedure.

Kolcaba (1994) developed a midrange theory of comfort while in graduate school and working on an Alzheimers unit. Unlike Morse, who approached the idea of enhancing comfort through comforting the sufferer, Kolcaba was looking for behaviors that residents would exhibit if the residents were functioning optimally with an absence of excess disabilities. After a concept analysis and development of a conceptual map, Kolcaba determined that comfort could be "defined for nursing as the satisfaction (either actively, passively, or cooperatively) of the basic human needs for relief, ease and transcendence arising from health care situations that are stressful" (p. 1178). In her midrange theory, Kolcaba specified the following definitions.

- Relief is the state of having a specified need met.
- Ease is the state of calm and contentment.
- Transcendence is the state in which one rises above problem or pain.

After completing the concept analysis, Kolcaba began to consider how to operationalize the concept of comfort using the following three questions:

- What makes patients comfortable?
- Why make patients comfortable?
- How do nurses know if their interventions (comfort measures) have succeeded?

The most important insight from these considerations was that comfort needs occurred in both physical and mental aspects. This led Kolcaba to recognize four different contexts in which comfort could occur. These are

- physical: pertaining to bodily sensations and functioning;
- psychospiritual: pertaining to bodily internal awareness of self, including esteem, concept, sexuality, and the meaning of one's life;
- environmental: one's relationship to a higher order or being; and
- social: pertaining to interpersonal, family, and societal relationships, including financial.

Placing these four contexts on a grid with the three human needs (Figure 11–2) allowed Kolcaba, other researchers, and practicing nurses to evaluate a person's

Figure 11–2   Kolcaba's Taxonomic Structure of Comfort

Type of Comfort

Context in which comfort occurs	Relief	Ease	Transcendence
Physical			
Psychospiritual			
Environmental			
Sociocultural			

Source: Reprinted with permission from Kolcaba, K. & Fisher, E. (1996). A holistic perspective on comfort care as an advance directive. *Critical Care Nursing Quarterly, 18*(4), 66–76.

level of comfort, design interventions to fit the appropriate context, and determine whether the interventions had been successful. Had the interventions led to relief, ease, or transcendence?

Kolcaba (2001) states that in her midrange theory of comfort, nursing practice is humanistic, needs-related, and holistic. Nursing interventions are defined as intentional care by nurses that are planned to meet the comfort needs of patients. Kolcaba believes that her theory relates nursing practice to both patient and institutional outcomes because understaffed units will not be able to achieve effective care. Thus, emphasizing comfort will enhance both patient and institutional outcomes. How Kolcaba envisions these outcomes as developing is clearest in the following propositions that she delineates for her theory of comfort:

- Nurses identify patients' comfort needs that have not been addressed by existing support systems.
- Nurses design interventions to meet those needs.
- Intervening variables are taken into account in designing interventions and deciding on mutually agreeable outcomes.
- If enhanced comfort is achieved, patients are strengthened to engage in health-seeking behaviors.
- As a result nurses and patients are more satisfied with health care.
- When nurses and patients in an institution are satisfied, the institution retains its integrity.

Both Morse and Kolcaba believe that nurses should focus on promoting patient comfort because it is a desirable state for the patient and, Kolcaba suggests, also for the nurse and institution. Additionally, both researchers have identified patient needs, examined patient cues, and developed ways to identify patient distress and measure patient comfort. With such tools, interventions or strategies aimed at enhancing comfort can be evaluated to determine the effectiveness of nursing care. Other researchers have examined those circumstances during which patients experience unusual distress and are most in need of comfort.

Patients' Comfort Needs

Schroepfer (2007) identified critical events when dying patients stated they were experiencing the most physical and/or psychosocial suffering. At these moments, the dying patients were most in need of a healer to provide them with comfort.

Although Schroepfer did not utilize Kolcaba's theory, the critical events fell into the four contexts Kolcaba identified. The first critical event, from the psychospiritual context, was "perceived insensitive and uncaring communication of the terminal diagnosis" (p. 140). The patients felt they were spoken to bluntly, did not have their questions answered, and were given insufficient information. They experienced such distress from the lack of information and emotional support at the time of diagnosis that they considered hastening their death. Comfort in the form of relief was obtained from other healers or family members who listened to the patients' fears and provided them with the necessary information.

The physical context was represented by "experiencing unbearable pain" (Schroepfer, 2007, p. 141). Patients experiencing pain with no relief also contemplated ending their own lives. The hallmark of this event was the healthcare providers' unwillingness to listen to or to believe the amount of pain the patients were experiencing. Comfort was obtained in the form of adequate pain management in a variety of ways for these patients. Some of the healthcare providers eventually noted the patients' suffering; one patient demanded to be transferred to hospice and once there found comfort. Another received comfort in the form of adequate pain management only after asking his physician to begin the process for physician-assisted suicide. In all these cases, comfort in the form of relief was eventually obtained, but only after a great deal of patient distress.

The physical context was also represented by patients who found the chemotherapy or radiation therapy they were undergoing to prolong their life was causing distress and reducing the quality of their lives. They eventually achieved ease after convincing at least one of their healthcare providers that they would be more comfortable without the therapy even though their life span would be a few months shorter.

The environmental context represented the final event identified by patients in the Schroepfer (2007) study. Sometimes, patients were extremely lonely; other times they found the hospital sounds, odors, and routines distressing. In any case, the environment was upsetting enough that some patients wished they would just die. Most of these respondents found relief with transfer to hospice.

Suffering from Care

What is most distressing about Schroepfer's (2007) study is that many of the patients were not suffering so much from their illnesses as from their care. Certainly, there are times, such as during endotracheal suctioning or insertion of an

IV, when care is unavoidably uncomfortable. However, it is disturbing when the patient is suffering as much from the care as from the illness and the suffering from care is preventable. Sundin, Axelsson, Jansson, and Norberg (2000) define suffering from care as unnecessary suffering that healthcare providers can eliminate. As in Schroepfer's study, the study by Sundin and others indicated that one of the major times patients suffered from care was when they desired to have someone stay with them, to talk with them about their predicament, and to console them (offer comfort). All too often, the healthcare providers would not or could not stay and listen. Similarly, patients in both studies reported that they suffered when they could not obtain enough information to make informed decisions about their care or could not influence the care that they were to receive.

Meeting Patient Expectations for Care and Comfort

But, is it likely that healers are intentionally so uncaring and do not attempt to reach their patients? Or is it possible that some patients and healers do not respond to each other, that the patient does not appreciate the healer's style of interaction or way of conveying comfort? Fagerstrom, Eriksson, and Engberg (1998) identified three specific types of suffering patients and ascertained the types of nurses and specific nursing behaviors that conveyed caring and brought comfort to each type of patient. The types of patients were satisfied, complaining, and complaining and dissatisfied. The types of nurses were competent and friendly, competent and contact creating, and competent and courageous. Although there were variations among patient/nurse combinations, for the most part in this study, the satisfied patient preferred a competent and friendly nurse; the complaining patient wanted a competent and contact creating nurse; and the complaining and dissatisfied patient needed a competent and courageous nurse.

Patient Preferences for Specific Types of Nurses

Satisfied patients represented the majority of patients in this study (Fagerstrom et al., 1998). They could be identified by their beliefs that they would be well cared for by their nurses and that their nurses were competent. Their comfort needs were usually met by nurses who were competent and friendly. Competent and friendly nurses

- paid attention to their patients' level of comfort;
- were able to identify when their patients needed help;

- were ready to help when their patients needed it; and
- gave guidance when physical help was not needed.

The complaining but satisfied patients still believed that their nurses were competent and wanted their nurses to have all of the attributes described above. However, they felt that the competent and friendly nurse did not meet their needs for dialogue and guidance. They needed a nurse that Fagerstrom and others (1998) called competent and communicative. Competent and communicative nurses displayed the attributes described previously but in addition they

- were willing to spend more time to establish contact and relationships with their patients; and
- allotted more time for discussion and encouragement.

The last type of patient in the Fagerstrom (1998) study, the complaining and dissatisfied patient, was usually anxious, insecure, and uneasy. These patients, representing the fewest patients in the study, were also the youngest patients in the study. They identified a lack of guidance from nurses and a need for closeness and dialogue. These patients felt they were neither noticed nor understood. They were more likely to suffer pain and loneliness than the other patients, especially at night. Most of the time, these patients needed what Fagerstrom and others identified as a competent and courageous nurse. The competent and courageous nurses displayed all of the behaviors the other types of nurses did but in addition, they

- had the courage to participate in their patients' suffering (embodied the patients' suffering);
- gave confirmation that they understood their patients' anxieties; and
- displayed hope and provided security.

Nurses' Inferences About Patient Suffering

What shapes whether nurses become competent and friendly or competent and courageous? One of the factors may be whether the nurses believe their patients are suffering. Davitz and Davitz (1980) studied nurses' inferences about patient suffering by asking medical-surgical, pediatric, and obstetric nurses to rate 60 situations of patients suffering from 1 to 7. Then they separated the nurses into how likely they were to infer that the patients in the situations were suffering. They separated the nurses who were most likely to infer patients were suffering (high inference group) from those who were least like to infer that patients were suffering (low inference group) and observed nurses from both of these groups in their clinical practice. They found significant differences in how the nurses approached their patients. The high inference group engaged in significantly more physical contact and direct actions than low inference nurses. For example, the high inference nurses would usually stand near the patient's head close to the patient's bed and would often reach out and touch the patient in a soothing fashion while attempting to maintain eye contact. These nurses corresponded to the competent and communicative nurses identified by Fagerstrom and colleagues (1998). In contrast, low inference nurses were attentive to their patients but behaved very differently; they addressed their patients from a distance (often the foot of the bed). Although they might straighten the bed, these nurses usually did not touch the patient. These nurses are comparable to the competent nurses in the Fagerstrom study.

In Chapter 9, The Nurse as Witness to Suffering, the issue of whether nurses could always embody their patients' suffering was briefly explored. The study by Fagerstrom and others (1998) seems to show that the majority of patients can perceive their nurse as caring and can obtain comfort from nurses who are not totally involved. However, there clearly are patients who require nurses who have the courage to enter into the patients' suffering in order for the patients to feel cared for and be comforted.

Comfort Strategies

As mentioned previously in this chapter, Morse (1992) believes that comfort rather than caring should be the primary focus of nursing. She notes that as healthcare professionals, we come in contact on a daily basis with people who have had catastrophic losses due to illness, injury, and disability. She believes it is nurses' responsibility to respond to the cues of suffering that patients display with appropriate, patient-centered comfort strategies (Morse, 2000).

Characteristics of Comfort Strategies

Using comfort as the primary focus of nursing, Morse, undertook a series of discrete studies to identify specific nursing strategies that promoted comfort for people suffering from a wide variety of causes. She discovered that the comforting response is focused on the suffering patient and that nurses either intentionally or intuitively assess the patient for behavioral cues of discomfort. The comfort strategy selected by the nurse also may be premeditated or almost reflexive. Morse, Havens, and Wilson (1997) classify comfort strategies as independent activities such as touching the patient, interventions such as repositioning the patient or giving a back rub, and collaborative functions such as providing pain medication. There are variations in the duration of the strategy from just a few moments to occurring over a much longer period of time. Finally, strategies may be direct, provided directly to the patient, or indirect, provided by manipulation of the environment. Morse, like Kolcaba, believes that manipulating the patient's environment by such activities as controlling light and temperature or ensuring appropriate visitation can help to assure patient comfort. According to Morse's research (1992), the domain of comfort has two main components: touching and talking, with the minor components of listening and posturing. In summary, nurses' responses

- are patient-led and distinct for the patient's state;
- have distinct and unique characteristics according to the relationship between the comforter and the person being comforted;
- are composed of two major and two minor components:
  - touching,
  - talking,
  - listening, and
  - posturing.

Morse (1992) defines patient-led as meaning that the caregiver observes a cue that the patient is experiencing discomfort and responds to that cue with a nursing strategy. This appears to be in part a refinement of a normal human response to suffering. Morse has determined that a comforting response is always led by the suffering person (the person demonstrates that she is in distress) whether the comforter is a professional or a layperson.

What is different is that although most people have learned and utilized a variety of comfort strategies, professional caregivers such as nurses have developed the use of comfort strategies to an art (Morse, 1997). The nurse selectively uses strategies, varying them until the patient displays less discomfort or distress. Although nursing students study these strategies in fundamentals texts and in classrooms, the strategies appear to be primarily acquired informally in the clinical setting by observing experienced nurses providing care and by gaining experience in which strategies are effective in which circumstances.

Dependence of Comfort Strategies on Patient Suffering State

The comforting strategies that the nurse uses are dependant on the cues the patient displays and the state of suffering the patient is experiencing. The states of suffering Morse describes are enduring and emotional suffering. These states are described in detail in Chapter 9. A brief definition and description of cues to those states as described by Morse (2000) follows: when patients are blocking emotional response so they can focus on what must be done in the present moment. Cues that a person is enduring are

- erect upright posture with shoulders back and head up;
- mechanical movements and a robotlike gait;
- lack of eye contact and an unfocused gaze;
- little movement of mouth and face while speaking and a monotone voice; and
- short sentences with many sighs.

Emotional suffering is a very distressed state in which emotions are released. The person is filled with sadness and displays the sadness by crying, sobbing, or moaning constantly. The emotionally suffering person may

- assume a stooped posture;
- have a face that is lined and a drooping facial expression;
- look as if he will fall apart;
- talk with whoever will listen, repeating his illness story over and over.

The comfort strategies used for the patient who is enduring need to be different from those used for the patient who is emotionally suffering. People who are enduring need to have their endurance supported whether it is by the presence of the nurse or the verbal reassurance from the nurse that the patient is "bearing up" well. Sympathetic statements and the use of touch may undermine the patient's ability to endure. People who are emotionally suffering, on the other hand, find touch to be helpful. Morse (2000) notes that when a caregiver holds the emotionally suffering person in his arms, he may literally be holding the sufferer together.

Comfort Strategies Used for the Suffering Patient

Morse (1992) found that touching is a very powerful comfort strategy. She observed that nurses used it alone or in combination with talking. Nurses tended to use

- touching alone if the person was perceived to be feeling alone or afraid;
- touching with a little talking if the person was ill, sick, or in pain;
- talking with a little touching if the person felt, insecure, afraid or depressed.

Why does Morse believe that touching is such a powerful and significant comfort strategy? She believes that "humans comfort others by directly touching the part of the sufferer's body that most expresses the pain" (Morse, 1992, p. 95). This obviously is most evident with physical pain. However, she notes that touch may be used to reduce distress when emotional pain is expressed somatically. For example, we wipe away a sufferer's tears or place our arms around those whose shoulders are hunched as if they cannot carry their load of suffering. Touch is a powerful tool; we allow those who are close to us to touch us. Yet, we allow only select strangers, such as nurses, to touch us and it is only appropriate for strangers to use touch in highly stressful situations.

To be certain that they have not crossed the boundaries and to see if they have been successful with their use of touch, nurses constantly assess the effectiveness of their interventions. They quickly shift to another strategy or combination of strategies if the first is not successful. Nurses videotaped by Morse (1992) caring for postoperative infants changed their pattern of touching sequentially from patting to stroking to rubbing within 10 seconds or less if the previous strategy was ineffective in comforting the infant.

In summary, during her extensive research with emotionally suffering patients and their nurses, Morse (1992) learned that experienced nurses

- read their patients' cues of distress;
- determine whether they have their patients' trust;
- select from a repertoire of strategies depending on the circumstance;
- assess the responsiveness of their patients to the interactions;
- are very versatile in their ability to switch strategies; and
- may use a combination of strategies.

Morse noted that at this point it is not clear how nurses read the patient. Their reading of patient distress may be intuitive or may be a subconscious recognition of patterns. Understanding this will help to further delineate how nurses can respond to patients' emotional suffering.

Morse believes that patients need to experience emotional suffering in order to reconstitute. A more detailed description of how nurses may help patients do that is located in Chapter 8, The Search for Meaning in Suffering. However, a brief summary of how nurses can help the patient search for meaning and obtain comfort is presented here from the perspective of Eifried (1998).

Nurses can help patients who are emotionally suffering by actively listening and encouraging patients to talk about their feelings. An intimate conversation is necessary, when patients can say anything that they want to say. The nurse listens to the patient's story and asks a few clarifying questions such as "How is this affecting you?" or "How do you feel within yourself?" When there is nothing that the nurse can say, the nurse helps the suffering patient just by being present and touching so that the patient feels the nurse's presence. The nurse can provide hope. This is discussed in more detail in Chapter 12 but praying with the patient or showing the patient what she can still do may begin to instill hope. Most important, as detailed in Chapter 8, the nurse can help suffering patients to call forth their voice. The nurse can listen and ask clarifying questions as patients try to integrate the illness experience into their life narrative. Sitting with patients as they reminisce may allow them to see that their lives have mattered and have value. Finally, the nurse can be a guide to the emotionally suffering patient. For example, the nurse may help the patient to look upon her body as a friend and consider symptoms as messages that she must care for herself in a different way in the future.

Comfort Strategies Used for the Enduring Patient

As noted previously, touch is not usually appropriate for patients who are enduring. Therefore, talking and listening are used more commonly as strategies with these patients. Morse (1992) researched types of comforting that nurses in an emergency department (ED) used to help patients endure during the first hours after their arrival at the hospital. Morse and Proctor (1998) believed that all of the nurses' types of comforting were aimed at helping their patients endure and were targeted to making the patients feel safe. The nurses' actions may appear small, insignificant, or a even a normal part of nursing care delivery. However, Arman and Rehnsfeldt (2007) verified that it is just such little extras that show the nurse is seeing and responding to the patient as a person and not as an object that alleviates suffering. There were eight types of comforting exhibited by emergency department nurses in Morse's (1992) study:

Keeping things cool: Nurses manipulated the environment surrounding the patient to keep it relaxed so that the patient would not experience undue anxiety.

They treated the patient's condition, whatever it was, as if it were normal. They used normal or even lighthearted talk to convey comfort to the patient.

Clicking through the assessment: Nurses assessed their patients quickly and competently but kept the patients involved in the diagnostic testing and distracted from the seriousness of their conditions. They used only enough touch and talk to gain the information they required but listened carefully to what their patients had to say.

Watching over: The nurses were constantly observing their patients so that any changes in their condition could be dealt with immediately. In acute illness, patients felt comforted knowing that they were being so closely observed.

Helping patients regain/maintain control and providing care within the patients' own comfort level: This comfort type included both touching and talking. Talk was usually soothing, distracting for the scared patient while touch might include stroking the patient's hand. If the patient was beginning to lose control, the nurse might use eye contact. However, each nurse checked each patient's response to her touch and changed strategy if the patient did not respond well.

Keeping the doctor on track: Nurses covertly and overtly made suggestions to the emergency department physicians intended to enhance patient comfort.

Bringing in and supporting the family: Nurses were very aware of the importance of family. They emphasized getting the family to the patient and providing support to both patient and family.

Reaching the person in the body: Nurses would speak to the patient even if the patient was unresponsive. Usually this meant speaking in short sentences and using the person's first name. This will be described in more detail later in the chapter.

Talking them through it: Nurses used specific patterned, rhythmic speech to help their patients through painful procedures. This is described in more detail in the section describing the "comfort talk register." Morse continued to look at how emergency department nurses maintain patient endurance. Although the ED nurses believed that they were too caught up in helping the patient survive, Morse and Proctor (1998) found that these trauma nurses did indeed comfort their patients. They discovered that the nurses used particular patterns of position, eye contact, and touch while talking their patients through painful procedures. These strategies encouraged patients to "hold on" and gave the message to the patients that they could endure the procedure.

Morse and Proctor (1998) identified a specific pattern to how ED nurses would position themselves to assist a patient through a difficult procedure. The nurse would:

- position herself at the side of the head of the bed so that her face was within intimate range of the patient (about 10 inches);
- turn to directly face the patient, thus demanding the patient's attention;
  - focus on the patient's eyes and search for cues in the patient's expression;
  - hold the patient's gaze if the patient's eyes were open; and
- use a constant, light palmar touch to maintain contact with the patient.

When nurses talked to trauma patients who were enduring, Morse and Proctor (1998) discovered that some of their vocalizations had some very specific characteristics. The vocalizations were

- on the patient's channel of communication—the loudest and highest pitch channel;
- loud and clear;
- patient-led, often acknowledging or reflecting the patient's voice;
- distinguished by a slow rate of speech, clearly marked utterance boundaries, short simple sentences, rhythmic pattern;
- sing-song in quality; and
- with a high frequency of tag questions when the nurse needed to verify something.

Comfort Talk

In fact, these communications were so distinctive and nurses used them for such a specific purpose that Morse and Proctor (1998) called them the "comfort talk register." Comfort talk was most frequently used with patients who were frightened. The patients might display crying, moaning, or other indications that they were not tolerating their pain or suffering. The comfort talk had four very practical functions: to help the patient hold on or endure, to permit the nurse to obtain necessary information from the patient, to provide information to the patient, and importantly, to communicate caring. In addition, comfort talk keeps patients focused on what is happening to them and helps them to prepare for what will be happening next. There is reason to believe that comfort talk has therapeutic value because it helps patients to remain in control despite catastrophic circumstances. Also, because the nurse is watching the patient so closely and reacting to what the patient says, the nurse using comfort talk may be the first to detect a change in the patient's condition. Morse and Perkins note that comfort talk is somewhat similar to the birthing talk that occurs in some cultures.

There were specific types of phrases associated with each of the functions (also called characteristics) of comfort talk (Morse & Proctor, 1998). The first function—holding on—was used specifically to help the patient stay in control and endure. To accomplish this, nurses might praise the patient, saying "You're doing a great job" or try to inspire the patient with courage by saying "You can do it" or "We're almost done." Nurses might support patients with their physical presence by holding their patients' hands or saying, "I'm right here with you." Nurses might command a patient to do something such as "Breath with me." Such a command might also serve as a distraction for the patient.

When the nurse is trying to gather information and assess the suffering patient, the nurse uses open-ended questions to gather information such as "Where are you?" It is particularly important that the nurse explain what is happening, including where the patient is and what is happening at the moment. The last type of question in this category is also crucial; the nurse validates her findings with the patient asking something akin to "How are you?"

The third characteristic of comfort talk is informing. Nurses warn their patients, telling them what to anticipate regarding procedures—for example, "You will feel a little prick now." Also included in this characteristic is explaining the procedure, the reason for it, and what the patient's likely response will be.

The final characteristic of comfort talk is caring. Nurses may use reassurance to calm a patient. To attempt to restore a patient's confidence, the nurse might say, "You're doing fine" or "There, there." The nurse might express empathy by saying, " I know." Or the nurse might make caring and consoling comments, acknowledging that the patient requires attention but not giving information. These comments often include the patient's name. For example, "OK, Sarah, all right."

Morse's findings with ED nurses validated what Davitz and Davitz (1980) had found years earlier about nurses' communication with patients who are about to undergo a procedure and were presumed to be suffering. High inference nurses (those who believed their patients might be suffering), when arriving to do a procedure, would do the following:

1. Introduce themselves.
2. Explain the reason for procedure.
3. Ask the patients if they had any questions and answer them.

4. Provide information as the procedure progressed.
5. Make an effort to express sympathetic understanding during the procedure especially when they caused discomfort.

In contrast, low inference nurses tended not to explain the procedure or discuss their actions as they proceeded. They were very matter-of-fact and usually did not respond sympathetically to the patient's discomfort. They related to patients as interchangeable prototypes and not as individuals.

Comfort from Doing the "Little Something Extra"

Arman and Rehnsfeldt (2007) found that when patients felt that their nurses saw them as people and interacted with them sympathetically as individuals rather than as prototype patients, their suffering was alleviated. Patients described this as being a patient and not a diagnosis. They appreciated their healthcare providers showing emotion and not just being matter-of-fact in response to their discomfort. Most of all, they noted that the nurse doing the little extra provided comfort. The little extra implied that the nurse had seen the patient as a person, recognized a unique need of the person, and had chosen to do something for the person that was small but highly personally significant. For example, a nurse's aide might provide a violet comfort shawl for a dying woman who loved that color, or a nurse might stay late to speak with a patient newly diagnosed with cancer. Arman and Rehnsfeldt noted that when patients felt most cared for, the caregivers cared for their patients less from the distance and the role of healthcare providers and more in the role of fellow human beings. Patients in their study were aware that caregivers had a choice. The nurses could choose to attend to routine and convention or they could choose to attend to their patients. The patients appreciated and found comfort in the fact that nurses chose to see them as people and took the time to attend to things that were very significant to them but might have seemed trivial in the rush of the healthcare system.

Comforting Interaction as a Model of Nurse–Patient Relationship

Morse, Havens, and Wilson (1997) studied how three separate levels of nursing actions, including comforting, combined to establish a therapeutic nurse–patient relationship. They called this the comforting interaction as a model of nurse–patient relationship. The three levels of nursing actions they described are

- comforting strategies such as comfort talk previously described;
- styles of care—how individual nurses combined particular comfort strategies into their particular way of providing care; and
- patterns of relating—normative professional behaviors such as how a nurse might distance herself from the patient.

Development of Nurse–Patient Relationship

Morse et al. (1997) described the following process of development of a nurse–patient relationship. A patient action, such as a behavioral signal of distress or discomfort (described in detail in Chapter 9) would call forth a comforting strategy in response from the patient's nurse (discussed earlier in this chapter). However, they believe that nurses do not rely on only one comfort strategy; instead, after assessing the patient, they combine several different strategies that they have used successfully in the past to form a specific style of care. The style is created in response to the perceived needs of the specific patient within some general patterned approaches. For example, Morse and colleagues note that while nurses may use humor to comfort patients with chronic pain, it is never used for patients with acute pain. Nurses' personalities, cultural backgrounds, level of experience, and whether they have a technical style of care or an affective style (as described by Davitz and Davitz, 1980) also have an effect on the style of care they utilize. Styles of care described by Fosbinder (1994) include

- translating: consisting of strategies of informing, explaining, and instructing;
- getting to know the patient: consisting of strategies of personal sharing, being friendly, and using humor;
- establishing trust: anticipating needs, being prompt, following through; and
- going the extra mile: doing the "little extra."

The final nursing action, the pattern of relating, becomes socialized as professional nursing behavior over time. The pattern of relating is taught to student nurses from their very first nursing course, but it is developed by each nurse as unique mannerisms and patterns during her student and nurse work experience. The patterns have been shown to vary with clinical specialty and nursing role. For example, Morse and colleagues (1997) note that the patterns of relating vary usually considerably between community health and emergency department nurses but do appear to be fairly standardized for such functions as counseling.

Dynamic Nature of Nurse–Patient Relationship

As the contact between nurse and patient evolves over time, they develop a nurse–patient relationship. Through the interaction of all three nursing actions and patient actions, the nurse–patient relationship is negotiated. That means that as the nurse begins to know the patient better, the nurse varies the style of care and pattern of relating to better suit the patient. Morse and colleagues (1997) note that "comforting becomes more adept, personalized, and caregiving more effective and efficient" (p. 338). However, the patient is always in control since she is the person who is guiding the nurse's response. So, if the patient begins to become more accustomed to the illness and its treatment and experiences less distress, the nurse will note that and alter the style of care and pattern of relating accordingly. "Thus the process of obtaining feedback, and reading patient signals of discomfort becomes a continual process, which makes the nurse–patient relationship dynamic and changing" (p. 338).

Morse, Havens, and Wilson believe that this model of the nurse–patient relationship is patient-led, dynamic, interactive, and context dependent. "Even though the model is driven by the patient's behavioral state, actions, and reactions, both the nurse and patient maintain control—the nurse selects the style or strategy to be used and the patient in negotiating, relinquishing and accepting care, maintains control" (1997, p. 321). Although they are using different words, Morse et al. are describing something quite similar to what Fagerstrom and colleagues (1998) found when they noted that patients behaving in different ways preferred nurses who were competent but varied in the distance they maintained from the patient and the amount of information they supplied to the patient.

Summary

For nearly 20 years, nursing theorists and researchers such as Janice Morse and Katharine Kolcaba have been advocating comfort as a major focus of nursing care and research. Morse (1992) has even argued that comfort should be the primary focus of nursing, with caring as a subset of it. Their interest in comfort has resulted in substantial theory development and research. The information in this chapter is largely based on their considerable body of research and the evidence-based interventions they recommend.

Key Points

1. Comfort is viewed as a major focus and outcome of nursing practice achievable for patients across a wide variety of conditions.
2. Nurses who infer that their patients are suffering are more likely to engage in comforting behaviors.
3. Although some of the comfort strategies that nurses utilize, such as administration of appropriate medications for pain and nausea, are learned in school, many others are learned through observation of experienced nurses and trial and error while caring for patients.
4. According to Morse, nurses utilize touch, talk, and position in specific ways to enhance patient comfort. The comfort talk register is an example of the way nurses use talk in emergent situations.
5. As a nurse develops a relationship with a patient, the nurse will usually change strategies and provide care in a style that is responsive to the patient's stated and inferred needs/desires for comfort.

Exercise: A Comfort Shawl Project

What Is a Comfort Shawl?

The comfort shawl programs began more than a decade ago following the experience of Janet Bristow and Victoria Galo, in a program in feminist spirituality at the Women's Leadership Institute at the Hartford Seminary in Hartford, Connecticut. Combining a desire to bring comfort and compassion to people who are suffering with a desire to be creative using two traditional women's art forms, knitting and crocheting, the comfort shawl project or ministry creates a bond between women's creativity and compassion.

The shawls go by a variety of names—comfort shawls, prayer shawls, peace shawls, and mantles depending on the people who are creating them. However, they have features in common no matter who is creating them. They are created out of soft yarns in soothing colors to provide visual and tactile as well as spiritual warmth and well-being. While knitting, the shawl maker either prays or meditates with the intention of bringing blessings and good intentions to the recipient. Usually a final blessing is offered before the shawl is sent on its way.

Figure 11–3   Prayer Shawl

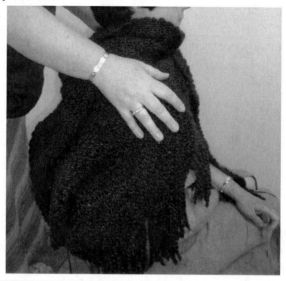

Source: Comfort Shawl Ministry at the Transfiguration Parish and the Parish Nurse Ministry, Manchester, NH, Dayle Moulton RN, MS, Director.

Some shawls are created to bring solace and strength to those in need, whether from illness, hospitalization, bereavement, or severe stress. Several hospital intensive care units have a supply of comfort shawls that are presented to their palliative care patients and their families. However, shawls may also be presented for joyous occasions such as marriage ceremonies and births or for transitions and natural events such as nursing a baby.

Whatever the reason, the shawls are meant to convey warmth, care, and compassion from the women knitting them to the recipients. The creators believe that anyone facing life transitions can benefit from being wrapped in the warmth and love of a shawl that was created with positive energy and good intentions. If a religious group has created the shawl, then prayers will have been said during its creation and may be said when it is presented. An example of a woman being presented with a prayer shawl is shown in Figure 11–3.

The following prayer is used at the presentation of a shawl by the Comfort Shawl Ministry at the Transfiguration Parish and the Parish Nurse Ministry, Manchester, New Hampshire, Dayle Moulton, MS, RN, director. It was composed from various sources by Sister Pauline Maurier and is reprinted with permission.

> This is a prayer mantle, a shawl of comfort. Wrap it around you when you are sad, happy, needing comfort, cold, ill, worried, at peace, needing answers, ministering, socializing or praying. Let it be God's warm embrace—a sacred place of security and well-being.
>
> The stitches have been knit in groups of three to represent the Trinity. It has been blessed by the hands and intentions of the knitters.
>
> Each time you wear this mantle, may you be cradled in hope, kept in joy, graced with peace, embraced with healing, and wrapped in love.
>
> May God bless and keep you; may God's face shine upon you and be gracious to you. May God lift you up and grant you peace.
>
> Amen.

How to Become Involved in a Comfort Shawl Project

1. Learn more about the comfort shawl movement by visiting the Prayer Shawl Ministry Home Page at http://www.shawlministry.com or by reading either of the following books:

   Izod, S., & Jorgenson, S. (2003). *Knitting into the mystery*: Harrisburg, PA: Morehouse.

   Bristow, J., Cole-Galo, V., & Hopkins, T. (2008). *The prayer shawl companion: 38 knitted designs to embrace, inspire, and celebrate life.* Newtown, CT: Taunton Press.

2. Locate a comfort shawl group nearby and become involved with the group.

3. Research the possibilities at the healthcare or other institution where you are employed and determine whether it would be possible to have comfort shawls available on appropriate units to provide to appropriate patients and families, such as palliative care patients, new nursing mothers, or bereaved parents.

4. Negotiate with a comfort shawl group to provide shawls for the unit.

5. Determine whether there are nurses on the unit where you are working who might be willing to knit or crochet to supplement the number of shawls needed for people on that unit.

Questions for Reflection and Journaling

1. Do you believe that providing comfort should be a more important focus in nursing than caring? Why or why not?

2. How do you know when patients are in discomfort or distress? Is it by intuition, observation of behaviors, or a combination of the two? Have you ever been mistaken about the amount of distress a patient was experiencing? When and how? What did you do to rectify the situation?

3. What do you believe your predominant comfort style is? Think about the most recent time when you used it intentionally to comfort a patient. What did you do and how well did it work?

4. Do you ever intentionally change your comfort style of relating to a patient? When did you first realize you did that? Did it work?

Case Study 11–2: Reflection on Comfort—It Is the Small Things That Are Truly Important and Comforting

Other people's words and actions make a huge difference, but the emotional tone underlying the words and actions is more powerful than either. During my brother's hospitalization for his bone marrow transplant, he found one of the most difficult times of each day to be the few moments following the morning conference at the end of the bone marrow unit when each patient's progress was discussed. After the conference the staff would leave the meeting and walk the length of the unit. He noticed that not just he but each of the patients in the unit would examine the faces of the staff as they walked down the hallway to try to determine what had been discussed about them during the conference. Most of the staff would hurry on past, intent on their next task. But one of the nurses would stop to speak warmly with each patient. She was not talking about the plan for the day or their current lab studies but just offering her presence and letting them know that she would be available for them throughout the day. He found this difficult time much more manageable on the days that she was working.

One of the most comforting responses to my diagnosis of cancer was from a colleague who worked as an emergency department (ED) nurse. She encircled me in her arms and said, "I just heard something. I want you to know that I will hold you in my thoughts and prayers until you are well again," and she held me close for a few moments. Her response embodied warmth of intent, action, and words as well as hope. It brought me comfort, and I remember thinking I hoped she was able to bring comfort to the patients and families in the ED in a similar way. I wondered when and how she had learned to be authentic and supportive.

Many other people in my life found ways to comfort me, even when they could not be physically present. I was heavily medicated during each of my chemotherapy sessions so that I was quite sleepy. My husband would bring me for treatment and sit until I was drifting asleep or I told him to leave; then I would rest with my eyes closed. When I opened my eyes one time, a social worker was sitting nearby. She moved over, obviously concerned, and asked if I wanted to bring a friend the next time so that I would not feel lonely. I smiled at her and said "I really don't feel like I could entertain someone at the moment—but I'm not alone. The warm shawl was made for me by a member of my church, the 'strong woman' bracelet is from a friend who recovered from breast cancer, the pillow is from a friend who is involved in cancer research, and the bear is from a colleague who wanted me to have something warm and fuzzy to hold. I'm surrounded by friendship, love, and support."

Questions on the Case Study

1. Are there any commonalities among the different ways that people conveyed comfort to this patient? If so, what are they?
2. How did the healers involved use touch, talk, and presence?
3. Why did it mean so much to the bone marrow transplant patient that the nurse stopped to talk—especially since she was not providing him with any new information or solace?
4. How have you responded when you were told of a person's frightening diagnosis? Did your response vary if the person was a patient, a friend, or a family member? Did your response vary depending on how the person responded to the news (e.g., with enduring or emotional suffering)?
5. Did the social worker verify that the patient needed support and comfort? How could the social worker have done that?
6. Do you believe the patient needed additional support?
7. What would you have done in a similar circumstance?

References

Arman, M., & Rehnsfeldt, A. (2007). The "little extra" that alleviates suffering. *Nursing Ethics, 14*(3), 372–384.

Davitz, L., & Davitz, J. (1980). *Nurses' responses to patients suffering.* New York, NY: Springer.

Eifried, S. (1998). Helping patients find meaning. *International Journal for Human Caring, 2*(1), 33–39.

Fagerstrom, L., Eriksson, K., & Engberg, I. (1998). The patient's perceived caring needs as a message of suffering. *Journal of Advanced Nursing, 28*(5), 978–987.

Fosbinder, D. (1994). Patient perceptions of nursing care: An emerging theory of interpersonal competence. *Journal of Advanced Nursing, 20,* 1085–1093.

Kolcaba, K. (1992). Holistic comfort: Operationalizing the construct as a nurse sensitive outcome. *Advances in Nursing Science, 15*(1), 1–10.

Kolcaba, K. (1994). A theory of holistic comfort for nursing. *Journal of Advanced Nursing, 19,* 1178–1184.

Kolcaba, K. (2001). Evolution of the midrange theory of comfort for outcomes research. *Nursing Outlook, 49,* 86–92.

Morse, J. (1992). Comfort: The refocusing of nursing care. *Clinical Nursing Research, 1*(1), 91–106.

Morse, J. (2000). Responding to the cues of suffering. *Health Care for Women International, 21,* 1–9.

Morse, J., Havens, G., & Wilson, S. (1997). The comforting interaction: Developing a model of nurse-patient relationship. *Scholarly Inquiry for Nursing Practice: An International Journal, 11*(4). 321–342.

Morse, J., & Proctor, A. (1998). Maintaining patient endurance: The comfort work of trauma nurses. *Clinical Nursing Research, 7*(3), 250–274.

Nightingale, F. (1859). *Notes on Nursing.* London, UK: Harrison.

Schroepfer, T. (2007). Critical events in the dying process: The potential for physical and psychosocial suffering. *Journal of Palliative Medicine, 10*(1), 136–147.

Sundin, K., Axelsson, K., Jansson, L., & Norberg, A. (2000). Suffering from care as expressed in the narratives of former patients in somatic wards. *Scandinavian Journal of Caring Sciences, 14,* 16–22.

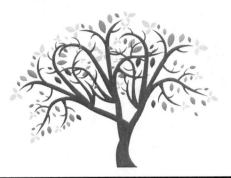

TWELVE

Inspiring Hope

■ **Caryn A. Sheehan**

Objectives

1. Compare and contrast varying definitions for the concept "hope."
2. Describe the components and sequencing of the development of hope identified by Morse and Doberneck (1995).
3. Identify how the development of hope relates to the states of enduring and suffering.
4. Discuss "hope" in the context of aging, disease, and suffering.
5. Review nursing research about hope.
6. Identify at least three nursing interventions that can be used in clinical practice to promote hope.

Student Project

Figure 12–1   Protected by the Sheets

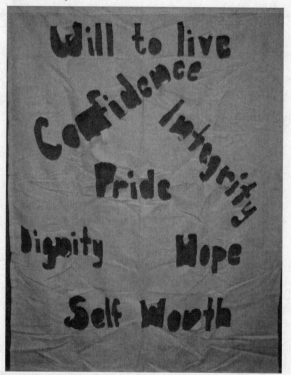

Case Study 12–1

Mr. Jackson had deformities of his face from his harsh experience as a soldier in the Vietnam war, though few people actually saw these deformities since he secluded himself in his makeshift home near the homeless shelter. Even Mr. Jackson, himself, did not observe these devastating physical changes to his face as he was permanently blinded from the original war injury. However, he could feel the physical changes to his face with his own hands and knew his appearance must be frightening. Years earlier, he had endured several reconstructive surgeries, but the injuries were so destructive that further plastic surgery would be futile. He knew he would never look "normal" again.

Mr. Jackson was devastated to learn that his infected foot was not resolving. He would require hospitalization for amputation of the toes on his left foot and further evaluation of his diabetes and declining kidney function. While the upcoming surgery did not frighten him, he hated the thought of having to go out in public again and allow so many strangers to see his deformed face.

In the hospital, Mr. Jackson made a habit of keeping his bed sheet pulled over his head at all times. Nurses, doctors, dieticians, and therapists all learned to speak to him "through the sheet" as they realized that he would not take the sheet down if someone else was in the room. While hospitalized, Mr. Jackson, once a brave and decorated soldier, had relinquished all hope of any normal life as he spent his days hidden in fear under a sheet.

A student nurse was working as the nursing assistant on his hospital unit the summer Mr. Jackson was hospitalized for his amputation. Each morning the same nursing student entered his room and talked to the man behind the sheet as if it was quite normal to have a conversation that way. Over time the patient developed a trust with the student nurse that he was not able to develop with the other staff, and quite surprisingly, one day when the student nurse asked if she could check his blood pressure, he actually pulled down the sheet instead of routinely sticking his arm out from under the covers. The sight of him was startling to the student nurse.

He surrendered and unveiled his broken body. I kept a straight face, though inside I thought I had seen a murder. I know it sounds awful, but this is honest and it hurts sometimes. I would never say this to a patient but I want to get my full story across without sugarcoating anything.

His face was deformed. His eyes looked like someone had ripped them out and carelessly sewed them back in. His skin was yellow and he barely had any teeth. I was shocked, and this was only what I saw above his neck. I attempted small talk. What else could I do? The awkward silence was killing me while I waited for the blood pressure cuff to inflate and slowly deflate.

He had a dialysis fistula in his left arm. He had many scars on his abdomen and a below-the-knee amputation of his right leg. I attempted small talk again. Surprisingly, he went along with me. Not only did I uncover him from his sheets, I uncovered the part of his past that had left his body here in front of me, deformed and destroyed.

I came to learn he was in a war and despite being injured, he returned safely home. He developed diabetes and eventually became homeless and could no longer take care of his health. As a result, the war and the disease had left his body severely damaged. He lost his eyesight, kidney function, and his lower right leg. This was not what mattered to him. He had lost his dignity, integrity, and willingness to live. This was the extent of his suffering. He was suffering so greatly he wished he were dead.

From that moment on, I realized why he shielded himself from the world with his covers. His sheets were the only thing that kept him sane. From the moment I entered his room, I was grappling with suffering. I felt nervous, scared, and helpless. I wanted so badly to give this man a second chance at a great future, knowing this was entirely out of my hands. I settled for the actions I was capable of. I listened to him, I held his hand, and most important, I treated him like a normal human being, not the monster he saw himself as. By the end of the day, I wasn't afraid to enter room 226. By the end of the day, I learned that times are going to be tough, and it helps to have someone present who is willing to listen and care. By the end of that day, Mr. Jackson no longer hid himself from the world. He no longer felt like a monster. He no longer wished he were dead. Listening and being present made all the difference that day.

By creating an environment of acceptance, trust, and kindness, this student nurse was able to offer hope to this patient. In this case, the hope was not about a cure or even related to his multiple medical needs; rather, the student engendered hope for normalcy. Mr. Jackson took a leap of faith in hoping he would not scare the student away, and in the end, pulling down his covers benefited both the patient and the nurse.

The picture in Figure 12–1 illustrates the relationship the student nurse and Mr. Jackson experienced. Getting past the sheets (in the presentation project, the sheet is literally cut through) resulted in positive characteristics (listed on the sheet) that were so foreign to him, such as hope, confidence, and self-worth.

Source: Courtesy of Jessie Cantone, student nurse.

Questions on the Case Study
1.   How is Mr. Jackson suffering (physically, emotionally, spiritually)?
2.   List three goals the nurse could talk about with Mr. Jackson.

Hope is the thing with feathers
That perches in the soul.
And sings the tune
Without the words,
and never stops at all.
Emily Dickinson (1830–1886)

Questions for Reflection and Journaling
1.   What is your personal definition of hope?
2.   Is hope the goal for all patients?

Introduction

Hope is such a fundamental part of human nature that it is often taken for granted. For ages, humans have thought about, written about, and even sung about the importance of hope to a fulfilling life. This chapter investigates the role of hope in relationship to suffering. The chapter concludes with discussing what role, if any, nurses can play in assessing and promoting hope among people who suffer.

Definitions of Hope

Hope can be an elusive concept to define because it is inherently subjective and dynamic. Often hope is easier to recognize and/or describe once it is low or lost.

One aspect that is often included in definitions of hope is its temporal relation that is future-focused. Research suggests that hope can be influenced by many factors such as age, health, level of activity, social support, and spirituality (Borell, Lilja, Svidén, & Sadlo, 2001; Chi, 2007; Duggleby, 2001). Because hope is subjective, it is often manifested verbally. Statements such as, "I feel like life has meaning" are easily interpreted as hopeful. But hope can also be manifested subtly by active participation in social events or by demonstrating self-confidence. Hope has been defined differently by many different theorists, most agreeing that it is a goal-oriented thought or emotion about future expectations (Lopez, Snyder, & Pedrotti, 2003). Characteristics of hope as cited in the literature (Duggleby, 2001; Kylma, 2005; Lopez, Snyder, & Pedrotti, 2003; Miller, 2007) include these:

- A feeling, thought, belief, emotion
- Important for taking action
- Related to motivation
- Future-oriented
- Goal/Outcome directed
- Dependant on autonomy
- Dynamic
- Concerned with what is possible
- Affected by interpersonal relationships
- Related to trust and faith
- Always possible

Related Concepts

Hope is related to several concepts. Optimism may be one of the closest relations, though it has a connotation of being more general in nature whereas hope can be very specific. One example of a specific hope would be when a frail elder wishes to maintain health long enough to attend her granddaughter's wedding. Hope and optimism need not occur simultaneously. The same grandmother who is hopeful about attending the wedding may demonstrate pessimism at the same time with a statement such as, "I hope I live long enough to attend the wedding, though I am sure I will be too weak to enjoy it." Other terms that are related to hope and may play a role in enabling hope include courage, strength, will, commitment, determination, enduring, hardiness, coping, acceptance, and resilience (Lohne & Severinsson, 2004; Miller, 2007).

Resilience is a related topic that has been the center of controversy. Typically resilience has been defined as the ability to reestablish equilibrium. Key concepts that can contribute to resilience after a tragedy are knowledge/information about the event, social support, appreciation of life, spirituality, reflection of the experience, and the use of active coping strategies (Chan, Ho, Fu, & Chow, 2006; Farley, 2007). Bonanno (2008) makes the argument that resilience is common, and humans are naturally resilient in the face of tragedy. Furthermore, he states that grief workers may actually hinder resilience by impulsively intervening to "help" people cope with crises when most people would recover without intervention. Bonanno's charge is that the concept of resilience has not been given the research or attention that dysfunctional coping disorders have. In opposition, others argue that resilience is a nebulous concept, nearly impossible to quantify as everyone experiences stressors in a different context (Roisman, 2005).

How can several people experience the same crises and have such different outcomes? When many people share a common stressor, such as surviving an earthquake, their responses will vary: some people may take immediate action and begin clearing a space to rebuild their home, others will cry and withdraw, others will relocate to another area far away. This complexity of human behavior is partly explained by the relationship of environment, support, past experiences, and past coping methods. The key is for nurses to tap into each patient's individual strengths that can best foster resilience. Wagnild and Collins (2009) encourage the use of the Resilience Scale combined with narrative assessment to identify and address resilience. The questions included are open-ended such as, "When you have experienced difficult times, how would you say you have gotten through them?" (p. 31) Other authors focus on fostering the interconnectedness of spirituality with resilience because both contribute to self-protection, positive growth, and hope (Farley, 2007).

Whereas the focus of this chapter is promoting hope, it is also important to acknowledge the normalcy of sorrow as patients deal with loss of health and loved ones (Herth & Cutcliffe, 2002). Hope may not be the actual outcome but may be the process by which people achieve peace, stability, and equilibrium. In this chapter, hope is viewed as a process that is important in helping those who are suffering to cope successfully.

Case Study 12-2

Mr. Johnson was an 83-year-old male patient who was admitted to the medical/surgical unit for dyspnea. He had advanced Parkinson's disease but was able to manage at home with the help of his spouse and the use of dopamine medications and assistive devices. For the past 3 months he had been noticing increasing difficulty with his breathing. His primary care provider attributed this change to a progression of intercostal muscle weakness related to his Parkinson's disease. Eventually Mr. Johnson had to call the ambulance because of his inability to breathe. In the emergency room, a near-obstruction of his airway from old food was observed and an emergency tracheotomy tube was placed.

The next day Mr. Johnson was all smiles. When being assisted from the bed to the bathroom, he would turn to (in what he termed) "dance" in a circle with his walker to demonstrate how pleased he was that he could now breathe so easily with his new trach in place. He repeatedly stated that he felt "like a new man" and he couldn't wait to learn how to care for the trach so he could go back home with his wife.

Mr. Johnson's outlook was indeed very hopeful. However, he was well aware that his new artificial airway would not impact his rapidly progressing Parkinson's disease. His source of hope focused on the increase in quality of life he would be able to enjoy during what was to be his last year of life; and he was not centered around curing his underlying disease. Mr. Johnson's case is an example of how hope can be preserved even in the midst of the most grim medical prognoses.

Questions on the Case Study

1. What risk factors for hopelessness does Mr. Johnson have?
2. What subjective and objective findings suggest Mr. Johnson is hopeful?
3. What nursing interventions would be appropriate to promote hope in Mr. Johnson?

Hope, False Hope, and Suffering

Hope is especially important in the context of suffering because it is a basic human need that nurses can address. So often nurses are frustrated that they witness suffering for which there is no cure. Indeed, hope has been criticized when offered or used inappropriately. Unrealistic hope can resemble denial and distort rational decisions (Baergen, 2006). Patients who are overly optimistic may not seek appropriate screening or treatment in a timely manner, which may result in worse outcomes (Schneiderman, 2005). For instance, a woman with aggressive metastatic lung cancer may be deprived of hospice support if she believes that cure and/or long-term survival are certain. Nurses need to be especially vigilant to steer clear of conveying false hope and consciously avoid saying unfounded responses such as, "It will be okay." For a patient enduring the deepest, darkest tragedy or loss, this statement may not only be false but it may also belittle the patient's profound feelings. Instead, the nurse can support the patient by using simple valid statements such as, "I will check in with you more often today" or "I will sit with you for a while so you won't be alone." Nurses need to be intentional when promoting hope so as not to mislead patients with false hopes.

One of the most important facets of this chapter is to help nurses recognize that even in the worst situations, while cure is not always possible, at least one pattern of hope is. Research has demonstrated that even in dire situations, such as complete spinal cord injury, hope remains (Lohne & Severinsson, 2004). Morse and Doberneck (1995) delineated four different patterns of hope although they noted there may be many more. The first was hoping for a chance for a hope. This type of hope might be seen in a patient with aplastic anemia hoping for a donor match so that she might receive a bone marrow transplant and then a hope for a chance to be cured. The second type of hope was incremental hope. An example of incremental hope would be a patient who was very slowly being weaned from a ventilator; each step in the weaning process becomes an incremental step toward the goal of breathing on his own. Hoping against hope can be seen in cancer survivors, especially those with recurrences, who find themselves hoping with each scheduled diagnostic test or each checkup that another recurrence will not be found. The final pattern of hope that Morse and Doberneck found was provisional hope. They identified provisional hope while studying breastfeeding mothers. There were so many factors that could get in the way of what the mothers were intending to do that the mothers created multiple contingency plans so that they could hope to accomplish what they had planned. Provisional hoping meant that the mothers hoped that at least one of the plans would work.

Thus, hope does not need to be centered on curing. The nurse plays an important role in assessing and pointing out areas for hope, be they as grand as hoping for a few months' remission from cancer, to hoping for the chance to plant in the garden for one more summer without pain, to hoping for a peaceful death. While nurses can impact the level of hope among people who suffer, often the need is not apparent until the patient experiences loss of hope.

Hopelessness

The various losses that have been described throughout this book resulting in physical or emotional suffering can contribute to hopelessness. Hopelessness is usually easier than hope for nurses to identify, and often nurses describe patients exhibiting hopelessness as "having given up." Symptoms such as lethargy, anorexia, passivity, and decreased affect may be apparent (Gordon, 2010). Feelings of hopelessness are closely related to depression and have been associated with physical illness and even suicidal behavior (Collins & Cutcliffe, 2003). Definitions vary, but hopelessness can be defined as the opposite of hope, or emptiness, indifference, despair, or loss of a reason to live (Kylma, 2005). Although identifying hopelessness is essential, nurses need not wait until patients exhibit such despair to intervene.

Development of Hope

Beginning in the 1990s, Janice Morse began to publish her investigations into the experiences of suffering patients. The result was the identification of two key behaviors of suffering patients: enduring and emotional suffering, along with the development of evidence-based nursing responses to patient suffering. Summarizing her findings in 2001, Morse described the state of enduring as the state of suspension of emotions that allows a person to get through a traumatic event. While enduring, the person is not able to understand or assimilate the event. As the person begins to be able to accept and understand how the event will change her life, she may enter the state of emotional suffering during which she laments, visibly suffers, and attempts to assimilate the event. Morse believes that it is essential to pass through the phase of emotional suffering to begin to experience hope.

In 1999, Morse and Penrod developed a model relating the concept of hope to previous studies of enduring and suffering. During that process, they recognized that an important state was missing from their model—the state of uncertainty. Morse and Penrod describe the state of uncertainty as being one when patients are just starting to realize what has happened to them but do not have "the information or the ability to weigh the odds or to understand the alternatives" (p. 148). Although they may know what they want, they have no idea how to achieve it. Morse and Penrod believe this is very significant because uncertainty paralyzes patients, preventing them from moving forward to suffering and, more important, to hope.

Morse and Penrod's model of suffering is a sequential model, they note that people move back and forth between contiguous states. They also note that while the states of enduring, uncertainty, and suffering are for the most part reflexive states, once people begin to enter the state of hope, they are usually thinking more clearly and their actions are usually chosen purposefully. They believe that people cannot begin to hope until they have entered the state of emotional suffering, the reality of the situation has begun to seep into the consciousness, and they have begun to develop a realistic appraisal of the situation.

In 1995, Morse and Doberneck elaborated a comprehensive model of the development of hope that they validated with four studies of completely different types of patients and supported with data from other researchers' studies. Listed here are the seven components of Morse and Doberneck's comprehensive model of the development of hope:

- *A realistic appraisal of the event and the threat to self*: As patients develop this realistic appraisal, they may say that they not only know intellectually what has happened to them but they also believe it. They begin to think about the possibility of adverse outcomes, not so much because they fear them but to begin to make alternative plans.
- *Envisioning of alternative plans and setting of goals*: When patients begin the process of thinking about ways to respond to what has happened to them and setting goals, they are entering the second stage of development. This has been called reality surveillance by some researchers because patients scan the environment for possible outcomes and actions. It is an active process because they are reviewing possible goals and actions and choosing the one(s) they find most attractive.

- *Bracing for negative outcomes*: In the third phase, people acknowledge the possibility of negative outcomes. Morse and Doberneck believe this phase is important in the development of hope because they believe that the patient's personal recognition of the potential for a negative outcome is often a motivating factor for the patient and a powerful force behind patient action.

- A *realistic appraisal of personal resources and external conditions and resources*: In this stage, because patients realize that a negative outcome is possible, they begin to assess the resources that are available for assistance so that they know how to locate them and can access them quickly if necessary.

- *The solicitation of mutually supportive relationships*: Morse and Doberneck learned that not only do patients need supportive relationships to develop hope but they actively seek out support from family and friends. The ability to reach out to others is a breakthrough in the process of suffering, indicating that they have become aware of the people around them and are able to ask for support. Patients at this stage discuss their goals with family and friends and mutually agree on goals. When one member of the group is discouraged, the other members will try to bolster the doubting person's hope.

- A *continuous evaluation of signs to reinforce selected goals and the revision of these goals*: During this phase, patients and their supporters continuously monitor the environment for signs that bolster hope. For example, hopeful results from a diagnostic test or a "good day" in therapy might be interpreted as positive signs that the chosen course of therapy is helping to achieve the identified goals. Morse and Doberneck note that superstition may surface at this time as well and patients and supporters may interpret a wide variety of omens as indicating that they have chosen the correct path.

- A *determination to endure*: There is usually a significant time lapse between the setting of the goal and its accomplishment. The final component of Morse and Doberneck's process indicates that patients need to use a considerable amount of physical and emotional energy to maintain their hope and to endure until the goal has been achieved.

Hope is a common term, yet nebulous to define definitively. Understanding the development of the concept of hope is essential in order for nurses to move forward with assessment and implementation of hope promoting strategies. The remainder of this chapter will be dedicated to addressing the concept of hope in clinical nursing practice.

Assessing Hope

Nurses can and should be including the assessment of hope as part of a holistic patient assessment. While many nurses complete a qualitative assessment of hope when it appears warranted, (with a simple, "how are you today?"), the use of formal hope scales can facilitate assessment and discussion. Some hope scales that have been used in the past include the Miller Hope Scale (1988), the Hope Index (1985), the Nowonty Hope Scale (1991), and the Hearth Hope Scale (1991) (Lopez, Snyder, & Pedrotti, 2003). The brief, six-item State Hope Scale has demonstrated good internal consistency and validity (Snyder et al., 1996). A 10-point Visual Analogue Scale (VAS) similar to the scale used to measure patient reports of pain can also be utilized to assess patients' perceived level of hope. Use of any scale to measure hope, including the VAS, should be repeated often so as to grasp the dynamic nature of hope. Because the concept of hope is illusive to define, finding the optimal assessment is challenging (Lopez et al., 2003).

Including Hope in Nursing Practice

Promoting hope is a complex and collaborative process. Nurses have been identified as both a source and a threat to sustaining hope (Bland & Darlington, 2002). The specialty area and nursing practice setting may also influence which nursing interventions to promote hope are utilized. Turner and Stokes (2006) observed that nurses in long-term care used more "hands on" hope facilitating techniques such as integrating touch and signs of love into nursing care; while nurses in acute care were more likely to use optimism and offer patients more choices in their care in order to promote hope. Many older adults never initiate or ask for involvement; they wait until they are asked to participate (Borell et al., 2001). Although some have argued that the research base on specific hope promotion strategies is weak, the research on developing evidenced based nursing interventions to promote hope is ongoing (Turner & Stokes, 2006). Overall, nursing interventions are generally congruent with the needs of their patients to sustain and engender hope (Holt, 2001).

Practice Suggestions

Often, providing usual nursing care and maintaining a trusting relationship can lay the foundation for promoting hope in patients in clinical practice. Nursing care should, at a minimum, provide for basic needs such as comfort, nutrition, security, safety, exercise, and sleep (Miller, 2007; Wake & Miller, 1992). As Maslow's (1943) hierarchy has proposed, some people may find it difficult to think of the future if their immediate needs are unmet. Utilizing therapeutic communication can also be essential for promoting hope. Active listening is not only a means for assessing the patient's current state of hopefulness; it can be a hope intervention as well (Herth & Cutcliffe, 2002). Turner and Stokes (2006) observed that nurses' ability to connect with patients and build trust were important facilitators of hope. Hope is closely related to social connection. Bailey and Snyder (2007) observed the highest levels of hope among people who were married or in a committed relationship when compared to people who were divorced, separated, or widowed. Social connectedness need not be solely based on the patient's family or friends. Meaningful relationships between patient and nurse can impact an elder's level of hopefulness (Herth & Cutcliffe, 2002). Therapeutic communication and cognitive behavioral interventions may even decrease the suicidality related to hopelessness (Collins & Cutcliffe, 2003). Primary nursing, or keeping the same patients assigned to the same nurses, can also facilitate the development of social connectedness/rapport and ultimately, hope.

Other interventions to promote hope include a focus on cognitive stimulation. The nurse can use storytelling or reminiscence in a therapeutic manner to identify what is important to the patient (Duggleby, 2001). For instance, an elderly female patient who constantly talks about her family may respond well to prompts when they are focused on family-centered goals such as "Let's set up a pain management plan that will allow you to stay for the entire birthday party for your niece next month." Encouraging patients to make choices and volunteer can also keep cognition active. "Do you think you will have the strength to get out of bed with physical therapy this morning, or would you rather get up later on today?" Keeping patients active in their own care decisions can create a more hopeful milieu (Borell et al., 2001).

Whereas Holt (2001) observed that nurses' actions to promote hope were quite congruent with patients' needs, one area of discrepancy was in supporting spiritual beliefs and practices as an important intervention to promote hope. Even though patients and families consistently rated "attending to spiritual care" as one of the most important nursing interventions to promote hope, only hospice nurses stated that they routinely address the spiritual and/or religious needs of their patients. Yet a review of research on hope and cancer patients revealed that religion was important to fostering hope and was significantly associated with better coping and adjustment (Chi, 2007). Family caregivers of patients with severe mental illness also identified prayer and spirituality as important to maintaining hope (Bland & Darlington, 2002). Spirituality may or may not include attention to religious needs, such as visiting with a church leader or participating in prayer (see Chapter 7 for a detailed discussion about spirituality and suffering). More often, spirituality includes identifying what is important in the patient's life.

Several other nursing interventions exist to directly address hope. A sample of palliative care patients and their spouses stated that frank discussion about hope actually lifted their burden and facilitated learning, healing, and trust (Benzein & Saveman, 2008). Herth (2001) has published several suggestions for research-based nursing interventions to promote hope. (See examples included in the exercise section at the end of this chapter.) With these, nurses are encouraged to have patients intentionally and actively nourish their hope reserves by participating in reflective thinking and writing exercises and creating physical reminders of hope. For example, the nurse might have a patient write down on different index cards words or memories that are personally significant. Then during a period of low hope the nurse can have the patient choose a card to read and think about. Nursing interventions to specifically address and promote hope have been identified as quite effective in a review of research related to levels of hope in patients with cancer (Chi, 2007).

The most important nursing intervention to promote hope is to help the patient set goals for the future. The ability to acknowledge that there will be a future is part of the definition of hope. Nurses are experts at mutual goal setting. Sitting for a moment to help a patient focus on what is truly important and write down some goals is a powerful nursing intervention. These points can be as lofty as "life goals" or as minute as goals for the rest of the day. Nurses are experienced in writing goals that are positive and feasible, and they can use this skill to assist patients to do the same. For an elder with congestive heart failure, a goal may be to play with grandchildren and experience minimal shortness of breath (Roberts, Johnson, & Keeley, 1999). Setting short-term attainable goals has been identified as especially important to fostering hope in terminally ill patients (Duggleby,

2001). For instance, a male patient in the final stage of life may be encouraged to set a goal such as to finalize wishes for his own memorial service or to call his daughter each day to tell her how much she is loved. Setting achievable goals reinforces the notion that a positive outcome in the future is possible.

Question for Reflection and Journaling

1. Can or should nurses promote hope in severely ill or terminally ill clients who are suffering?

Conclusion

Even in the grimmest situation, some aspect of hope is possible. A hope for a patient who is actively dying may be for a peaceful death. A hope for a woman suffering with major depression may be that she can get out of bed the next morning or that she can muster the strength to hug her son before he leaves for school. Hopes need not be grand or elaborate, just personal and possible. Nurses are in the ideal position to help patients who are suffering to find hope again.

Key Points

1. Hope requires some future-oriented vision.
2. Nurses play an integral role in assessing and promoting hope for their patients.
3. Being obvious and intentional about fostering realistic hope is good nursing practice.
4. Hope can be large or small in scale—but always possible.

Inspiring Hope Exercise (Based on hope interventions of Herth, 2001)

Making hope tangible:

1. Create a personal treasure chest of hope materials.
2. Decorate a box (shoe box works perfectly) with colors that remind you of hope.

3. In the box place pictures of two people you perceive as role models of hope.
4. On the back of each picture write a phrase about why each person inspires you.
5. Write on three index cards memories or beliefs that remind you of hopeful times, or experiences when you have been hopeful in the past.
6. Include two physical items that remind you of hope. (For instance, during the depth of winter, a tissue paper flower might remind you of blooming gardens to come in the spring.)
7. Open the "Hope" chest when you have a day that is particularly frustrating. Take out one item and reflect on its meaning for you.

Case Study 12–3: Hope

My sister and her husband had been married for nearly 3 years when they finally sought medical evaluation to find out why they had not yet conceived a baby. After numerous invasive tests they were diagnosed with "unexplained infertility," meaning there was no clear reason to explain why my sister was not able to get pregnant. Although we were all greatly relieved there was nothing wrong, this cause of infertility was the source of great frustration as there was "nothing to fix." Upon hearing this news, a barrage of comments from well-meaning family and friends told the couple to "just relax"—that somehow their anxiety was the real problem. These comments stung, insinuating that again, the cause of their infertility was their own fault.

Now, if you have ever known a couple suffering with infertility, you will know that the experience becomes all-consuming. Their crisis was exacerbated by fear, the lost dreams, the lost potential to experience the amazement of pregnancy and birth, and the irony of feeling "sick" with infertility while living in a perfectly healthy body. While they tried to be supportive of each other, thoughts about blame and questions about why they were being "punished" often arose. My sister often commented to me that dealing with the emotional consequences and the invasive physical testing for infertility was as consuming as having a part-time job. Soon after the diagnosis, the couple met with several specialists to discuss treatments to help them to conceive.

Since the couple was desperate to have a baby, the decision to pursue treatments with medication was straightforward. However, after several months of hormonal manipulation, the couple still had not conceived.

In my role of sister and friend, I did my best to remain as supportive as possible and tried to come up with the right words whenever another disappointment arose. But as my sister continued to struggle, something quite unexpected happened: I became pregnant with my first child. As soon as my husband and I finished celebrating, I was overwhelmed with guilt and sadness that I would have to break this news to my older sister. I waited as long as I could before finally sharing the news of my pregnancy. Of course she was supportive and happy for me, but I couldn't help thinking that I had contributed to her suffering.

While I was busy with a new infant, my sister's struggles with infertility continued and eventually the physicians recommended in vitro fertilization as the couple's last hope. The procedure is invasive, expensive, and psychologically exhausting. No one enters into that treatment lightly. Hope was the foundation of their in vitro procedure. Each time the couple would wait and hope they had enough eggs, then hope that enough would fertilize, and then hope the embryos would survive long enough to be implanted, and then the ultimate hope—the pregnancy test. The entire process required so much energy and hope, and after several failed attempts, there was yet another negative pregnancy test.

How long could the suffering last? My sister's battle with infertility was nearing the 5 year anniversary and her doctors warned that the treatments were rapidly accelerating her body's aging and decreasing her chance to conceive. At this point my sister tried to protect herself from pain; she avoided baby showers and pregnant women, and her heart was particularly heavy around Mother's Day. When it seemed that her situation could not be more bleak, another blow came: I was pregnant again. How could I possibly tell her once more? I knew she was very vulnerable, more than when I was pregnant with my first child 2 years earlier. I kept quiet about my pregnancy until it was obvious because I was so scared to tell her. Her response was much more kind that I could have been in her position.

As I neared the delivery day of my second child, my sister and her husband were at a turning point. They began to seek information about adoption as they readied themselves for their last attempt at in vitro fertilization. But they were told the embryos were poor quality and the chance of success was unlikely. Waiting 2 weeks for the pregnancy test seemed like an eternity. There were tears as they prepared themselves for the same outcome they had heard so many times over the past 5 years. On the day of her pregnancy test my phone did not ring as usual in the midafternoon. For a moment I thought the change in routine may have meant that the test was positive, but I convinced myself their changed response must have been because this was their last hope, and their last hope was lost. I left my usual, heartfelt message of support on their answering machine.

I was busy feeding and burping and bathing and changing a newborn— caught up in the very activities my sister had worked so tirelessly for, when my phone rang that evening. My sister's tone of voice was so foreign, I hardly recognized what she was saying; the test was positive. She was pregnant! The power of hope had sustained her through years and years of disappointment. Remarkably, my niece was born healthy the next summer, and they named her, Camryn Hope.

But the story doesn't end there, for it was nearly 3 years before my sister could even think about having another child. She and her husband knew that more in vitro would be too difficult to begin again. This time their infertility journey took them to an adoption agency where they waited to adopt a special needs child from China. It happened that their adoption procedure was delayed because of changes in regulation of overseas adoption. The waiting was extremely difficult and frustrating. While news of available children trickled in to her adoption agency, the plans and referrals always fell through for my sister. Three years into the process, a picture of a child who was available for adoption pulled at my sister's heartstrings and she e-mailed me her photo and medical record to review. In reading about the child's developmental delays, her cleft palate and lip, and possible physical and growth problems, my response was hesitation, "How will you be able to provide all of the care she needs?" Quite surprisingly my sister, who usually shared my trepidation and practicality responded, "Sometimes you need to take a leap of faith and do what you think is right." I was shocked. I almost began to talk her out of moving forward with the adoption. But she was wise beyond her years from all the suffering she had been through with infertility. It was my turn to have faith and hope.

While my sister waited anxiously to see if her application for this child would be approved, I received the news that I was pregnant for the third time. The uncertainty of the adoption still weighed heavily, but telling my sister felt different this time. She had been a mother for 6 years, and she knew she would eventually be matched with a child to adopt. Once she learned that the adoption was indeed moving forward, we were finally able to enjoy being "expectant mothers" at the same time.

Remarkably, with less than a couple pages of poorly translated information to base a decision on, my sister and her husband journeyed halfway around the world to meet their new daughter in a very remote part of China. Little Lily Mei jumped head first into their lives. To all of our amazement, she did not have a cleft palate or lip, and it was clear she did not have developmental or learning delays. She has been living in the United States for about 6 months and her ability to spread joy, speak English, and grow accustomed to such a new way of life has exceeded all of our wildest hopes (see Figure 12–2).

It is true that hope can sustain us through the darkest times, if we allow it.

Figure 12–2 Sisters

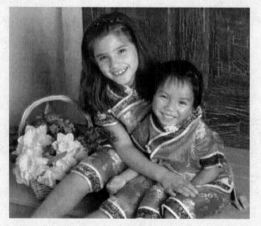

References

Baergen, R. (2006). Pediatric ethics, issues, and commentary. How hopeful is too hopeful? Responding to unreasonably optimistic parents. *Pediatric Nursing, 32*(5), 482.

Bailey, T., & Snyder, C. (2007). Satisfaction with life and hope: A look at age and marital status. *Psychological Record, 57*(2), 233–240.

Benzein, E., & Saveman, B. (2008). Health-promoting conversations about hope and suffering with couples in palliative care. *International Journal of Palliative Nursing, 14*(9), 439–445.

Bland, R., & Darlington, Y. (2002). The nature and sources of hope: Perspectives of family caregivers of people with serious mental illness. *Perspectives in Psychiatric Care, 38*(2), 61–68.

Bonanno, G. (2008). Loss, trauma, and human resilience: Have we underestimated the human capacity to thrive after extremely aversive events? *Psychological Trauma: Theory, Research, Practice, and Policy*, (1), 101–113.

Borell, L., Lilja, M., Svidén, G., & Sadlo, G. (2001). Occupations and signs of reduced hope: An explorative study of older adults with functional impairments. *American Journal of Occupational Therapy, 55*(3), 311–316.

Chan, C., Ho, R., Fu, W., & Chow, A. (2006). Turning curses into blessings: an Eastern approach to psychosocial oncology. *Journal of Psychosocial Oncology, 24*(4), 15–32.

Chu-Hui-Lin Chi, G. (2007). The role of hope in patients with cancer. *Oncology Nursing Forum, 34*(2), 415–424.

Collins S,, & Cutcliffe, J. R. (2003). Addressing hopelessness in people with suicidal ideation: Building upon the therapeutic relationship utilizing a cognitive behavioural approach. *Journal of Psychiatric and Mental Health Nursing, 10*(2), 175–185.

Duggleby, W. (2001). Hope at the end of life. *Journal of Hospice and Palliative Nursing, 3*(2), 51.

Farley, Y. R. (2007). Making the connection: Spirituality, trauma, and resiliency. *Journal of religion and spirituality in social work, 26*(1), 1–15.

Gordon, M. (2010). Manual of Nursing Diagnosis (12th edition). Sudbury, MA: Jones and Bartlett.

Herth, K. (2001). Development and implementation of a hope intervention program. *Oncology Nursing Forum, 28*(6), 1009–1017.

Herth, K. A., & Cutcliffe, J. R. (2002). The concept of hope in nursing 4: Hope and gerontological nursing. *British Journal of Nursing, 11*(17), 1148–1156.

Holt, J. (2001). A systematic review of the congruence between people's needs and nurses' interventions for supporting hope. *Online Journal of Knowledge Synthesis for Nursing, 8*(1), Retrieved from CINAHL with Full Text database.

Kylma, J. (2005). Dynamics of hope in adults living with HIV/AIDS: A substantive theory. *Journal of Advanced Nursing, 52*(6), 620–630.

Lohne, V., & Severinsson, E. (2004). Hope during the first months after acute spinal cord injury. *Journal of Advanced Nursing, 47*(3), 279–286.

Lopez, S., Snyder, C., & Pedrotti, J. (2003). Hope: Many definitions, many measures. In S. Lopez & C. Snyder (Eds.), *Positive psychological assessment: A handbook of models and measures* (pp. 91–106). Washington, DC: American Psychological Association.

Maslow, A. (1943). A theory of human motivation. *Psychological Review, 50*(4), 370–396.

Miller, J. (2007). Hope: A construct central to nursing. *Nursing Forum, 42*(1), 12–19.

Morse, J. (2001). Toward a praxis theory of suffering. *Advances in Nursing Science, 24*(1), 47–59.

Morse, J., & Doberneck, B. (1995). Delineating the concept of hope. *Image: Journal of Nursing Scholarship, 27*(4), 277–285.

Morse, J., & Penrod, J. (1999). Linking concepts of enduring, uncertainty, suffering, and hope. *Image: Journal of Nursing Scholarship, 31*(2), 145–150.

Roberts, S., Johnson, L., & Keely, B. (1999, July). Fostering hope in the elderly congestive heart failure patient in critical care. *Geriatric Nursing, 20*(4), 195–199.

Roisman, G. (2005). Conceptual Clarifications in the Study of Resilience. *American Psychologist, 60*(3), 264–265.

Schneiderman, L. J. (2005). The perils of hope. *Cambridge Quarterly of Healthcare Ethics: CQ: The International Journal of Healthcare Ethics Committees, 14*(2), 235–239.

Snyder, C. R., Sympson, S. C., Ybasco, F. C., Borders, T. F., Babyak, M. A., & Higgins, R. L. (1996). Development and validation of the State Hope Scale. *Journal of Personality and Social Psychology, 2*, 321–335.

Turner, D., & Stokes, L. (2006). Hope promoting strategies of registered nurses. *Journal of Advanced Nursing, 56*(4), 363–372.

Wagnild, G., & Collins, J. (2009). Assessing resilience. *Journal of Psychosocial Nursing & Mental Health Services, 47*(12), 28–33.

Wake, M. M., & Miller, J. F. (1992). Treating hopelessness: Nursing strategies from six countries. *Clinical Nursing Research, 1*(4), 347–365.

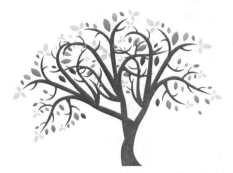

Index